The Joy of **Gay Sex**

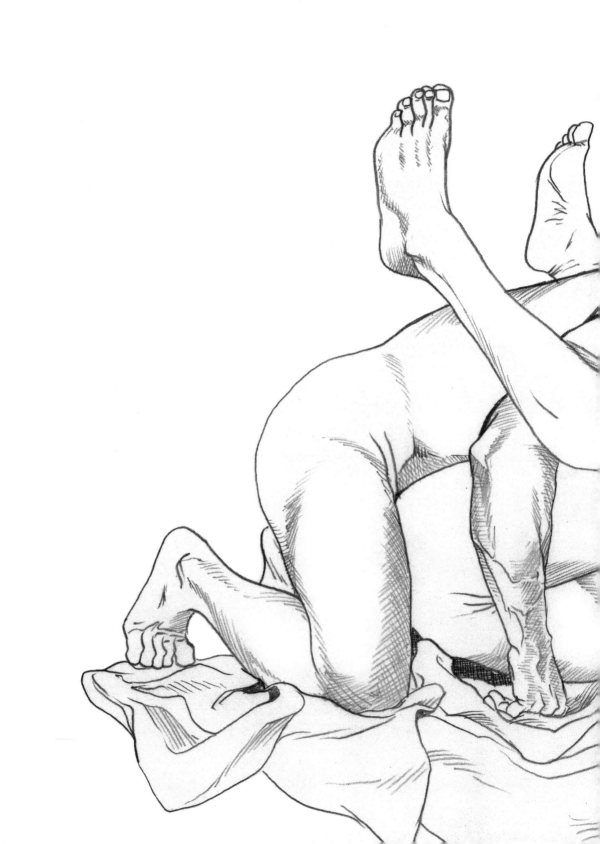

The Joy of **Gay Sex**

Fully Revised and Expanded Third Edition

Dr. Charles Silverstein
and Felice Picano

Illustrations
by Joseph Phillips

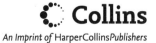

Collins

An Imprint of HarperCollinsPublishers

THE JOY OF GAY SEX. Copyright © 2003 by Dr. Charles Silverstein and Felice Picano.
All rights reserved. Printed in Canada. No part of this book may be used or reproduced in any
manner whatsoever without written permission except in the case of brief quotations embodied
in critical articles and reviews. For information address HarperCollins Publishers, 10 East 53rd
Street, New York, NY 10022.

HarperCollins books may be purchased for educational, business, or sales promotional use.
For information please write: Special Markets Department, HarperCollins Publishers, 10 East
53rd Street, New York, NY 10022.

First Collins edition published 2006.

Designed by Ralph L. Fowler

The Library of Congress Cataloging-in-Publication data has been applied for.

ISBN-10: 0-06-001274-9 (pbk.)
ISBN-13: 978-0-06-001274-8 (pbk.)

06 07 08 09 10 WBC 10 9 8 7 6 5 4 3

PRINTED IN CANADA

This book is dedicated to

Mama Albina

ACKNOWLEDGMENTS

Various people advised us on technical aspects of this book. We thank them all, including Joe Arkins, Bill Bartelt, Carlos, Barry Cream, Betty of Boston, Brian King, Tony Neto, Barry Nevins, Robert Padgug, Dan William, M.D., and Les Wright.

CONTENTS

Introduction   xv

List of Entries

A Brief History of *The Joy of Gay Sex*

It has now been more than a quarter of a century since the original edition of *The Joy of Gay Sex* was published. When we (Silverstein and White) first wrote the book, we had no idea it would become the cultural barometer of gay life it has become. It's not that oral sex, say, has changed. That's probably been the same since cavemen started drawing pictures. What has changed is the place of gay people in society, our relationship to the straight world, and consequently, how we feel about ourselves.

The book was first published in 1977. It was to be the first illustrated gay sex manual published by a mainstream publishing house. We decided to write the kind of book that we would have wanted to read ourselves as adolescents, a guide for men coming out. We also reasoned that the book should have a wider focus than just sex, that it should also advise the reader about life in the gay community and ways of fighting homophobia. Therefore, the majority of passages in the finished book were of a nonsexual nature.

We also agreed that the book should be sexually stimulating. Toward that end we wrote six masturbation stories that we peppered throughout the book. They were the usual porn stories, such as the young athlete in the locker room getting banged by either his teammates or the coach. We also wrote about "kinky" sex, such as bondage and water sports, and tried to be wise older brothers to teenagers who were struggling with homophobic families.

But the publishers heavily censored the book. It was, after all, 1977, only four years after the American Psychiatric Association had removed homosexuality as a mental disorder, and the straight world was not yet ready to accept an open celebration of gay sex. Most publishers were still terrified that illustrated sex manuals would be removed from bookstore and library shelves, and the owners and librarians arrested for peddling pornography, or what was then called smut. The publishers were worried that the public outcry against gay people created by Anita Bryant would seriously affect sales, and that local police officials and governmental customs would confiscate the books. Attorneys on both sides of the Atlantic, therefore, scrutinized the manuscript and forced the authors to defend their text on many occasions.

Worries about censorship and confiscation of copies led to the removal of all the masturbation fantasies. The lawyers also objected to the word *shit*, and they went ballistic over the essay on bondage, which they pared down to only one short paragraph.

The editor in chief of Crown Publishers objected to the frequent use of the word *cock*. He called the authors into his office and asked, "Why can't you use the word *penis* instead?"

"Because," said one of the authors, "your *penis* is part of your anatomy, but your *cock* is what you fuck your wife with." The shocked editor in chief relented.

The English publisher requested that we change the entry on teenagers to say that an adult having sex with a teenager is mentally sick, perverse, and belongs in jail. We refused his demand, but the conflict ended by having no entry regarding teenagers at all. We simply believed that omission was better than lies.

The publishers' fear of legal troubles over the book was not unfounded. In the United States, chain stores carried the original edition under the counter, so that straight customers wouldn't be offended by it. Some libraries bought the book to a chorus of objections by the religious Right, who often had it removed. (As late as December 1995, the presence of the book in the Clifton, New Jersey, library was challenged by the religious Right.)

In 1977, a French Canadian firm translated the book, titling it *Les Plaisirs de L'Amour Gai*. The publisher sent thousands of copies to Paris, where French customs seized and shredded them. Thousands of copies of the American edition were also imported into Britain, where they were seized by Her Majesty's Customs and burned. (The 1977 edition was eventually translated into German, Italian, and Danish.)

The book had a particularly hard time in Canada, where local police and governmental customs tried to suppress it. In Winnipeg in 1980, for instance, a newspaper reported that a woman rushed into a bookstore looking for a copy of *The Joy of Cooking*. She picked up *The Joy of Gay Sex* by mistake, or so she claimed. When she got home, she opened the book (to *F*, in order to make a fricassee?) and was profoundly embarrassed by what she saw. She called the police, who, upon her complaint, raided the store and confiscated all copies of the book. The police had trumped up the whole affair. Fortunately, the court ordered the books returned because homosexuality was legal in Canada.

Two years later, in Hamilton, Ontario, *Joy* was removed from the McMaster University bookstore and transferred to the medical bookstore, as a result of a complaint by an anthropology professor. Of its illustrations, he said, "I've never seen anything to equal them. They are definitely the most disgusting things I've ever seen on sale anywhere." Censorship of the book sparked a heated controversy on campus about free speech. The president of the university stepped in and announced that moving the book "struck at the very nature of the university as a center for free inquiry." He then ordered that it be kept in the *medical* bookstore.

Banning books is a complicated matter. When a book is prohibited from being published or distributed in a country, the publisher and the bookstore are both liable for criminal prosecution. Even if a book isn't banned for publication *within the country* (as *Joy* wasn't in Canada and England), and homosexuality is legal there, the book can be declared "obscene" by the customs office. In that case, it cannot be imported *into the country*.

When Jearld Moldenhauer, owner of the Glad Day Book Shop in Toronto, ordered copies of *Joy* from the United States, Her Majesty's Customs confiscated them, even though homosexuality, including anal intercourse, was legal in Canada. At great financial risk, Moldenhauer sued for the return of the books. Silverstein volunteered to testify at the trial that was held in Toronto in March 1987, where the customs officer testified that pictures and descriptions of anal intercourse were on the prohibited list for entry into Canada. When asked if he'd considered the educational or cultural value of the book, he responded, "That's not my business."

In his testimony, Charles gave the history of the book and the reasons for writing it. The Crown pointed out that there were nine pictures of anal intercourse in the book. It was all quite polite, the Canadians not being given to dramatics in the courtroom as we are here. In what must be counted as one of the finest legal decisions for gay people, Judge Hawkins wrote on March 20, 1987: "To write about homosexual practices, without dealing with anal intercourse, would be equivalent to writing a history of music and omitting Mozart." The books were ordered returned to the Glad Day Book Shop. You can read Judge Hawkins' full decision at: www3.sympatico.ca/toshiya.K.ncl/joy.htm.

Even with these legal wins, a system of de facto censorship existed almost everywhere in the United States. Many gay men were simply too intimidated to ask a clerk for the under-the-counter book.

Even though a British firm held the copyright, *Joy* was never published in England. *Gay News*, a London-based gay newspaper, had published a poem in which the author imagined giving a blow job to Jesus on the cross. Mary Whitehouse (their Anita Bryant) sued the paper for blasphemy under a law that hadn't been invoked for ages. The paper was subsequently closed down, and gay people came in for a great deal of criticism. The publisher was understandably afraid that the same thing would happen to them if they published *Joy* in Great Britain.

Ironically, it was the case of a heterosexual man that resulted in overturning British customs laws against pornography. Around 1987, he bought a mail-order life-size, inflatable female sex doll. Customs confiscated it. The man turned to the European High Court to rule on the dispute. Since Great Britain was joining the European Common Market, it was ordered to apply the same liberal standards for importation as the rest of Europe. The straight man got his fuckable doll back, and it meant the end to the censorship of gay materials.

But gay people everywhere loved the book because of its permissive tone about sex. For years afterward, the authors met people who said how favorably it had affected their lives. The book turned out to be a monumental achievement in a post-

Stonewall era, raising public awareness that gay life was alive and well, and that wanting to have sex with another man was more than okay; it was wonderful.

By the late 1980s, the AIDS epidemic had already killed tens of thousands of gay men. The original *Joy of Gay Sex* was out of print, and we thought that a new edition, updated for the 1990s, might influence young gay men to avoid unsafe sex. Felice Picano agreed to coauthor the book. Felice is a novelist who founded the Seahorse Press in 1979 and cofounded Gay Presses of New York in 1980, publishing the works of other gay writers at a time when mainstream publishers refused gay manuscripts.

The authors had not been spared the devastation of the AIDS epidemic. Within a year after publication of *New Joy*, both Felice and Charles would each see his lover die of the disease. Edmund's lover had died a couple of years earlier.

Young men coming out today have been spared watching the slow and painful deaths of lovers, friends, and colleagues—and their own, for that matter. How different gay life was in the eighties and early nineties. Some HIV-infected gay men preferred a Pollyanna-type physician who might say, "Don't worry, everything is going to be fine," while a different gay man preferred the direct approach: "Sorry, son, you're going to die soon." No matter what anyone said, they all died anyway.

The medical establishment was not very sympathetic in those days either. They were terrified of being infected by being in close proximity with an AIDS patient. Some wore full gowns, masks, and gloves when they walked into the hospital room of an AIDS patient. Some doctors actually refused to walk into the room at all. In some cases hospitals refused to admit AIDS patients, actually paying transportation costs to get rid of them. And after death, most funeral homes refused to accept the body and hold a service.

Desperately ill gay men mixed herbal formulas in their blenders, products claiming to be "natural," the buzzword of the period. Some felt like medieval witches brewing potions from spiders and the wings of bats. Some turned to eating only vegetables, others to high colonics. Still other dying men paid for unorthodox but expensive "treatments." Frightened gay men, with no hope for salvation from traditional medicine, ate the foods and had the treatments. No matter what they ate, they died.

It was in that social milieu that Felice and Charles decided to write the second edition of *Joy*, calling it *The New Joy of Gay Sex*. Some gay and straight editors were repelled by the idea. "How could we publish a book about gay sex when sex is killing the gay community?" they asked. But a virus, not sex, was the villain. And perhaps grandiosely, we thought that we could save lives while at the same time maintaining a permissive attitude about gay sex.

There was no censorship at all the second time around, no topic too hot to handle. Our editor's only interest was to help us to make the manuscript as clear as possible. He only raised an eyebrow over one illustration, which was intended to illustrate a fetish. Ron Fowler, one of the illustrators used, had drawn a picture of an erect cock around which (and the balls) was wrapped barbed wire. No blood was pictured. We had it changed because the publisher had generally been so accommodating to our text.

HarperCollins published *The New Joy of Gay Sex* in November 1992, with a new set of illustrations. In July 1993, a Japanese publisher published it in Japan. But the book was text only. "No pictures of organs allowed in Japan," they said. We thought that ironic since Japanese pornography has been famous for centuries. The Japanese publisher invited us to help publicize the book in Japan. We were to spend a week in Tokyo. It was one of the perks of publishing.

Ni-Chome (nee-show-may) is the name of Tokyo's gay ghetto, to which we went on our first night of the book tour—and virtually every night thereafter. The streets there are even narrower than in Greenwich Village; the place blazes with neon lights and is crowded with gay men of every nationality and the gay Japanese boys who prefer them. "Are you rice queens?" a wide-eyed young Japanese man asked us. "I'm a potato queen," he announced. "I'll show you the bars in Ni-Chome." And he became our guide for the night.

We attended a panel (held in a discotheque) about sexuality organized by the Japanese publisher, after which the throng attending the evening's activities danced. That included two men dressed as condoms. Before the week was out, Felice modeled for a Japanese sweater company (and met another American), while Charles, with the help of a friend, learned how to cruise a Japanese bathhouse. Grabbing genitals or asses is too aggressive in their culture. One must use indirection, no small task for an American and, especially, a New Yorker.

* * *

By the turn of the millennium, gay life had changed so dramatically even from the previous decade that a third edition of *Joy* was deemed necessary. What were those changes?

They began in 1995, the year of the "cocktail," the first really effective treatment against the HIV virus. Protease inhibitors were used for the first time, and they were combined with other drugs. It was called Highly Active Anti-Retroviral Therapy, or HAART. The dying stopped almost completely. AIDS became a manageable, if still incurable, illness.

The spectacular rise of the Internet around the same time was a second major change in gay life. Most gay men seem to use it to trick with other men. Tricking is hardly a new idea, whether by walking the streets, using phone lines, or connecting via modem. But the gay men who are aided the most through the Internet are those who are minorities within the gay minority: men who are turned on by kinkier kinds of sex. Before the Internet, men into a fetish, for instance, or water sports, often had a hard time finding one another. Now there are on-line bulletin boards and clubs devoted to these sexual activities. It has made life much easier for them.

Another major change is many younger gay people's drive to become assimilated into mainstream America. Wanting to marry legally and adopt children are prime examples of this change. But not all gay people like the idea that gays are just like straights. To them, there's a certain cachet in being disreputable, an advantage in being a member of an underground society. They fear that the "ethnicity" of homosexuality will be lost forever, as for example camp, the gay "secret language" from the earlier part of the century, seems to have been lost.

These changes are reflected in *The Joy of Gay Sex: Fully Revised and Expanded Third Edition*. While still not encyclopedic, the book is far more comprehensive about sex than the previous two editions, and at the same time, with extended and in-depth entries on growing older, teenagers, married men, bisexuality, homophobia, and transgenderism. We hope it better reflects the changing sociopolitical landscape of gay men's lives in the early twenty-first century. Naturally, we've also written up-to-date, fuller sections on HIV disease, sexually transmitted diseases, barebacking, and drug use, topics that continue to be of great importance to gay men.

Two generations of gay men have already come out utilizing *The Joy of Gay Sex* and *The New Joy of Gay Sex* as user-friendly books. The nonsexual entries in those books identified how the outside world discriminates against us. While this new edition is not a critique of gay life per se, we haven't shied from identifying potential problems within our community: how gay men harm themselves through self-destructive behavior. The obvious examples are drug and alcohol abuse, barebacking, and new HIV infections. We hope that our third edition will assist another generation to fight what homophobic institutions still exist, as well as the internal problems that a small but significant part of the gay community still suffer.

Anus

Culturally induced fears have given many people phobias about their assholes. This bias against the anus is unreasonable. True, it is used for elimination, but so is the penis—yet that objection has not made the latter organ any less attractive. The anus is not only an avenue for elimination but also a sexual organ. It is highly sensitive, as it is lined with particularly responsive nerve endings. Moreover, the anus is close to the prostate gland, and its stimulation is highly pleasurable.

All trace of shit can be banished if one takes an enema before intercourse. Every drugstore sells disposable enemas or convenient bulb-shaped plastic ones. Most men who use them regularly keep them in their shower. Daily use of enemas, however, should be avoided, as it could create psychological dependence and/or physical damage to the small intestines. People who are just beginning to experiment with anal sex sometimes fear that sticking a large cock up the anus will tear the skin; proper lubrication and relaxation, however, will prevent pain or damage (see *First Time*).

More experienced men often worry that by repeatedly getting fucked they will lose muscle tone in their asshole. There is no research on this problem, but it seems that many of these worries are probably unfounded and may cover up feelings of guilt (see *Guilt*). One occasionally finds gay men who disparage achieving sexual pleasure through their anuses. This might be a result of low self-esteem caused by the archaic notion that only women get fucked. This is both an insult to their own bodies and historically wrong, since men have found pleasure in their assholes since the time of the cavemen, as we've learned from pictographs.

Barebacking

Barebacking—fucking without a condom—is the single most dangerous sex practice there is (see *Dangerous Sex*). As a method of sexual gratification, it's as old as recorded history. Until the arrival of AIDS, gay men never used condoms when fucking. In fact, pulling out before you came was considered rude. Until the mid-1980s, condoms were deemed kinky, a sex toy among gay men (see *Condoms*). The AIDS epidemic caused a change in our way of having sex. As of December 2000, 775,000 people in the United States had been diagnosed with AIDS (the figure for HIV disease is much higher). One-half million have died (see *HIV*

Disease). The worldwide statistics are even more alarming. Since we know so much about the transmission of the virus, fucking someone without a condom is equivalent to two men playing Russian roulette with each other.

Younger men seem to be more attracted to barebacking. Perhaps these risk-taking men haven't watched the slow death of lovers and friends. For them, AIDS is history, like their learning about the Vietnam War. It's simply not in their experience, as it is for an older generation of gay men. That's too bad, because it's a statistical certainty that some of them are going to pay a price—the diagnosis of HIV disease.

It would be a mistake, however, to look at barebacking only from a moral perspective. Recent research informs us that emotional problems influence a gay man's sexual behavior, including his contribution in transmitting the HIV. Depression is the main culprit. Gay men who are depressed, including both acute and chronic depression, are far more likely to participate in unsafe sex (see *Depression; Safe Sex*). Men with impulsive personalities, especially excitement seekers, are another category of psychologically impaired gay men. They generally describe themselves as "spontaneous," a claim that is untrue. A man who is spontaneous can make voluntary choices about his behavior; an impulsive man cannot. Both depression and impulsiveness can be effectively treated by both medication and psychotherapy.

If you have a friend who is endangering his life by barebacking, ask yourself whether psychological problems might be the cause. If so, taking a moral approach won't change his behavior (nor will accusing him of stupidity). Help him to make an appointment with a shrink, but only one well versed in gay sex and HIV research.

How does a responsible gay man (like you) fulfill his sexual desires, but not endanger himself and other gay men? If you're going to fuck, carry condoms. Have them in your night table in your bedroom. Insist that your sex partner use one if he's going to fuck you—"Put the condom on or put your clothes on." Ignore the entreaties of a man who says, "You can fuck me without a condom," especially since you can be sure that he said the same thing to the man who fucked him last night, and the night before, and . . . (see *Sexually Transmitted Diseases*). If, for some reason—either you are under the influence of alcohol or recreational drugs or a mix of both—you do bareback, be sure to get tested about *a month later* (see *Booze and Highs; Drug Abuse; Drugs and Sex*). If you test negative, get tested again in two more months. If you believe that the man who fucked you might be HIV-positive, treatment with AZT is available.

There may be a day when condoms are no longer necessary because AIDS scientists have successfully produced a vaccine. That's still years off. In the meantime, lovers who are both HIV-negative and who *never* trick out need not worry about the HIV or STDs.

Bars

In a small town there may be only one gay bar. If you go to it, you're making an open declaration of your homosexuality. The straight townspeople may see you entering, and the gay clientele will immediately recognize you. The bar itself will probably be more chummy than sexual. There will be a regular crowd night after night, joking and socializing, and the atmosphere is likely to be warm, permissive, and lively.

In smaller towns and cities there may only be one bar catering to gay men, lesbians, bisexuals, transsexuals, and transgendered people. These bars generally have a cozier, homier scene and might be more frequented by younger gays still feeling out their precise sexuality. These bars usually combine the resources and assets of a cruise bar, dance bar, and coffee shop.

In a big city, gay bars are far more numerous, anonymous, and specialized. A young dance crowd will go to one; older men will frequent another. In one, the latest fashions are on display; in another, outfits will be more casual or punkier; in another, body piercing and tattoos will predominate and be deemed erotic; while another bar may be given over to chaps, engineer boots, and black motorcycle jackets (see *Body Decoration*). There are also neighborhood bars somewhat like the ones in small towns, bars for post-retirement-age men, bars arranged around a piano where a singer belts out musical numbers and others join in, bars kept dim or with specific darker rooms where men can neck and grope each other, in effect "trying out the merchandise" before leaving together. If you're just entering the bar scene or if you've just moved to a new city, you'll need to scout around. Local gay newspapers ("bar rags"), the *Gayellow Pages*, and *Damron's Guides* usually list bars, along with codes explaining any specialization.

There's not much to do in bars except drink, talk, and in some cases play pool, watch old movies, and dance. And, of course, cruise (see *Cruising*). Once you become known in a bar, people will probably gossip about you; you'll find you have a reputation, and even your sexual tastes will become common knowledge. Though this may strike you as intrusive, it does have a practical advantage: The men who approach you are more likely to be compatible. If the typecasting becomes annoying, move on to a new bar (see *Types*).

If you're traveling, it pays to visit a gay bookstore first and buy an up-to-date bar guide. Visiting gay bars in other countries or communities is fascinating: It's the fastest way to learn different gay customs. As a foreigner, you are often at a distinct advantage in gay bars, being exotic, as well as a new face. Local gay men interested in trying new sexual experiences will attach themselves to you, knowing that their experimentation will probably not become known to their friends. It used to be that gay

Europeans pounced on gay Americans because they were said to give better blow jobs. That's less true today, but often Americans abroad find themselves enlisted into kink, which they're supposedly more open to and experienced in (see *Kinky Sex*). Likewise, Germans and the Dutch have a reputation for S/M and leather. Many Mediterranean gay bars have back rooms similar to those in the USA in the 1960s and 1970s where men have sex together on the premises. Be aware of personal and sexual safety in these back rooms (see *Dangerous Sex*). They're rife with pickpockets. In Asia, Africa, and South America, foreigners in gay bars should be advised on specific local customs, counseled against accepting drugs or drinks from locals. Horror stories about being doped, robbed, beaten, and worse are not uncommon. Of course, one advantage to being gay is that it doesn't matter where you go. You can establish an almost instant rapport with others like yourself.

Baths

In the "good old days" (i.e., a few decades ago) before the AIDS crisis, no visit to another city was complete without checking out its best-known "tubs"—Denver's Ball Park, Beverly Hills' Club 8709, and San Francisco's Ritch Street Baths were the equivalents of the Rockies, the Hollywood sign, and the Golden Gate Bridge as must-see spots. Baths or bathhouses (known in Europe as saunas) were one of the most popular meeting places for gay men, and one of the few places where sexual contact was, if not guaranteed, at least expected.

Which was pretty much their undoing. During the mideighties, political forces both within and outside the gay community decided that bathhouses were loci of unsafe sex practices. Compromises were attempted in some cities: Literature about AIDS was strewn all over the bathhouses' public areas, and machines selling condoms and spermicidal lotions were placed next to those selling Dr Pepper and Sprite. In some cities, doors were removed from the rooms, and in San Francisco, "monitors" were appointed to rove the baths checking that people were not fucking or sucking without condoms. But as the death toll from AIDS rose dramatically, these half measures came to seem less attempts at preserving civil rights than a way of preserving a lifestyle—glamorized in the seventies—that seemed fatally outmoded. Some gay bathhouses do still exist and are, oddly enough, more prevalent in smaller cities than in larger ones, and mostly in the American South and Midwest and in Europe. (Although recently the few remaining in large cities have expanded as a result of increased popularity.) Lately sex clubs have replaced them (see *Sex Clubs*). Should you find yourself near a bathhouse, you may want to go in and at least look around.

Lockers (cheaper) and rooms (more expensive) are usually available, the former often in a gymlike changing-room area. The rooms are usually small plasterboard cubicles containing a bed, a lamp, a tiny shelf, and nothing else. Bathhouse amenities generally include a pool or Jacuzzi that can hold anywhere from four to twelve people. Also likely are showers, saunas, and steam rooms; sometimes there's a dormitory area or a small gym or workout room; also there's a lounge with a TV or video screen for porn flicks or even old movies.

A night at a bathhouse can be a boring or an eye-opening experience. And who knows? You might even meet someone you'd like to see again. If you decide to have sex, be certain it's safe sex. Even before the AIDS crisis, sexually transmitted diseases were a constant bathhouse problem. The same caution should be exercised in sex clubs (see *Saying No*; *Safe Sex*; *Sexually Transmitted Diseases*).

Bears

B4 c+ d+ e+ f+ g++ k- - m q r s++ t+ w.

Huh! What's going on here? It's "bear code," a highly developed lexicon of the personal and physical characteristics of a gay man who identifies as a "bear."

The "bear movement" began in the mid-1980s as a rebellion against the dominant gay culture, which overwhelmingly idolized chiseled gym bodies as the standard of gay male beauty. Trim, neat, and well-styled haircuts characterized the most visible gay men then—and now—while the predominant gay body, as featured in gay magazines and in porn videos, displayed full heads of hair, a neat little bush of pubic hair above the cock (with balls shaved), but no hair at all on the chest, back, or legs. An unshaven chest or back, an evident tan line, or love handles were viewed by many gay men as signs that one simply didn't care about one's appearance.

But bears beg to differ. Bears are hairy (everywhere) and big, although not necessarily overweight. Bears think of themselves as highly masculine, real men, and they don't wear drag or anything in the least bit feminine. They don't mind smelling like men, which doesn't necessarily mean they have strong body odor—but no colognes or moisturizer aromas, please. And while many gay men with gym bodies often consider themselves social climbers, or at least they try to Keep Up with the Bruces, most bears reject financial standing and social status as goals. As a result, many gay men find them to be a particularly open, friendly, social group. That is not to say that one can't find an occasional muscle bear or cover bear who is as narcissistically fastidious as the most dedicated circuit boy (known as twinks, by bears). New York

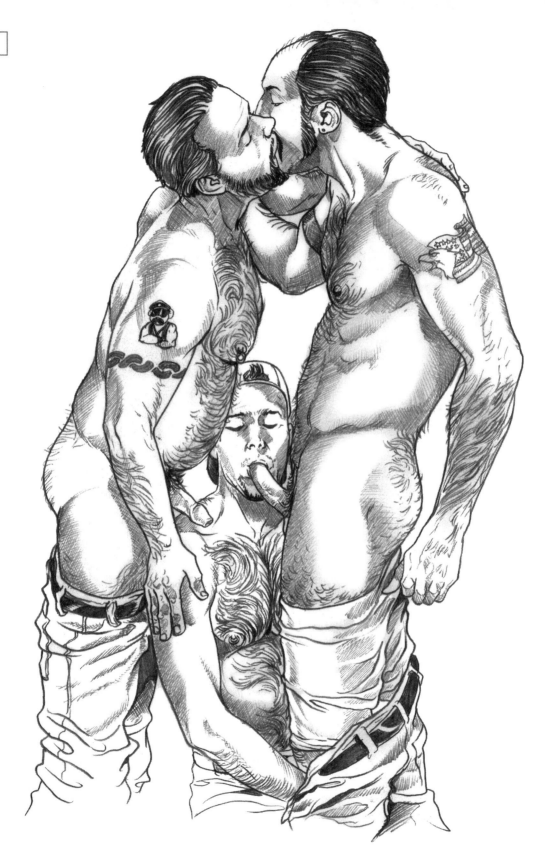

City and San Francisco, we're told, now even have their own steroid-enhanced muscle-bear culture.

The typical bear can be identified by three major physical characteristics: facial hair, body hair or "fur," and a heavy or "husky" build. Nit-picking bears sometimes argue about how much hair is required to be a member of beardom (could there be a hairless bear?). But many bears also claim that physical characteristics take a backseat to a certain set of attitudes about gay masculine behavior, adding up to an entire "bear culture."

There's also a distinct stratification of bear types. Subcategories include grizzly bears (older or grizzled-looking), Santa bears (white hair), panda bears (Asian descent, with or without chest hair), and black bears (African-Americans). No polar bears? Younger, or less husky, less hairy gay men, who are often sexually submissive to other bears, are usually called cubs. *Cub* is the term often used by a bear to describe himself when looking for a daddy or a top (see *Daddy/Son Fantasies*). A slimmer-built bear is sometimes called an otter—essentially, a thin bear. The appellation *wolf* is a latecomer to the bear totemic system, meaning someone who is a loner, perhaps an independent-minded otter not as integrated into the gay scene as those in mainline bear culture. While bears reject the queen culture with its nod toward effeminacy, a few have slipped in anyway. We're informed that they're called cha-cha bears behind their backs. While many bears wear lots of leather, they're not necessarily into S/M. For some, it's part of their masculine image.

There are over 140 bear clubs, often called dens, throughout the United States and internationally. They have newsletters, meetings, social gatherings, and national conventions such as Octobearfest in Denver, Orlando Bear Bust, Bear Pride Weekend in Chicago, and the national annual Bear Rendezvous in San Francisco. They even have their own flags. Most of these clubs have Web sites, where membership is welcomed. There you'll find profiles of individual members, each identified through the bear code. Remember the profile mentioned at the top of this entry? Here it is again, this time with its "bear code" deciphered.

> A *mostly full beard; a definite cub; a definite daddy-type (although it conflicts with being a cub); a big dick; above average fur; loves to grope ("paw") another bear; totally vanilla sex (no kinky stuff); has some muscle definition; is out in public; the outdoor type; only interested in open relationships; is taller than the average man; and has a tummy.*

Other aspects of the bear code inform the reader of more subtle physical and personality characteristics of the bear. Some bears have tuned the code with shades of meaning so fine that it equals the sophistication of *The Oxford English Dictionary*. Because of its tolerance and its reputation for sociality and friendliness, we believe the bear phenomenon is a healthy addition to the gay community. Bear culture simply allows some otherwise isolated and underappreciated gay men to relate to other gays with whom they feel most comfortable, providing for greater diversity in our population, and with the added benefit of fighting straight stereotypes, both from within and outside the gay community.

Bisexuality

Perhaps no other word in the area of human behavior is used with such imprecision. First let's talk about what bisexuality does not mean. In the classical culture of ancient Greece and Rome, many adult men were bisexual in that they were married to women and had adolescent boys as lovers. This arrangement was probably responsible for some of the great epic and lyric poetry of Hellenic times. There was always an age difference between the males, and the older man had to play the "active" and "masculine" role in intercourse. If he wanted to play the "passive" or "feminine" role (he wanted to get fucked), he became an object of ridicule. This kind of sexual arrangement is generally considered pederasty (sex with adolescents) and should not be confused with the sort of bisexuality we want to discuss.

Similarly, we're not talking about sex between men who are normally heterosexual but because of sexual deprivation (in prison, say) turn to one another. Nor would we call a man bisexual who has sex exclusively with men although he is capable of great emotional intimacy with women. We do not subscribe to Freud's theory of bisexuality, that everyone is bisexual at birth but at a certain point is unconsciously forced to choose either heterosexuality or homosexuality. Freud, like many of his age and culture, believed that the only correct choice was heterosexuality.

Nor are we talking about the so-called bisexuality of closeted gay men. Many homosexual men pose as bisexuals though they have sex only with other men. Their "bisexuality" is a convenient if dishonest passport into heterosexual respectability: It's often assumed for business or social reasons.

What, then, is a bisexual? A bisexual is someone who has sexual relationships with both sexes. A bisexual can have affairs with men and women simultaneously. Other bisexuals have long homosexual affairs that may last for years; the bisexual will then enter into an equivalent long-term heterosexual relationship. Obviously these arrangements may be fraught with complications.

One great advantage to bisexuality is that it enables someone to play very different emotional and sexual roles. With a woman, the bisexual might be fatherly and assertive, and with another man, childlike and passive. With a woman he might be open, cheerful, and confiding, a true partner in the complex relationship, and with a man he might be impersonal, anonymous, and passionately animal. Or he might be tender and supportive with a younger man and rather rough and competitive with an older woman. Homosexuality might be reserved for lasting relationships and heterosexuality for occasional thrills, or vice versa.

The possibilities are various, and not all of them entail a clear separation between sexual and psychic response. Some bisexual men have arrived at the blend of the traits usually considered "masculine" and "feminine." They react to members of either sex in much the same way.

There are some problems in this polymorphous paradise. Truly bisexual men and women belong to one of the most persecuted groups in society. Both gays and straights find them confusing, and their very existence threatens widely held preconceptions. Many heterosexuals secretly believe that if a homosexual could know the joys of straight life, he would be an instant convert. Conversely, many gay men consider their own lives so clearly superior to the "dullness" of heterosexuality that they ascribe bisexuality to hypocrisy or cowardice. And bisexuals are more often accused of being "promiscuous" than straight or gay men (see *Promiscuity*).

Gay life constitutes a genuine society complete with its own slang, humor, mating rituals, and gathering places—even, in larger cities, its own economy. Such ready-made institutions do not exist for bisexuals. They must carefully pick and choose straight and gay friends to shape a life tolerant of their catholic tastes.

For some men, bisexuality is simply a transitional stage between heterosexuality and homosexuality. The joke goes like this: A bisexual is a guy who is cuter than his (female) date. Bisexuality can provide a resting place for assessing one's feelings and values, as well as the reactions of one's friends and family. But if the pose is maintained too long, it can become an act of bad faith, of self-deception, and the source of pain.

What if a man who has been happily homosexual for years finds himself attracted to a woman? Should you have an affair with her? If there's a real sexual attraction, why not? Should you tell her about your homosexuality? Most men won't, but then most men seldom talk about their past with women they have just met. But should you continue the affair, and if she begins to become emotionally attached, you should tell her. She may back out; she may try to "cure" you, in which case set her gently but firmly in place. If you're lucky, she may simply take you at face value and your relationship moment by moment. What if you enter an affair with a man who has been heterosexual till now? From time to time straight men, especially if they are sophisticated and live in big cities, do develop a crush on a man they know to be gay (see *Married Men; Sex with Straight Men*). If you find the man attractive, there is no reason not to go ahead. But if you know his wife or steady woman friend, you may find yourself entering a romantic triangle not very different from an all-straight or all-gay one. Be prepared to lose both his friendship and hers.

Once you have your new bisexual male in bed, you'll probably be surprised by how gentle he is. Many women train their male lovers to be tender and romantic, and the result can be something of a shock to a gay man entertaining fantasies about a tough, brutal straight guy. Especially because, having already done the macho act, he may want you to fuck him or he may want to suck you off. He may not be good at either (after all, he's had no experience), but his secret reason for trying homosexuality may be to experiment in precisely these new areas. He might also be frosty with guilt the next time you meet. Don't worry that you're "corrupting" him; he's going into this sexual encounter with his eyes wide open. But don't expect a lasting relationship, no matter how much fun he is in bed. The main rule in dealing with straight men is to be discreet. They worry more about their reputations than Spanish virgins.

Blow Job

At some point in almost every gay encounter someone will probably offer his partner a blow job. This is nothing more or less than sucking cock, not as foreplay, but as a complete sexual act, including orgasm. The blow job is naturally the preferred method for quickies or when there is a danger of discovery, but its attractions are by no means merely functional. As a prelude to anal intercourse, as the same in the duet of soixante-neuf (see *Sixty-Nining*), a good blow job (which despite its name does not require blowing) is the ideal technique.

Until recently in many European countries, blow jobs were virtually unheard of between men and considered demeaning—they were performed only by women and usually only prostitutes. In the older and non-Judeo-Christian cultures of the East and in societies of Asia, Africa, and South America, blow jobs are acceptable for everyone regardless of gender. Cleopatra of Egypt, for instance, is reputed to have sucked off one hundred Roman noblemen in Rome in one night, and a thousand Roman soldiers back home, but this is probably exaggerated.

It's difficult to say how it happened, exactly, but the United States has become the blow-job capital of the world: Men from all over the world vacation here, often traveling across the country to experience the superb technical prowess of American cocksuckers.

The blow job is also the preferred and sometimes the only method of sexual contact of some men. Guys otherwise indifferent and even hostile to gay sex will, on occasion and in the right mood, eagerly look for or at least accept a blow job from a gay man.

A good blow job should be a pleasure rather than a task. And it can be pleasurable

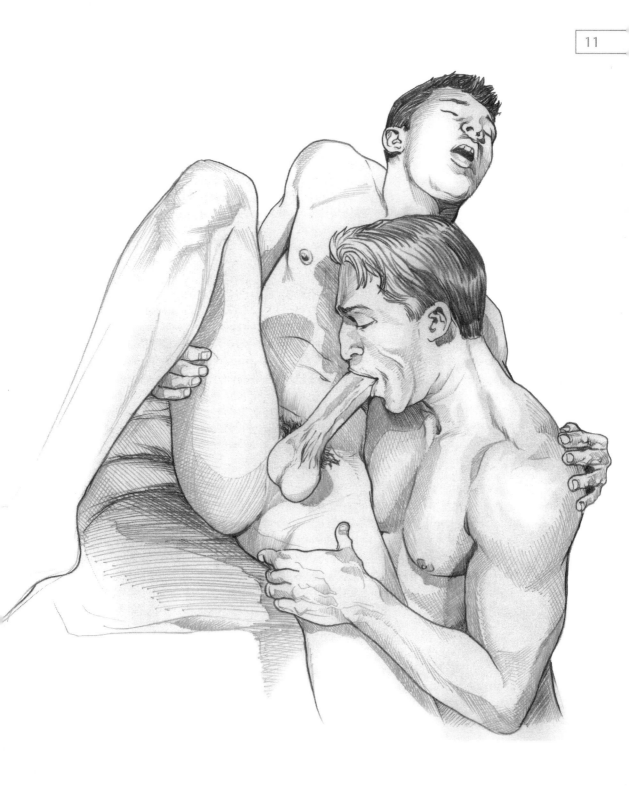

for the one sucking as well as for the one being sucked. Few who have experienced the subtle yet complete control of another's body and pleasure through his cock, and the thrill of carefully gliding that cock and that man to sexual fulfillment, consider the experience "demeaning"—or "passive."

Body Decoration

Piercing body parts has a long history. For example, Caesar's bodyguards were said to have worn nipple rings as a sign of their virility. In ancient America, the Maya and other cultures practiced ritual piercing. Sculptures show cords studded with thorns being passed through the tongue or penis. This was a religious rite related both to fertility and penitence.

Seventeenth-century buccaneers often pierced their ears and wore a gold piece, sometimes a coin taken from the treasure hold of some hapless galleon that had fallen captive. Each earring commemorated a ship the pirates had helped capture. German U-boat sailors during World War I also marked their "kills" in this fashion.

Piercing is but one form (albeit the most common) of body decoration, a practice that also includes tattooing, scarification, and more lately, branding. Devotees of piercing explain that it is like tattooing, whose practitioners treat the human body as a canvas upon which colorful art is etched. In piercing, the human body serves as an armature to which metal sculpture is attached.

Earrings have traditionally been considered a "sign" of homosexuality in our society, where any adornment on men was suspect. Then rap singers and people in the punk movement began wearing them, but on either ear. If a straight man wore an earring, he put it on his left ear. An earring on the right ear was reserved for gay men. During the eighties, earrings joined tattoos and wildly carved and dyed hair as signs that set one apart from the common herd. Of all the punk body-fashions, piercings, rings, and tattoos have been assimilated by the larger society. In gay urban centers, men wear a single ring or stud in one ear. Two, three, or more rings are common, either thin gold rings an eighth of an inch apart near the center of the lobe, or a series of rings around the entire curved edge of the ear. In these examples, piercing is a fashion statement. Earrings, nose rings, lip rings, eyebrow rings, and in some cases even tit rings have no sexual meaning. As in all fashion, wearing earrings waxes and wanes. They're not quite as popular today as they were a decade ago.

Sexual piercing, on the other hand, is generally a component of S/M sex (see *Sadomasochism*). Most S/M piercing is done on and around the cock. In the popular *Prince Albert*, the head of the cock is pierced through the urethra, and a ring is inserted. The *guiche* (pronounced "geesh") is a piercing through the perineum, the space between the balls and the asshole. Locking a Prince Albert to a guiche can make a neat chastity device. The *frenum* is a piercing through the frenum of the cock (the loose piece of flesh beneath the cock head). Tit piercing is also extremely common. There are other variations of cock piercing and ball piercing, and a sophisticated terminology is associated with them.

A variety of jewelry-like devices can be placed through these pierced holes. Rings and barbell studs are probably the most common. D rings, clamps, and locks are other forms of adornment. Most of this jewelry is made of surgical steel, although some men prefer the luxury of gold. Some gay couples symbolize their relationship by means of a ritual piercing. They wear their rings on their cocks or belly buttons instead of on their fingers.

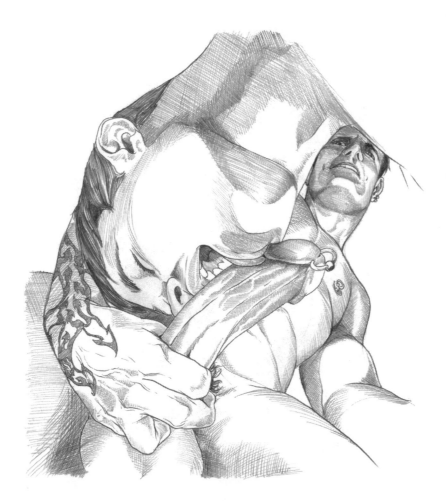

The act of piercing or the use of rings or studs may be the whole of the sexual experience between the partners. Sucking and fucking, so common in most other forms of sex, may not be part of the piercing scene. Some men will jerk off; others may not come at all.

Piercing may also be temporary, in contrast to the placement of rings and studs. For instance, one expert places needles in the body of his partner, then connects them with kite string to form a frame above the body. Combining piercing with bondage, he then "plays the instrument," plucking the strings to create pain in different parts of the body. The object of this, according to S/M experts, is to reach what they call the pleasure/pain threshold. This is the point at which the body changes the perception of pain to a perception of pleasure. There is not yet scientific evidence to confirm or refute this claim.

There are obvious dangers to be avoided. Never pierce yourself, and never allow a stranger to pierce you. Piercing should only be done by professionals who have the proper sterile equipment and who can advise you about aftercare, which can last from two to six months.

Tattooing is almost always done for aesthetic reasons. A small (but obvious) tattoo on one's ass cheek or just above the bathing-suit line is certain to be an icebreaker on the beach, or in bed. More serious tattoos cover more than half the skin of the body. Some of the newest tattoo art has elaborate science fiction themes consisting of fantastical figures. Tattoo artists who design them have become quite famous, particularly at tattoo conventions.

For a small minority of men, piercing and extensive tattooing are not enough. Usually aficionados of heavy S/M sex, they move on to scarring their bodies in particular patterns. An even smaller subset will get branded.

Body Fluids and Disease

The HIV is transmitted by "body fluids." The fluids are blood, semen, and (to a lesser extent) saliva. It is absolutely certain that the HIV can be transmitted by blood, mostly ass-fucking. It is less certain to what extent semen (or pre-come) ingested during oral sex can transmit enough of the virus to cause infection.

There are only a handful of documented cases of men who claim to have been infected through oral sex, and as a result, most gay men don't use a condom when sucking cock. The problem here is that while sucking is obviously much *safer* than fucking, it's not 100 percent *safe*. We advise you not to suck cock if: (1) you have been to a dentist for any reason within forty-eight hours, (2) you have an open sore of any kind on the inside of your mouth or severe gum disease, or (3) your partner has any kind of lesion or sore on his cock. In all these cases, it's best to wait until healing is complete before engaging in oral sex. And any of the above require extra caution if you or your partner has AIDS or is HIV-positive. Should you forget these rules or only notice an open sore after you've sucked cock, immediately gargle with a mouthwash with 18 percent or more of alcohol or a suitable solution of hydrogen peroxide and water. Since several cases of men infected orally may have occurred as a result of particularly rough oral sex—also known as irrumation, in which one man fucks the other man's mouth rather than having him suck—you might want to consider carefully before getting into this kind of a scene (see *Kinky Sex*).

Few (if any) medical authorities believe that tongue-kissing (or French-kissing) can transmit the virus, but you can get other STDs such as herpes that way. Feces, not strictly a body fluid, are not implicated in HIV transmission, although they can transmit other sexual diseases, such as hepatitis, that are as dangerous. If you have a friend or lover who is HIV-positive or has AIDS, you should use caution in cleaning any of his body fluids (see *Condoms; HIV Disease; Safe Sex; Sexually Transmitted Diseases*).

Body Image

There's a character in *War and Peace* who never realizes how beautiful she is. Her most dazzling attribute is her glance, her wonderful spiritual eyes, but when she studies herself in the mirror, her eyes go dead. She becomes rigid and disapproving—and she remains in ignorance of what everyone else knows, that she is the woman with the beautiful eyes.

Many people fail to perceive their looks clearly. We all carry around in our heads a sketch, if not a finished painting, of how we appear, and too often the sketch is unflattering. Sometimes the sketch may be redrawn along more attractive lines if we've been cruised heavily in the streets. But the next time we are ignored or rejected, the sketch turns into a caricature. Not everyone goes through these agonizing fluctuations in self-esteem about his body, but there's bound to be some correlation between the way people react to your body and the way you regard it. If everyone tells you that you look terrific, you'll begin to believe it—at least until the next time you face a mirror or have to choose some clothes or decide whether to grow a goatee.

It's not bad to be affected by what others say, but it's terrible to be ruled by it. This is especially important today, due to the increased display—some say exhibition—of nude and nearly nude male bodies, not only in gay magazines, but also in mainstream media, movies, on the Internet, in billboard and newspaper advertising. In recent decades, women were regularly subjected to such objectifying display, but not men. But for better or worse, men have caught up, and we are daily subjected to seeing handsome, tall, slender males with wide shoulders, huge arms, muscular legs, large rear ends, and small waists: Adonises. The working out of the male abdomen has become such an obsession that the muscular "six-pack" shape now seems to be required of any male appearing in public.

This is, of course, as unfortunate for many men's body image as a generation of so-called supermodels has been for women's self-image. Our bodies are defined primarily by genetics, secondarily by health, and thirdly by exercise. No matter how healthy and exercised you may be, by virtue of your ethnic heritage or hereditary assets, you may never be able to fit into what has become almost a stereotypical male physique. However, it's worth remembering what you consider your worst feature may strike others as your best.

Men with a poor body image convey a sense of insecurity to the people they meet. Their insecurity is off-putting and their fear of being ugly, self-fulfilling. A few use their poor body image almost deliberately to keep other men at a distance. The scenario goes like this: "I'm ugly; he couldn't possibly like me; no one could like me; therefore I needn't risk getting close to anyone." Quite neat, really, but an awful way to live.

A poor body image can be improved. One way to let the light of reality invade this murky business is simply to ask a friend what he likes about your body. You will be surprised when your partner praises your small ears or the "butch" veins on the back of your hands (Butch? Your hands?). Or the rivulet of hair running from your navel into your crotch—features you've never given two thoughts to, since all you can think about is your giant nose or your forlorn buns.

If there's someone you trust completely, you might ask him to join you in an experiment. Have him sit in a chair and look at you while you stand and study yourself in the mirror. Tell him all the things you like about yourself—your wry smile, your big eyes, your powerful neck, your skin color, even the chipped tooth that you secretly pride yourself on. Naturally this orgy of self-regard will embarrass you at first, but it is curative. You could look at yourself in the nude or clothed. If you don't want to do all this in front of someone else, do it alone, but make sure that you say the complimentary things about yourself out loud. Why this *viva voce* approach should make a difference is not certain, but it does work. Perhaps people need to hear positive things about themselves, and not just think them.

If you wish to do something to improve your body, don't just talk about it: Do it! Swim, take up a new sport, or join a gym. When you begin to show physical gains, show them off with more revealing clothing by going to a pool or a beach; give people a chance to tell you about yourself. All too often false modesty or anxiety causes us to cut off compliments. Attend to other aspects of your appearance—your clothes or your hair; change any part of you that will give other people and you a visible sign you're feeling better about yourself. Even if it doesn't significantly change your looks, it will improve your health, place you alongside other physically healthy men, and it could alter your attitude for the better.

And don't let anyone put you down!

Our advice boils down to setting your own standards for your looks rather than submitting to the standards (either real or imagined) of others. You must begin by yourself. After that, the good feelings you radiate will be magnetic to other people.

Bondage and Discipline

Bondage always implies domination, but not necessarily S/M. Some men like the sweet agony of being tied up and then subjected to a long blow job to which they can respond only with groans; or to having their body licked and caressed until they're mad with pleasure; or to being fucked in the mouth or in the ass while they writhe, unable to do anything to stop the action.

Other men prefer being the dominator. They like nothing better than to handcuff their partner or tie him tightly to the bedpost or bed board to feel complete control over him; the domination can then be teasing, gentle, or rough.

When it is a part of S/M sex, bondage is an extreme dramatization of the master-slave relationship: The master is in such total control that obedience is no longer an issue. The thrill for the slave comes from his being completely dependent on the master (and the complete trust this dependence signifies).

What to use in bondage? Women and some men prefer softer ties—silk, satin, chamois, any material that is completely pleasurable to the touch. Others prefer leather thongs and wear them wrapped around their neck (or a dog collar) when they go out at night, as advertisement and inducement. Still others use anything handy— telephone and electrical wiring, bedsheets, towels, metal and plastic police restraints—just as long as it fits into the roles being played.

The biggest turn-on, and conversely the biggest problem, in bondage is control— and the lack of it. While the master's control is crucial and indeed desirable to some degree, the exact degree of control ought to be decided upon in advance by both parties. This will keep the bondage a sexual turn-on and keep it from becoming a dangerous, frightening experience.

We assume you've chosen someone trustworthy to tie you up. To do otherwise is to place yourself in a particularly dangerous position. For example, a friend of the authors' was sitting at home one evening. His doorbell started ringing and didn't stop.

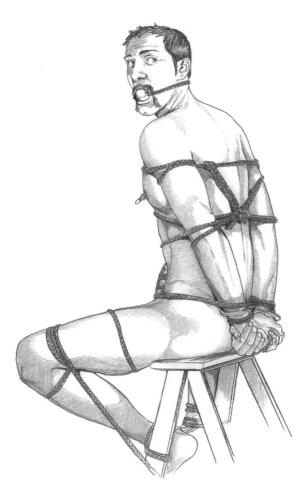

When he opened the door, he found his next-door neighbor on his knees, naked, arms and legs bound by rope, ringing the bell with his nose. After having sex, his trick had left him bound and robbed him (see *Dangerous Sex*).

Since the wider publication of Robert Mapplethorpe's photos of rubber- and leather-encased men, and the film *Pulp Fiction*, with its examples of the same, other kinds of bondage and discipline have become more popular, e.g., sheathing your body with a full rubber or leather "body-glove." Some of these are artistic, expensive, made-to-order items. They can be tailored to fully enclose the body except for a few breath holes, with zippers over the mouth, eye, penis, and anus slits. Often, the encased man is stood up in a corner of a room, then hung from (carefully) set up wires and/or set upon shelving, in effect becoming an exhibit, a piece of human decor. Or, opposite to being exhibited, he might instead be hidden away, further encased in coffinlike boxes and closets. Obviously this is a fairly esoteric way to get your kicks, and definitely not for the claustrophobic or easily bored. Still it has its devotees.

The bondage scene in gay life can go beyond sexuality in other, even more arcane ways. The famous Mineshaft in New York City used to hold its Bondage Club's meetings on Sunday afternoons, and it wasn't surprising to walk in on a half dozen young men tied up in heavy hemp rope in all sorts of positions, and to have a lecturer in full British Admiralty dress explaining the intricacies of the nineteenth-century English marine knots being used, a lecture that—save for the naked, writhing bodies—might be held in any museum, with precise terminology, wooden pointer, and avid listeners (see *Body Decoration; Sadomasochism*).

"Discipline" used to be considered intrinsic to bondage and paired with it, the two shortened to read as "B&D." This is less true today, partly due to the huge growth of the gay leatherman scene, with S/M now such a large and complex sector of the gay community. Discipline can consist of anything from insults and verbal abuse by the master to his slave, to the most brutal kind of physical torment. All of it must be acceptable a priori to the slave being disciplined, or it has no meaning or context within their relationship.

Should you find yourself in a sexual situation with a stranger who tries to talk you into bondage or discipline, or who, without asking your permission, begins to tie you up or "discipline" you verbally or physically, stop him immediately and tell him you are not interested. If he persists in the behavior, instantly get yourself away from him and out of the situation. Don't bother explaining yourself or defending your position. Even if he's merely insulting you, you don't need the abuse, and you don't deserve it.

Booze and Highs

By the age of thirty many gay men have had the following experience. You wake up one Saturday or Sunday morning, only to find a naked man in bed with you. His head is on your chest and he's licking the hair around your nipples. You look at him and haven't the foggiest idea who he is or how he (or you) got there. "Hi, honey," the naked man says as he nuzzles your ear. "Would you like me to make you breakfast?" Only then do you realize that you also don't know *where* you are!

Amusing stories like this (and many variations) are often told in the gay community. As a unique experience it retains its humor. When it occurs more than once, it's a sign that you're having "blackouts," a sure symptom of alcoholism.

Alcoholism is widespread in the gay community. There is also evidence that the incidence of alcoholism is greater in the gay than the straight community, and that this difference gets larger yet when comparing gay and straight teenagers.

Gay men subject themselves to the devastation of excessive drinking for many reasons. In an earlier edition of this book we said that the insidious effect of homophobia was the primary reason. For most of the past century gay men could meet only in seedy, Mafia-owned, police-controlled bars in large cities, or furtively during late-night encounters in parks or woodlands, or in public toilets (tearooms). As a result, gay men were forced to socialize in bars and around liquor. Gay men were subject to capricious interrogation by police, to entrapment, and to seeing their names published in local newspapers under the headline PERVERTS ARRESTED. Little wonder gay men invariably felt ashamed of their sexual orientation and guilty over their sexual desires. Still, with the advent of gay liberation and its successes, homophobia can no longer be identified as the *primary* reason gay men become alcoholic (see *Drug Abuse; Homophobia; Guilt; Tearooms and Back Rooms*).

Drinking has always been used to oil our social inhibitions. A drink or two gave a man more courage to ask another man to dance or for a date and made rejection of the offer less painful. Repeated rejections often led to repeated drinks, or worse yet, ingesting other drugs together with alcohol (see *Drug Abuse; Drugs and Sex*).

Feeling yourself a part of the special crowd of gay men is another reason some men become addicted to alcohol. In time, and after a night of excessive drinking, you wake up in the morning only to discover you've traded your sense of inferiority and fear of rejection for a troublesome chemical dependency.

Many men start drinking when they are teenagers. Some are the children of alcoholic parents. A considerable body of research shows that alcoholism runs in families. Children of alcoholic parents tell stories of violence in the family, times when the child came to the rescue of his mother, who was being beaten by a drunken father. All the more of a surprise that these teens often become alcoholic themselves. Some alcoholism specialists believe that the tendency toward alcoholism is inherited and that a gene in our bodies predisposes some of us to it. Others think it is learned as a way of coping with stress and conflict.

Almost everyone drinks on occasion, and few gay men can claim to have lived a totally alcohol-free life. Experts generally call these people drug users. You probably are one. Most of us are. "Users," however, do not have problems with chemical dependence.

The next category is "drug abusers," including those who cannot perform sexually without alcohol or drugs or both. Drug abusers also suffer other bad consequences from their drinking or drug taking, such as poor judgment in choosing sex partners, spending money stupidly, or falling down on the job. The first stage of abuse is often hard to detect. Since your ostensible purpose in frequenting bars is to search for romance or sex, you'll scarcely notice that your tricking has declined and your drinking has increased.

Drug addiction occurs when you lose the power to make choices about your drinking and drug taking. Chemical dependence becomes what's most important in your life: more important than sex, friends, family, your job. People who abuse drugs find that, in time, how good you feel from taking the booze or pills evaporates and is replaced by how badly you begin to feel and how completely you screw up your life.

Alcoholism specialists now describe alcoholism as *alcohol myopia*. The abuse of alcohol narrows your sense of self and your social judgment, creating a form of near-sightedness, or what is called *disinhibition*. Most people feel inhibited and shy at times; alcohol and drugs remove those inhibitions, making them feel bolder. But inhibitions (and caution) are sometimes good, sometimes appropriate to a situation.

Alcohol myopia leads to many problems. The use of alcohol and drugs is the primary reason gay men practice unsafe sex and become infected with the HIV. Disinhibition also leads to other unsafe practices in which physical harm or illness may occur (See *Dangerous Sex*; *Fisting*; *HIV Disease*). Men under the influence of alcohol choose riskier and more promiscuous men for partners when drunk than they would when sober.

A problem for HIV-positive men is that alcohol interferes with the effectiveness of protease inhibitors, since both drugs are metabolized in your liver.

When combined with another disinhibitor such as the social environment of a dance club, alcohol can lead to your ingesting one or more party drugs whose contents may be unknown. Be particularly careful about drinking alcohol and taking ecstasy (X) in the same evening, since both cause dehydration, an even riskier prospect. Combined with your water loss from sweating on the dance floor, dehydration becomes triply hazardous. Deaths have resulted from the combination of alcohol and ecstasy. While dancing, you should drink water (or soft drinks or sports drinks) constantly.

In addition, men under the influence of alcohol or recreational drugs may easily be robbed, beaten up, or sexually assaulted (see *Rape*). Most men don't talk about these experiences, and the gay press seldom writes about them, adding to this conspiracy of silence.

And if these problems weren't enough, alcohol and drug abuse inhibit your immune system and can lead to an additional decline in T cells, another danger.

If all this sounds grim, and it is, there is help. If you have an abuse or addiction problem, you should join Alcoholics Anonymous or Narcotics Anonymous (listed in the phone book). Most large cities have gay AA and Al-Anon meetings. You'll meet other people who are also seeking to cope with alcoholism. And because anybody can have a booze or drug problem, you may end up meeting people at these meetings who become important in other personal and career ways.

Some people seek help through psychotherapy in conjunction with AA, which may be beneficial. Therapy alone, however, has *not* been very successful in dealing with alcoholism. Too many therapists regard alcoholism as a symptom of a neurotic disorder and will not treat the so-called symptom directly; and therapists cannot provide the round-the-clock support that most alcoholics need.

What if your boyfriend, best friend, or lover is a substance abuser? You may be in for a series of problems that may make you feel helpless and impotent to make changes. If your lover or a family member is an addict, don't make the most common mistake in the book: Don't try to change him or make him go to AA. While you have every right to express your concerns, try to avoid blaming him or being self-righteous about the problem. Avoid increasing guilt, shame, or anger in your lover, and in yourself as well.

Don't do this alone. There are organizations for people whose family members are alcoholic. Join Al-Anon or Nar-Anon. You'll find them listed in the phone book. Their support may be vital for your own self-esteem in this difficult period. Psychotherapy may also be useful, especially if you are deciding whether to continue the relationship.

Bottom

As you become more sexually experienced, you'll discover you prefer certain sexual activities and positions. You may find that you prefer getting fucked, no matter the time, place, or partner. You may also have begun to find yourself evaluating the men you meet by a new index: the size, shape, and the hardness of their cock, how much they check out guys' buns, and how often they come on by talking about fucking or saying they're interested in "getting ass."

When this happens, you have become a bottom, or bottom man. The name, of course, derives from the placement of the person being fucked—i.e., on the bottom.

Being a bottom doesn't mean that you always have to be fucked in the missionary position. That can get boring. There are other positions (see *Bottoms Up; Face-to-Face; Sitting on It*). Nor does being a bottom make you less desirable than a top. It also doesn't mean that you can't fuck another man if that's what you and your partner choose. Assuming you practice safe sex, feel free to fuck your lover or trick or take turns fucking each other. Many bottoms claim that they are the only gay men who really know how to fuck; they know what feels best. Being known as a bottom can be useful in meeting potential sex partners, in that if your reputation precedes you, people not interested in being tops automatically eliminate themselves from a potential sexual adventure. Identifying yourself as a bottom is useful when placing ads in newspapers or profiles on the Internet (see *Sex Ads; Profiles*).

But it would be a distortion of reality to suggest that being a bottom is merely a matter of who fucks whom. It is, more importantly, a state of mind, a feeling that one has about oneself in relationship to other men. It is best typified by a line in Richard Burton's translation of the *Arabian Nights*. "Rise, doff thy clothes and take thy pleasure." In some men "bottom" denotes wanting to be taken care of, being protected by a more powerful man, as if there is safety in standing under his psychological umbrella. Another bottom may like humiliation and a top who will treat him roughly, perhaps tie him up and smack his ass hard before (and during) fucking (see *Top*; *Spanking*; *Bondage and Discipline*). In some men being a bottom reflects an important streak of passivity, as if to say, "I want to give myself up to you." But don't take "passivity" too literally. Every gay man knows that the world is populated with very pushy bottoms.

Some bottoms are particularly turned on by large cocks, actually, huge donkey dongs, not only large, but really thick. They answer ads and profiles of men who claim extraordinary endowments—and sometimes it's true. This prize is the visual

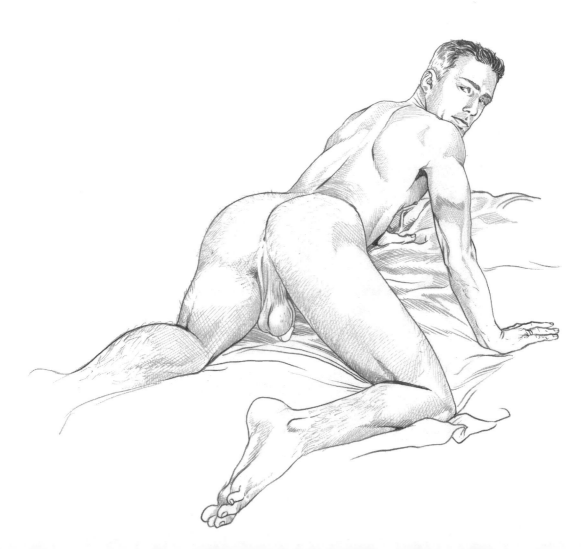

ambrosia of some bottoms. A cock's length is rarely a problem; its thickness may be. If an exceedingly thick cock fucks a bottom hard, the two sphincter muscles may get torn (see *Male Sexual Response*). Still, we know of men who have been damaged this way and, after recuperating, go back for more. We recognize the excitement of being plowed hard by a huge symbol of masculine authority. We suggest, however, that if it's your fantasy, place your trick on his back and sit on his cock. That way you'll have a better chance of avoiding physical damage. And be sure that you use an extra large condom (see *Cock Size; Condoms*).

Psychologists have no idea how these preferences develop, nor how and why they change. It's probably best to indulge them as long as one makes decent choices in men, avoids heavy drugs and alcohol, and has safe sex (see *Booze and Highs; Drug Abuse; Safe Sex*).

Bottoms seem to predominate in gay life, or so they complain. Paraphrasing Mae West, bottoms are heard to say, "A hard man is good to find." The predominance of bottoms was demonstrated during "Underwear Night" in a South Miami club. Perhaps a thousand men checked their clothes and danced in their underwear. During the entertainment, the emcee (for reasons unknown) asked all the bottoms to collect on one side of the dance floor and all the tops on the other. If the dance floor had been on a ship, it would have capsized! Almost the whole of them were bottoms, and it made for a dreary night.

What happens if you (a bottom) go home with a trick who also turns out to be a bottom? It simply won't work to have two submissive men in bed together unless one of you is willing to take charge. Many bottoms are capable of "topping" another man when need be; others can't get hard if asked to fuck. Still, there are lots of other things to do in bed. But in the end, if no one is willing to make a move, you may just as well get dressed, go home, and go on-line (see *On-Line Cruising*).

Bottoms Up

For the man turned on by the touch and sight of buns, nothing is more exciting than to see a partner lying on his stomach, legs spread apart, waiting to get fucked. In this position the buttocks seem rounder, their texture smoother and more cushiony. Sometimes when fucking someone who's lying on his back, you slam into nothing but hard bone and taut muscle (which, granted, can be a pleasure, too). But if your partner's on his belly, his buns are curved and supple and susceptible. A pillow under his pelvis will make his ass more prominent and adjust its angle.

Some men like to fuck guys draped over the broad arm or low back of a sofa or a

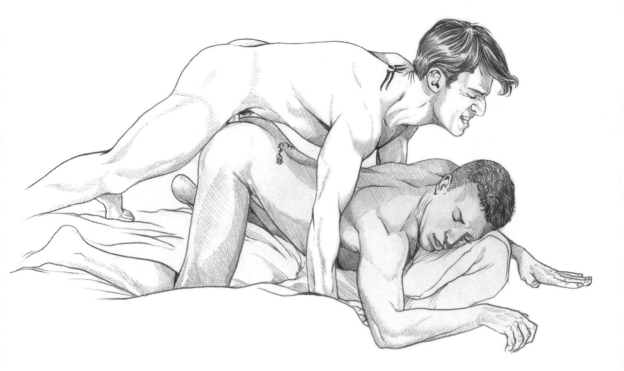

well-upholstered chair. Others like them standing against a wall, a window, even a mirror, while still others prefer the classic simplicity of their lovers facedown, spread-eagled on the mattress (see *Mirrors*).

For the man getting fucked, the very passivity of these positions can be a turn-on or a bore depending on one's mood and general sexual makeup. They're not very good positions for kissing or for watching the action or even for jerking off. You can reach around to steal an occasional sidelong kiss, you can watch yourself in a mirror, you can dry-hump the mattress or work your hand—or better yet, his—under you and beat off. But the real appeal of the position is its passivity.

For guys attuned to S/M, the appeal can be the submissiveness of the slave (see *Bondage and Discipline*). For the majority of gay men, being covered and surrounded by another man can feel comforting and secure. For everyone, the sense of being entered and massaged from within, over and over, without control, is primary, perhaps even primal.

• • •

Buns

They come in all shapes and sizes, and there is an admirer for each variety. They are among the main attractions of the male body. Buns are versatile and beautiful—cushiony when relaxed, firm when flexed: at once soft and hard, smooth and strong, plush and steely. No wonder the world is filling up with replicas of Michelangelo's *David*; even in soapstone or Styrofoam, the rear view is beguiling. David's weight rests on one leg, which accentuates the roundness of that cheek and

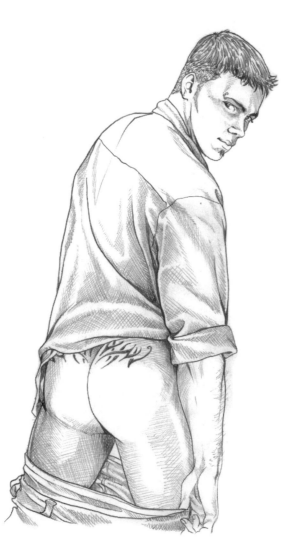

hollows out the dimple. The other curve is relaxed and the corresponding bun describes a gentler curve. And no wonder we now get to see men in underwear ads with excellent buns. Certainly those who wonder at the benefits to mankind wrought by gay liberation (or by Calvin Klein, for that matter) need only look as far as their local newspaper or billboard. Two decades ago it would have required special efforts—e.g., going to a beach or to a shower room—to see what's now displayed daily and everywhere for all to enjoy: nubile, young male buns everywhere you turn, perfect in close-fitting undergarments or bathing suits.

If jeans show off the ass, genes dictate its size and shape. There are many exercises for reducing but few for building up the gluteus maximus, the largest buttock muscle; only those who do a lot of kicking (soccer players, swimmers, and dancers) are likely to improve noticeably on what God gave them. But there are a couple of exercises for transforming apples into cantaloupes.

Stand upright, step forward as far as possible with the right foot, bending the knee but keeping the torso straight. Your left leg will then be stretched out straight behind you; do not let the knee touch the floor. In one motion, push up with your right foot and return to a standing position. Repeat exercise, bending the left knee. Do three sets of twelve repetitions each. At first you will have trouble maintaining balance; hands on your hips will help, but practice will make perfect. After you have become used to the exercise and have done it for several days, do it with a light barbell on your shoulders.

Another exercise is this: Stand straight, holding on to a bar or shelf at hip height. Kick straight back with one leg as far and as often as you can. After you are sore, switch legs and do the same with the other leg. This tightens the bottom muscle and keeps the buttocks from sagging.

Camping

Camping is a form of pretense and humor that attributes—and then comments with much embroidering upon—effeminacy in a person or a group of people. Camp is opposed to seriousness, antithetical to tragedy, and represents the triumph of style over content. A bunch of gay men camping can, for instance, spend hours "dishing" (gossiping) one another and swapping insults ("You're secretly butch? Well, honey, you'll die with that secret!"). In this guise camping tends to sound quite bitchy, even vicious, but outsiders often fail to pick up that the insults being traded are all in good fun. During one such session, someone might say to another, "Miss Thing, you're the absolutely, drop-dead most vicious queen on this green earth!" and mean it as a great compliment.

Camping is a form of gay humor that is dying out. True, it may well have been the by-product of oppression, secrecy, and self-hatred, and now that gays are more self-accepting, as well as more accepted, they may have less of a need to camp. But the demise of camp is not altogether a cause for celebration. Camping was and can still be terribly funny and it does have one merit: It prevents gay men from becoming too pompous or serious in discussing their problems. One example of camp dialogue supposedly overheard during a police raid on "the trucks," a preliberation sexual gathering area in Greenwich Village: "Run, Mary! It's the cops!" To which someone else responds, "Please, no names!" At its best camp can be rebellious, elusive, Dada, an anarchic force in gay life.

The word itself is odd; it may derive from *army camp*, where prostitutes gathered, including male homosexuals. Or, it may come from *kemp*, which in English dialect means "impetuous rogue."

Whatever its origins, *camp* is an extremely versatile word, a noun ("He's such a camp"), a verb ("Don't camp on me"), and an adjective ("His apartment is so camp: the interior of St. Lucy's, complete with confessionals!"). As a noun it means a funny, effeminate, or outrageous person or happening. As a verb it means "stop putting me on." The adjective signifies "amusing," even "preposterously amusing," and generally evokes a nostalgic interest in other periods, especially in bygone fads and follies.

Many women are insulted by the application of the feminine gender and exaggeratedly feminine qualities to men. This is understandable, but it misses the point. Camp seeks to disarm its enemies by identifying with the oppressors. If straight society accuses us of being women, we'll turn the accusation into a compliment. In fact, we will show them we're more outrageously feminine than they imagined. As blacks tease each other by calling themselves niggers, thereby defusing the insult hurled by whites, so gay men make a virtue out of the vice attributed to them.

Homosexuals eager to maintain a highly masculine image also object to camping, on the grounds that a conspicuous display of effeminacy only blackens the already tarnished picture straights have of gays. This objection seems misguided; bigots do not make distinctions between shades of effeminacy or masculinity. It's enough that you're gay for them to hate you.

Ever since 1964, when Susan Sontag first wrote her "Notes on Camp," Camp has taken on another, more specialized sense, as a sensibility peculiar to gay men. Fascinated by pop culture, by aging divas, failed movie stars, all the absurd pretensions of the past. This fascination, Sontag points out, is not cruel curiosity but an affectionate regard for "failed glamour."

> The experiences of Camp are based on the great discovery that the sensibility of high culture has no monopoly on refinement. Camp asserts that good taste is not simply good taste; there exists, indeed, a good taste of bad taste. . . . Camp taste is, above all, a mode of enjoyment, of appreciation—not judgment. Camp is generous. It wants to enjoy.

At least, that glamour conscious enough to be ironical about itself. Thus all the Tallulah Bankhead jokes. Example: The well-known actress with the deep voice is in a public john and notices there's no toilet paper. She asks for some from the occupant of the next booth, who reports she's used the last piece. Tallulah meditates, then replies, "Well then, dahling, do you have two fives for a ten?"

Celibacy

Celibacy simply means refraining from sexual activity, but over the centuries a great deal of fact, myth, and fallacy have attached themselves to the word and the practice. Those who are celibate because it is required by a religion or sect usually refrain from any sexual activity, including masturbation. In some religions—Catholicism, for example—even sexual thoughts are prohibited by the clergy. Nonreligious, less strict interpretations of celibacy do allow sexual thoughts, erotic fantasies, and daydreams along with masturbation, but do not allow sexual contact with another person.

But why, you might ask, would a sane person think of practicing celibacy?

The answer is that while it may be unusual for most adults, celibacy is not bad for you, even mentally or physically. The male body has a built-in method for ridding itself of semen (hence, nocturnal emissions), and in some cases celibacy can actually be refreshing. For example, gay men undergoing psychotherapy because of troubled romantic relationships often end them and avoid new ones, remaining celibate while they sort out their life. One also finds celibacy as the choice of some men who are either HIV-positive or symptomatic (see *HIV Disease*). In these men, celibacy may result either from depression or the fear of contaminating another.

What most discover when they become celibate is a surprising lack of pressure and stress in their life. They feel relieved, relaxed, and capable of being more objective about themselves and their relationships with others. Without the constant need to be sexually desirable, they begin to recognize abilities and values in themselves that may have been overlooked or underrated: charm, a sense of humor, psychological penetration, conversational ability, creativity. Work on these areas (free of sexual pressures) can lead to a fuller sense of yourself, providing a new confidence that ultimately makes you even more desirable should you decide to end your period of celibacy.

And of course if you are inexperienced with homosexuality and are not exactly sure how deeply you wish to engage in gay sex, it's probably a good idea to remain celibate until you find the appropriate person or until you feel completely certain you want to begin having sex.

Chat Rooms

The types of chat rooms are as various as the people who use the Internet. Sometimes these groups of people (called clubs or rooms, depending upon the server) are listed geographically by city or state, or by age groups from young guys to "silver foxes" (see *Teenagers; Growing Older*). You'll also find rooms based upon ethnicity. Or there may be a room with guys who are into a particular sexual variation that interests you, such as slaves or fetishes (see *Bondage and Discipline; Fetish*). You all may be fans of the old TV show *The Brady Bunch,* or into snowboarding, or followers of J. R. R. Tolkien's fantasy *The Lord of the Rings,* or interested in leather and tit torture. The only thing that matters is that you all share something of interest (see *Sadomasochism; Sex Toys*).

Let's go back to your screen name or at least the one you've chosen to use in chat rooms. Few guys will use their regular e-mail address in what could be a sexually exciting Internet connection. So you might as well take some time and figure out what name you're going to use. If all you're going to do in a chat room is discuss eighteenth-century Moulton china, then having a screen name like Sweaty-from-the-Shower is probably not the best idea. If instead you intend to use chat rooms to meet guys for on-line sex or to meet guys in person after you've "talked" on-line, then that could be a terrifically appropriate name. They may even have profiles available for each name. What do you do? You can stay in the room and follow the conversation and see if you're enjoying it. You don't have to say anything. You probably don't even have to acknowledge a greeting from someone who may have noticed you "enter" the room. Or you could jump right into the chat. It may be three-thirty in the morning where you are and there's no one "in" the chat room. Or there may be dozens of guys present, mostly from somewhere distant, where it's only 7 P.M. Or 7 A.M. for that matter; the Internet is, after all, global.

Inside chat rooms, there is usually a topic, or topics, though distractions are frequent. There's often a specialized argot or slang—you will quickly notice. There are various shortcuts people use there called "emotions"; for example, to signal that you're happy with what someone just said, keyboard a colon followed by a closing parenthesis, :) and you have a smile; do it the opposite way, :(, and it's a frown. Other common contractions include LOL for "laughing out loud," ROF for "rolling on the floor," RT for "real time" (getting together right now), DL for "down low" (use discretion/meet in private place), pvt for "private," vgl for "very good looking." The language of the chat room murders spelling and punctuation, and literary skills take a backseat to marketing. The whole message, conveyed in one line, must include physical descriptions (yours and his) and sexual proclivities. You'll soon pick it up.

If you're enjoying your back-and-forth with someone else in the room and want to "meet" him privately, you may want to open a private channel only to him. Say he responds to your instant mail, and you decide you want to talk privately. You can click your way out of the chat room altogether and remain in private or instant-mail communication. Say you discover he lives nearby and you want to speak to him one-on-one. You'll end up exchanging phone numbers, signing off the Web, and telephoning each other. And move on from there.

On the other hand, the guy may have a video-camera hookup on his computer, set up so that you can receive real-time videos of him in his room (see *Webcams*). This is a great way either to meet someone or to check out someone you're talking to, and if you're into having sex that way, it can be extremely hot watching someone via his video hookup while he watches you via your video hookup, while on other, dedicated phone lines you are talking dirty to each other while, say, jerking off.

As a general rule, people come and go in chat rooms quickly without them or others remarking upon it. But sometimes a more elaborate courtesy is involved. Play it by ear—or in this case, by eye. And of course, it's probably a good idea to treat someone on-line as courteously as you would like to be treated. If not, he might easily come back under an unrecognizable name and snub you when you are most looking for contact (see *Etiquette*).

Warning: If you're at work or at school and using their on-line hookup and they have restrictions about its use and chat rooms, your employer can identify that while you're supposed to be doing an assignment or weekly accounts, you're "swishing" around a Transvestites Anonymous chat room (see *Transgender*). Employees have been fired for as much. Also be forewarned that if you are in a relationship and using chat rooms without your partner's approval or knowledge, he can infiltrate your favorite rooms and harass you, bad-mouth you to others, or in a particularly ingenious case of friends of the authors, he could go into the chat room under another name, "meet" you, successfully seduce you away from others, and have you all to himself—and only reveal it later on, that night, in bed (see *Couples*). Many couples have broken up this way.

Civil Rights

What do these people want?" ask some uncomprehending heterosexuals about the civil rights demands of gay activists. "The same rights you have," we answer, "no more—no less!" In almost half of the United States and in many of the cities and towns across the United States, we gay people are still not protected from discrimination. Whereas African-Americans, Latinos, Asians, and Jews face dreadful discrimination, they at least have the possibility of legal recourse. Gays, however, cannot always fight discrimination in the courts.

Civil rights remain the most important continuing issue in the gay liberation movement (see *Gay Politics; Gay Liberation*). In almost every state, and in many municipalities, gay groups are lobbying for laws forbidding discrimination in employment and housing, as well as demanding equal protection under the law, and calling for equal partnership rules that will allow visitation to those institutionalized (in hospitals and prisons), as well appealing for financial, health insurance, and other social benefits for gay spouses. For decades, bigots have argued that gay firemen and policemen will have a natural tendency to seduce their colleagues, and gay teachers will corrupt their students. Now that gay people have come out and have openly served in those positions for decades in many larger American and European cities without any such problems arising, this argument has largely been defused.

In the European Union, gays can and often must also serve in the military, and any nation wishing to join the EU must have an open-admission policy for gay men and women. All of the Scandinavian countries now recognize gay marriage, although not all of them have legalized gay adoption. In the United States, meanwhile, the Don't Ask, Don't Tell policy set up during the Clinton administration has been a stunning failure. Gays continue to be hunted out of the armed services, and incidents of gay bashing have not abated. While many gays don't see this as an important issue, the truth remains that for many rural and urban gays, for women and for gays of color, the armed forces represent one of the few legitimate avenues through which they can hope to better themselves socially, educationally, and financially.

More than half of the states have repealed their sodomy laws, but many remain on the books. Although statutes vary greatly, they generally prohibit a number of sexual practices performed by both homosexual and heterosexual consenting adults. These include anal intercourse and oral-genital sex. The same strictures that penalize homosexual sex also forbid a husband and wife to sixty-nine. As a result, groups like the American Civil Liberties Union have placed legislation against these ordinances high on their agenda.

Another area of gay legal struggle involves children in divorce cases. In the past, judges routinely refused to award custody to a gay parent and sometimes even forbade visiting rights to the gay parent. In the past decade we have seen an enormous increase in gays parenting their own and adopted children, and studies have concluded that gay parents are as good as, or better than, heterosexual parents at child raising (see *Gay Families*).

These studies have also assisted gay parents who want to adopt, which in the past was another area of conflict. Today, even single gay male parents adopting are common in larger states and cities, although this of course depends upon the discretion of your locality.

Insurance companies have traditionally prohibited gay men from naming their lover as the beneficiary of their life insurance policy (see *Insurance*). But many national and international corporations (among them Walt Disney and IBM) have changed their in-house benefit policies, extending health insurance and other spousal benefits to one's lover. Therefore, some gay people may be able to choose anyone as their beneficiary; but most gay people still don't have this right.

Domestic partnership bills now exist in dozens of American and foreign cities (Boston, Seattle, Portland, New York City, Providence, West Hollywood, Beverly Hills, Los Angeles, San Francisco), and even in a few states. Vermont recently passed its own version of a spousal law that all but equates gay marriages with nongay ones. And while passage of a similar state bill appeared close in Hawaii, the vote was postponed. However, in a knee-jerk reaction, many other state legislatures with more conservative members have attempted to ensure that no such law can be passed in their own areas, and when these have failed to get out of committee, they have tried to pass other "marriage-protection" (actually marriage-discrimination) laws in which Vermont's or any other state's legal gay marriages will not be recognized. These issues remain "hot," and it seems that it will require more time and lawsuits before they are settled.

AIDS discrimination used to be severe everywhere, but as the disease spread during the 1990s into the nongay population, many of these practices fell into desuetude. However, AIDS discrimination in most jailhouses and prisons across the country continues unabated, with AIDS and HIV-positive patients regularly subjected to segregation, abuse, substandard health treatment, and an almost complete lack of social equality. And AIDS discrimination worldwide continues unabated as the plague rages on, especially in so-called third world countries. A recent world AIDS conference encountered substantial resistance to ensuring help and education to homosexuals, even when the United Nations secretary-general stepped in and chastised the recalcitrant countries.

Immigration authorities continue to have the legal right to forbid entry to the United States to any person who is HIV-positive, and immigration laws against gays are still on the books and still utilized, although in several recently publicized cases, "political refugee status," based on the peril to the immigrant's life back home due to his homosexuality, has been successfully utilized to allow gays to enter the United States. Fortunately, homosexuality is no longer cited as grounds for denying citizenship.

There have been many gains and losses in the civil rights struggle. The gains have generally come about because gay people became more militant in their demands, and more efficiently organized. But for many gays, earlier generations' struggles seemed either already fulfilled or, more flippantly, old-fashioned and passé. Until, that is, several heinous incidents during the mid-1990s reminded a new generation that none of us is safe until all of us are safe, and that none of us can rest until all of us enjoy fully equal rights. Wyoming college student Matthew Shepard's death at the hands of gay bashers electrified and nauseated our nation and the world; his grisly death scene, iconized on the cover of many magazines, with its inescapable allusion to the original Christian martyrdom, alarmed many devout Americans who had previously accepted antigay discrimination as a religious duty and brought about a new and ongoing debate about bigotry that significantly aided the gay rights movement. We cannot and we should not expect another such sacrifice to secure our gay rights. We believe that each of us owes a responsibility to those gay men who preceded us as well as to those who will follow us, a responsibility to make gay lives a bit easier than our own.

One way to fulfill this responsibility is to join a gay rights organization. It may be militantly political or it may quietly serve the community. Some think that such activity is the true final stage of coming out. It is an enriching experience.

Clubs

Your friends invite you dancing at a club. It's probably not an all-gay club; possibly only on a Saturday or Sunday night is it a "gay" or "all-men" night, while during the week it caters to all comers, or conversely, it may be gay only on a Thursday or Friday night and open to regular customers all other nights. In smaller towns or foreign destinations, it may be "boys' night." You pay at a booth or hand in your complimentary tickets. The entrance may be up a long escalator past palm trees and mirrored walls, or down a twisting staircase into a neon extravaganza, or you're whisked in an elevator up to a high floor, and when the doors part, you are in a long corridor, pools of light shining on the carpet. The main room is huge. Hundreds of men (and a few women) are on the dance floor gyrating under a medley of shifting lights and booming sounds. The dancers seem to be mostly in groups; a few in couples. When you and your group take to the floor, you affect nonchalance, though you might actually be thrilled to be surrounded by so many different men.

Another scenario: You arrive at a location outside the local suburb following a map printed from an e-mail invitation; or perhaps it's closer to home, behind a small door in a mostly boarded-up block in a questionable area of town. There could be a heavyset, large, maybe older guy at the door, checking ID and taking door money. You enter a short, dark hallway, into a series of fairly dark rooms that, if the light ever went on, would be revealed to be cinder block and concrete or peeling paint. But there's an area for getting drinks and standing around, and a tiny dance floor, where a bunch of guys dressed like you and your buddies are dancing like mad. You surge into them en masse, meet and greet other pals, and you're in. Maybe later on somebody done up in a heavy "alternative" outfit or with so many piercings and rings they'd never get through an airline terminal checkpoint without setting off alarms will get up on the tiny corner stage and begin screaming and ranting and, occasionally, even singing. That's the "talent."

Whichever place you're at, after ten or a hundred songs have seamlessly blended into one another and you're quite exhausted, you desert your group and enter the bar area. A porn flick or perhaps an old movie may be shown against the wall, over and over without the sound. You sit down beside some perfect strangers, who smile and offer you a joint. Although they seem pleasant enough, you don't know them (or their level of drug usage) and you're already a little stunned from the music and the exertion. Perhaps you only take one tiny hit, or you decline altogether. You want to experience everything, not get where you're too high to enjoy yourself. You return to the dance floor. Strobes are flashing, the speakers are belting out the latest club hit; the next thing you know your feet have a will of their own. Gay people, you decide in a burst of chauvinism, really are better dancers than straights.

There is no better proof of the emergence of gays from their closets than the continued existence of such clubs. Gays had few choices before gay liberation. They could only gather in sleazy, hideaway bars buried in basements and as hard to gain admittance to as speakeasies. Now hundreds of gays troop into big, spacious, luxurious clubs where the dancing, the sounds, the lights, and the company are great. And when bars open that are reminiscent of the older kind, they usually make that a point of interest, calling themselves the Dungeon or the Firetrap. During the heyday of club dancing in the late seventies, the main problem the gay clubs faced was how to keep straights from moving in and elbowing out the original gay clientele. At gay resorts and many urban centers, the favorite gay hangouts are usually "tea dances," held in the afternoon and early evening on weekends, with fewer drugs, less drinking, but often the same good music.

A new generation is trying to retain most of the best aspects of the traditional older gay clubs, while updating them to meet their own needs and interests. Many newer clubs are smaller than the dance palaces of the past, far less glitzy, homier; they are located not in the usual gay ghettos, but in working-class, mixed, or ethnic neighborhoods. This reflects a desire both to strike out on their own and to be more politically aware. As a rule, the young men filling these clubs have specific interests in fashion, politics, and music. The latter ranges from the salsa and merengue found in Latin clubs, to hip-hop, techno, and "house" music. Other clubs stress an interest in gender-bending and cross-dressing, with performances from drag queens and other artists (see *Transgender*).

Some gay men become so attached to going out clubbing that they can't fathom a weekend without at least one night at their favorite hangout. That's fine as long as you are having a good time and going for the socializing and the exercise. For others, it's a once-in-a-while kind of thing. And for still others, it's a cruising ground. They go through one club after another looking for sex partners. Of course, a side benefit of the closed or membership club is that whomever you trick with is a known entity. His reputation—your own, too—is on the line every time you enter the club. A less beneficial aspect is that member clubs invariably limit their membership, "card" non-members, and generally prefer a fairly homogeneous clientele (see *Racism*).

There is one serious problem in going to a dance club: drug taking. More than in any other place where gay men congregate, you're likely to find drugs at clubs; drugs such as Special K, coke, crystal, and ecstasy are used not only as a social lubricant, but to help one enjoy the music and to provide the energy to dance until the wee hours of the morning. For many gay men in urban centers, the club culture and the drug culture are synonymous. Quite a few gay men, especially those going to "circuit parties," indulge in a combination of party drugs, some of which could be lethal (see *Drug Abuse*). The combination of drug use and the charged sexual atmosphere also leads some gay men down the path to unsafe sex afterward (see *Safe Sex; Drugs and Sex*).

Cock Size

A scene in Petronius' *Satyricon* takes place at the Roman baths. Speaking about a naked youth, he writes: "He was soon surrounded by a thronging multitude, clapping their hands and showing the most awestruck admiration. The fact is, he possessed virile parts of such enormous mass and weight, the man really seemed only an appendage of his own member."

Perhaps we inherited our fetish of the cock from the Romans, but what a tiresome obsession it's become! The man with a big cock feels that he is valued for his appendage alone. The man with a small cock is embarrassed by it and feels that he is spurned because of it. Size queens turn down a lot of sexy men because they fall a millimeter short of the desired length. Most men fear that their cocks are not large enough; the fear is often a cover-up for other insecurities.

The truth is that cocks vary greatly in length, width, and shape. Some are straight when erect; others curve back or sideways. A particular cock can also appear small when soft and surprisingly bigger when hard. Conversely, some cocks that are large when flaccid become only slightly longer when hard. But an obsession with size—your own or someone else's—only serves to reduce you or him to a statistic, and society is already too preoccupied with quantifying human beings.

At the end of the nineteenth century, a French physician, Dr. Jacobus (the nom de plume of Jacobus Sutor), made a survey of cock size in Africa. He was a French army surgeon assigned to various colonial outposts, where he conducted research. Part of that research was to run from village to village measuring the dick of any man who consented; it's unclear whether the French government authorized the project.

Jacobus claimed that Sudanese Africans have the largest cocks, with Arabs running a close second. (He didn't measure those of the French soldiers in Africa.) The largest cock he encountered belonged to a Sudanese and measured twelve inches in length, with a *diameter* of two and one-quarter. "The unfortunate Negro who possessed this 'spike,'" said Dr. Jacobus, "was an object of terror to all the feminine sex." (But what a hit he'd be at a gay sex party.)

If you think your cock is too small, don't fuss with vacuum pumps or hormones or other contraptions, because they don't work for enlargement—although they have

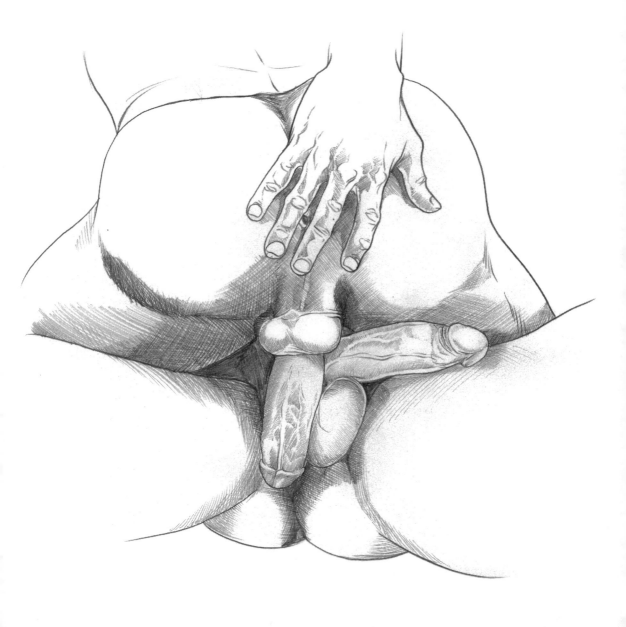

other uses (see *Sex Toys*). Nor should you pad your crotch; false advertising will hardly make you feel more secure. And now the Internet is filled with "spam," e-mails about how to "enlarge" your penis. Delete them immediately. Do not believe that you can increase the length of your cock by attaching weights to it. Ads in the gay press tell about a new form of surgery that promises to increase the size of your cock by cutting some of the muscles that attach it to the bone and by inserting tissue in it to increase thickness. Please don't do it because the results can be disastrous; some men end up with lumpy dicks that face due south (instead of north) when hard.

Realize that your cock has many other aspects than size alone. A lover or fuck buddy can give you feedback—you may be surprised to learn he likes the way it curves up when hard or the way that large blue vein zigzags down its length; he may like it just because it's fat and stubby. He may think that your cock is in perfect proportion to the rest of you; he may be glad your cock is no bigger than his. You're probably aware of the various attractions of other men's cocks, but in contemplating your own you may make the mistake of seeing its size alone. If you like another man's cock, be sure to tell him about it; he, too, needs reassurance (see *Foreskin*).

Coming Out

Coming out is not only the first time one has sex with another man. It is also the psychological, social, and even the public stance that someone takes toward his homosexuality. In the past, few people were lucky enough to have come out in a relaxed way. Perhaps today fantasy and reality seem to be a little closer.

You've gone to the far end of the beach (where you know men in pairs and groups hang out) just because . . . well, just for fun. You don't really give it much thought, wanting to sun with these guys, but you do notice your mounting excitement. They all seem to be having fun. In the water two slender fellows are sitting on the shoulders of beefier guys and playing war. Near you, another group, all well built and methodically tanned, are playing cards on a blanket and listening to a radio.

Right next to you is a man who appears, like you, to be alone. The sun is so glaring you turn on your stomach and rest your head on your arm. You close your eyes and listen to the waves, the war cries, the transistor radio—and your own pulse throbbing in the ear pressed against your biceps. When you open your eyes, you let them travel up and down your neighbor's body. His oiled flank has picked up orange dye from his beach towel. His profile glows in the bright, white light. His chest is almost hairless except for a wisp of hair around each nipple. His legs, however, are luxuriously furred and powerful. In a rush, that forbidden desire to touch his body comes over you.

Your neighbor has now turned on his side. The sun is so bright and strong you're not certain if his eyes are trained on you. Now you can see how broad his shoulders are, and how narrow his hips, from which his muscular thighs project like arrows from a quiver, bristling with golden feathering. He *is* looking at you. He comes to your towel and asks you to oil his back.

He's staying at the hotel down the beach, and after you've sunned for hours and jumped into the breakers and laughed and looked at each other and applied still more lotion to each other's body, he asks you up to his room for a coffee or beer. You feel you should tell him you're not . . . not what? Not attracted to him? Then how do you explain the embarrassing mound swelling your swim trunks? Sure, you'll come up for a drink.

He's very casual as you stroll through the lobby and ride up the elevator, and you wonder whether you've been mistaken about him. After all, he is from out of town. He may just have stumbled by accident on the "wrong" end of the beach. You realize he's not feeling guilty—a realization that makes you recognize that you are. No matter. He's a really good conversationalist, knows a lot about movies and music, has a great smile, a great . . . body.

Even in his room, once he's closed the door (at last!), he's still casual; never more so than when he steps naked out of his swimsuit and announces he's going to take a shower. "Want to take one, too?" he asks.

"Sure," you say with a nonchalant shrug and a throat dry enough to grow cactus in.

"Well then, come on." He leads the way.

You follow impatiently, reluctantly, gracefully, clumsily, happily, fearfully, as his brown body, with its band of white around the center, shimmers in and out of focus. Once you're both in the shower, nothing could seem more natural than scrubbing his back and, as he slowly revolves, his chest. Some nagging little martinet in your brain keeps shaking his finger at you and gasping in shock, but you ignore the reprimands and move smoothly into his arms. His body is still hot from all the solar energy absorbed that day, glassy from the thundering water. Now his hair is wet and pressed against his skull, which turns out to be surprisingly delicate and finely shaped. He pulls you still closer, kisses you, and you're not certain whether you're drowning or in something very much like ecstasy. No man has ever kissed you before, and you feel that bristly day's growth of beard above the smooth lips. He backs off a second and says, "You're okay?" All you can manage to do is nod and hope he knows the nod means "Yes."

In bed you're so happy and so *relieved*—relieved of a cumbersome burden of yearning you've been shouldering too long—that you run your hands through your damp hair and just sigh.

"What's wrong?" he asks.

"Nothing," you tell him. "Everything's right. But I should tell you something. This is my first time with a guy."

"You could have fooled me. Do you want to stop?"

"In about two days."

He does think you should take a breather. Then you talk about your past. You remember the years you jerked off to porn magazines and videos; lest you be ostracized by your peers for being a fag, you never showed too much attention to a friend in school. Your new friend has lots of interesting things to say, and his story is not too different from yours. That nagging in your brain is less insistent. The talk is great, but what you really want is to get back into bed. At last you just say so and he says, "Sounds good to me."

He takes the lead in sex, and you don't explode, nor does the devil rise up out of the mattress to claim you. In fact, it feels good, but what feels best is this *freedom* to be next to another man. You can't believe you are finally free to touch him everywhere, to lie under him and on top of him, to kiss that sandpaper beard. Will it leave a beard burn? you wonder in panic. Will people be able to *tell*? The panic gives way to a surge of pleasure, the pleasure of inhaling another man's aroma, for surely that's what you're doing, that's what this freedom is, the freedom to breathe in the smell, the touch, the reality of an affectionate and sensitive man who seems to like you.

His jacket and slacks fit you, and after you're both dressed, you go down to the dining room (no, the people can't tell, but, oddly, you wish they could). You feel a little formal and tired and relaxed after the sun and the sex—and the drama, taking place mainly in your head. Not much gets said over dinner, but looks are exchanged, and during coffee he squeezes your hands under the table. "I never thought," he says, "I'd be the one to bring someone out."

"To do what?" you ask.

"I just brought you out. Coming out. That means having your first gay experience."

The label sounds strange to you. You thought the word should be *freedom* or maybe *graduation*. But of course that is what they—no, *we*, you suppose—yes, we gay guys call it: coming out.

*   *   *

The earliest urges toward homosexuality are usually exercised in adolescent fantasies. The homosexual aspect of some boys' fantasies may be disguised—a boy may masturbate while imagining a man and a woman having sex and may scarcely notice that most of his attention is focused on the man, zooming in for more close-ups of his anatomy than of hers.

Although some boys conjure up scenes of deep love and affection with members of the same sex, for most the fantasies are distinctly sexual. At puberty, boys think constantly about sex and generate powerful fantasies through masturbation. Society condemned masturbation for so long that even liberated people said little in its favor beyond assuring us there's nothing "wrong" about it. This latent Puritanism has concealed what is very much *right* about the masturbatory fantasies through which adolescents explore which kinds of physical types and psychological characteristics are exciting (see *Sex Phobia*). The jerk-off fantasy is a rehearsal, a preview of coming attractions, and it is a crucial learning experience (see *Masturbation and Fantasy*).

At some point the neophyte gay will have his first homosexual experience in the flesh. All the horniness held in check and vented only during masturbation will be released in a flood of desire. The initial sexual experiences are something very special. A few gays coming out confuse good sex with love. With maturity they learn that sex is not always a measure of love or intimacy.

After one or many experiences, someone coming out will have to say to himself, "I'm gay." To ever greater numbers of men entering gay life, this statement comes naturally and easily. Others find self-acceptance harder to achieve, and coming out takes longer. They may have sporadic sexual contacts, but they shrink from admitting their homosexuality even to themselves. Others think of themselves as gay, but refuse to let anyone else in on the secret (see *Homophobia*).

Of those who do come out publicly, some tell only one or two friends, others only members of their family; a few are open with everyone. Most often we disclose our homosexuality to parents, brothers and sisters, intimate friends, and lately, employers, because we want no artificial barriers to stand between us and the people who are important in our lives (see *Out on the Job*). If we come out to them with love, they are unlikely to remain distant for long, although some parents demonstrate neurotic behavior when they learn of the son's homosexuality (see *Parents*). Even so, despite the risk, many sons feel the temporary stress is worth the bother if it eliminates the more insidious stress of always lying to others.

Perhaps the most harrowing part of telling others about our homosexuality is having to face our own doubts and fears. If a gay man says, "I can't tell my parents because they believe homosexuals can never be happy," he may simply be attributing his own misgivings to them. It's easy to assign our own doubts to our parents, and it can be significantly counterproductive and downright wrong to do so. Many gays finally get up the nerve to come out to their folks only to hear them say, "We've known it for years. We were wondering when you were going to find out yourself."

Coming out often proceeds through stages, from fantasies to the first same-sex experience to acknowledging it to yourself and then telling others that you are gay. A final step is often at last identifying with the gay community (see *Gay Liberation*). How someone moves through these stages will differ from individual to individual and will be determined by various factors. How old you are and where you live will definitely make a difference. If you live in a small town, far from the big cities where homosexuality thrives openly, or in a religious or other kind of sex-restricted environment, you may find little support in your efforts to come out. If you are a young man still living at home, or an older man whose whole mature life has been spent in the straight world—say in the armed forces—coming out can be baffling and even painful and you may want to look for guidance and help from gay organizations and from friends.

A homophobic religious background is another important determinant. Those who grew up as Mormons, Orthodox Jews or Muslims, fundamentalist Protestants, or strict Roman Catholics often have especially difficult coming out experiences. Other ethnic and sociocultural factors can also influence coming out, both positively and negatively.

The AIDS crisis of the past twenty years can also be another strong impediment to young men coming out. More than one child has grown up hearing from parents and family that sexual excesses reward gay men with life-threatening illnesses—who could blame someone for turning away from gay contact out of anxiety and confusion? Men, young men in particular, searching for love and to satisfy their healthy sex drive, rightly fear that their inexperience or foolishness could destroy them (see *Saying No; HIV Disease*).

Gays just coming out have responded to HIV disease with a number of sexual strategies: Some act as if they are omnipotent, totally invulnerable to human illnesses. This grandiosity is dangerous to you and to your sex partners. At the opposite extreme are men who have pretty much taken vows of chastity, not because sex is immoral, but from the belief that any gay sex is dangerous (see *Celibacy*). Most gay men try to remain midway between these two extremes by meeting their sexual needs with responsibility (see *Safe Sex*).

AIDS has highlighted the responsibility we have as members of the gay community. Our first responsibility is to be informed about and to practice safe sex. The second is to encourage friends, lovers, and tricks to protect their own health. Finally, many gay men find that involvement in the gay community can provide sustenance and meaning in their life. Consider joining an AIDS service organization and working with gay political groups that are fighting for our civil rights (see *Civil Rights; Gay Politics*). It'll help you feel part of something larger and more important.

Compulsive Sex

One gay man wishes he had more sex. Another complains that he has too much sex. What's ironic about this disagreement is that both men may be having exactly the same kind of sex and with the same frequency. Perhaps that's to be expected in a Judeo-Christian society with its ambivalent (at best) atti-

tudes toward sexuality. Propagation, yes; pleasure, no. It's hard to find anyone brought up in America who hasn't been adversely affected by it, and it's the reason why places like Brazil (even though Catholic) and Thailand are so appealing to us. Men in these foreign countries impress us as being better in touch with the sensuousness of their bodies and more relaxed about sex as a natural behavior.

The controversy over the American concept of compulsive sex began in Minnesota in the 1980s with the invention of "sexual addiction" as a diagnosable and treatable abnormality. It is not, however, approved as a diagnosis by the American Psychiatric Association. This diagnosis was first applied to straight people. It was claimed that to these people sex had the same uncontrollable, addictive qualities as heroin to a heroin addict.

Shortly thereafter, a few gay therapists claimed that gay men suffered from the same problem, but to distinguish gay from straight men, they changed the diagnosis to "sexual compulsion." The main characteristic of sexual compulsives, they claim, is their discomfort and guilty feelings about the nature and frequency of their sexual behavior. These men feel guilty about jerking off too much, cheating on their lover, having anonymous sex, and participating in kinky sex, particularly S/M, water sports, and scat (see *Kinky Sex; Sadomasochism; Scat; Water Sports*). The treatment usually offered is participation in a twelve-step group called Sexual Compulsives Anonymous (SCA). These groups use the customary AA model as their guide, and men are supported by the group in ending their "compulsive" sex and substituting "normal" sex.

Many people and many gay mental health professionals abhor the concept of "sexual compulsion" for historical as well as clinical reasons. For many decades homosexuality itself was diagnosed as a mental illness because it was said to be compulsive. Psychiatrists and psychologists used the words *homosexual* and *compulsive* interchangeably until the 1973 deletion of homosexuality as a mental illness by the American Psychiatric Association. Most gay mental health professionals reject the sexual compulsion diagnosis because it sounds too much like a return to the days when gays were taught to feel guilty because of their homosexual fantasies and behavior.

The authors do *not* believe that being made to feel guilty about their sexual behavior advances the rights of gay people. We, like other critics, note that the complaints of gay men are a reflection of the strict behavioral code of our repressive society that goes something like this:

1. You shouldn't jerk off too much (whatever that means).

2. You should be in a monogamous relationship only.

3. You should not have sex in tearooms, the bushes, or dirty-book stores.

4. You should avoid kinky sex, especially if it is "disgusting" and not egalitarian (see *Bondage and Discipline; Kinky Sex; Sleazy Sex*).

We do not agree with any of the above-noted "shoulds" and "should nots." They are highly intrusive and have little or nothing to do with good gay health, mental or physical.

It's important that a gay man distinguish between his actual sexual experiences and his feelings about them. A man may feel guilty about jerking off and call it compulsive if he does so every day (even two or three times a day), while another man may jerk off equally often but consider it normal and healthy. Another man may feel guilty about tricking out on his lover and call that compulsive. The sex itself isn't necessarily compulsive. The label he's applying reflects the power of guilt in our repressive society.

The authors see the concept of "compulsive sex" as yet another technique by which our society is trying to make gay men feel guilty about their sexual behavior. Those mental health professionals who advocate the diagnosis of "sexual compulsion" seem to us to be cops in the service of a heterosexual society that wishes to control our desire. That's the last thing gay people need.

This is not to say that gay men have it all together, either. Like our straight counterparts, we sometimes have sexual problems and dysfunctions (see *Drugs and Sex*; *Impotence*; *Problems of Ejaculation*). We sometimes don't know how to channel our desires. We're often hesitant in our approach to fulfilling sexual fantasies and make some serious mistakes along the way, usually hurting ourselves rather than others.

The authors believe that the main sex problem is guilt, just as psychiatrists tried to make us feel guilty for being homosexual in the first place. Perhaps a gay man should not be tricking out when he's in what's supposed to be a committed relationship, but we believe that this man would be ill-advised to confess it to a group of people who reinforce feelings of guilt about sexual behavior. Our belief is that it is a problem in the development of attachment and intimacy, not sex. Instead, he should be encouraged to discuss his obviously unfulfilled sexual and/or emotional needs with his lover—possibly in the presence of a skilled couples therapist. If unattached, the gay man should seek a therapist in whom he can develop feelings of trust. While we have long been encouraged about the healing properties of AA and NA, which seem to be effective for substance abusers, we remain skeptical about the efficacy of twelve-step groups regarding sexual problems.

There are probably gay men who feel that SCA groups have helped them. We do not wish to create further conflict within them because of the choice they've made. They should act in their own self-interest. We merely suggest that they look at the alternatives and make an informed choice.

Condoms

It's not known how long condoms have been in existence. Some scholars claim to have found allusions to them in the works of Virgil and the Roman satirists. Condoms (and dildos) first appeared in England by 1660, supposedly brought over from Italy, and were in wide use by the eighteenth century, when sexually transmitted diseases had become rampant in Europe. By then they'd become so common that they were manufactured, openly sold, and even advertised in Paris and London as "implements of safety which secure the health." A certain Mrs. Lewis held the London monopoly in the 1740s. By 1770 the monopoly had passed to Mrs. Phillips, who became famous for her products. We find many references to condoms in the literature of the day: Samuel Johnson's biographer James Boswell casually writes in his journals of sexual encounters in which he was "unclad"—i.e., not wearing a condom. The young author agonizes over whether he's contracted a venereal illness and will have to undergo a protracted and painful cure for "the clap" (see *Sexually Transmitted Diseases*).

Early condoms were expensive, if natural, products, usually made of lengths of sheep intestine sewn closed at one end and colorfully secured at the base with a red ribbon tied around the balls. Often ill-fitting and strong smelling, they became increasingly expensive, rare, and difficult to obtain as rural areas shrank and sexual hypocrisy grew in strength during the industrial revolution. Late in the nineteenth century, rubber replaced animal gut as the condom material of choice, but these early products broke easily unless they were made so thick that most pleasurable sensations were completely dulled. The perfection of vulcanized rubber in the beginning of the twentieth century not only made possible the durable rubber tires that assured the ascendancy of the automobile in America, but also allowed for the cheaper, safer, thinner, and more pleasurable latex condoms so often found strewn around parking areas in various lovers' lanes.

By World War II, every kit handed out to the millions of men in the U.S. armed forces contained its share of "rubbers"—as latex condoms had become known—for protection against venereal diseases. At the same time, the discovery of penicillin and antibiotics seemed to promise a future free of the worries that had afflicted our ancestors' sexual lives. Up to about 1970, young men still carried fold-up wallets indelibly deformed by the impression of a rolled-up Trojan, Sheik, or other brand of condom, but with a somewhat different intention: birth control. With the advent and instant popularity of the oral birth-control pill taken daily by women, condoms all but vanished from American life.

Condoms weren't in widespread use among homosexuals. When they entered gay sexual life at all, it was usually as a curiosity, a sex toy. Especially among those gay

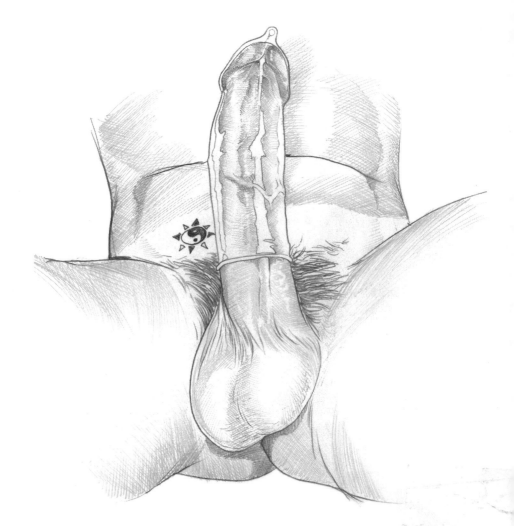

man who'd come out since the Stonewall rebellion of 1969 or who'd never had any heterosexual experience, condoms—if they were thought of or used at all—were considered kinky, something a little daring. Now, however, with the spread of HIV disease, condoms have become mandatory in our lives—truly a matter of life or death—although some gay men adamantly reject them (see *Barebacking*).

Also known as a rubber, a safe, a sheath, a come bag, a scumbag, a hat, a cap, a coat, or a capote, a condom is nothing more than a tube, usually made out of extremely thin latex rubber, with one end closed or slightly extended into a receptacle tip. Condoms are used during fucking, sucking, jerking off, and other sexual acts to receive and hold the come that shoots out of the cock opening (the urethra) (see *Male Sexual Response*). They provide an effective barrier against disease organisms.

Usually condoms are sold rolled up flat; they are about the size of a Susan B. Anthony dollar coin, and one condom is sealed per package. Latex rubber, rather than "natural" or sheep-gut, condoms are the least permeable by bacteria and so the only safe type. Many condoms are sold prelubricated. You'll also find them in different colors, tastes, and sizes.

When buying condoms, you should read the information on the outside of the package and inspect the package to see that it's sealed tight. Most condom packages are dated. Check to see the date is current. Old condoms can easily break. To put on a condom: Remove it from its package. Check the condom for any rips, tears, or perforations. Obviously this isn't always possible without breaking the mood established between you and your partner. Some men "wet" instantly, which is to say that they exude a lot of precome as soon as their cock gets hard. If you're one of these, skip the following few sentences. For those who are dry when hard, you might want to put a dab of lubricant on the inside of the condom. This makes it go on easier and helps stimulate you during sex. Use only water-based lubricants such as K-Y or ForPlay. Don't use Crisco, baby oil, Vaseline, or any petroleum-based lubricants (see *Lubricants*). These work chemically against the latex and can make it degrade and tear. You can, however, use them for jerking off.

Holding the condom, place the head of your cock into the condom's opening and then slowly unroll it back along the cock shaft toward the body until it's on fully. It should fit snugly but not too tightly. It's important to hold the condom by its tip to prevent air from being trapped inside, as this causes the condom to balloon out and rip. Condoms can catch painfully on genital hair, so go slowly.

When removing the condom, roll it over the head and off. Should you lose your hard-on when inside someone's ass, hold on to the base of the condom while pulling out. Some men "double bag," use two condoms, one on top of the other. Those who use condoms while sucking prefer condoms without receptacle tips, as tips can get caught in teeth and tear. Most condoms are made in one size. If your cock is too thick to fit into standard condoms or so narrow it flops around in them, you can find specially made condoms. Larger and wider sizes are known as Max. Check in specialized sex shops, which often have names like Leisure Chest or Tool Chest. If you live in a rural area, look for condom ads in the pages of gay periodicals or straight sex magazines.

Be aware that condoms can break during long and rough bouts of ass-fucking. This is one area where it doesn't pay to be economical. Only use a condom once! Even if you didn't come in it, throw it out and put on another. It's a good idea to keep condoms handy. Those men who complain that putting on a condom "breaks the mood" obviously haven't tried having their sex partner put it on for them. If at the same time you lubricate each other and talk about your sexual fantasies, this can be a terrific turn-on. If you've never used a condom before and are uncertain about using one, try it out alone, jerking off. Do this several times until you're comfortable with putting it on and taking it off after you come.

HIV disease is believed to be transmitted mostly through ass-fucking, and safe sex guidelines recommend a condom even for sucking. This can be a problem because many men complain about the lessened sensation while wearing a condom, and few but rubber fetishists are interested in sucking a cock covered with one. Many get around this by not sucking or by not allowing their partner to come in their mouth. However, if you're someone who has a lot of precome, be safe and always use a condom while being sucked. And naturally it's always better to be safe than sorry. Don't, however, use a prelubricated condom. It tastes awful.

Some gay men who are into getting fucked have begun to buy and use women's condoms, either because they don't trust their partners to provide their own condoms, or because they want to double their safety from infection. These are vaginal condoms, used by women for decades to prevent pregnancy or the transmission of STDs. They are generally cone-shaped, wider at the lip, and narrower the deeper it goes in. Unlike women's genitals, however, most anuses don't have labia, natural protrusions that can hold this kind of condom from slipping in during intercourse. So it's usage for anal sex can be limited. However experimental you want to get around this issue, always wear a condom for ass-fucking unless you know your partner has tested negative for HIV.

Cosmetic (Plastic) Surgery

According to recent statistics, 1 percent of Americans will undergo some form of cosmetic surgery. It has become a $20-billion-a-year industry in the United States and is growing fast in Scandinavia, Germany, England, and South America.

The most common cosmetic surgical procedures over the decades have been facial. Among those, rhinoplasty (a nose job) and surgeries on the upper and lower eyelids and on the chin remain the most common. Some of these can have medical purposes. Nose jobs, for instance, can effectively treat a deviated septum and/or crooked nasal passages that block breathing or make it more difficult. But most people—including gay men—have these operations not for medical reasons but to make their noses smaller and more shapely, to enlarge or close up their nostril cavities, to enlarge or cut back their chin, and especially when removing fatty deposits around the eyes, to make themselves look younger and more attractive.

Recent facial procedures that are almost as popular include laser surgery for the eyes to alter the shape of the cornea and make wearing corrective lenses unnecessary, cheek implants that "lift" and reshape the face by raising cheekbones, and lipid implants inside the lips to make them larger and fuller. The last is not permanent and may need to be redone. We don't yet know about the other two over the long haul, as they're only a few years old. They, too, may require upgrades.

The rest of the body has also come in for plastic surgery, and with certain exceptions most of this is for cosmetic and not health reasons. The most popular surgeries for men target a few specific areas. First, the upper chest, where the pectorals may be too fat-filled or otherwise have problems. Some males—both gay and straight—retain vestigial mammary glands, and some of these men, upon reaching manhood, find that these may on occasion "leak" or in effect lactate around the areola and nipple area. This can be painful, embarrassing, and at times can lead to infection. Vestigial mammary glands are also prone to developing masses, both cancerous and benign (yes, men can develop breast cancer). Surgery removes the glands, and usually the supporting fat.

For other men, there is no medical cause for removing the fat from a pectoral area. It's merely to achieve a flatter, more aesthetic chest. Other men with already fairly well developed muscles in this area, contrarily, have fat implanted into the pectorals. Like many weight lifters, they will discover later in life that they'll have to continue a rigorous pectoral muscles regimen to prevent their pecs from becoming all fat when natural male musculature declines with age.

Second, and also common, is the cosmetic removal of lipids from around the lower chest area, waist, and hips, an expensive procedure, which is generally accomplished in a few hours. Males tend to develop and carry fat differently than women—generally, more in front, between the sternum and the lower groin, and in a more or less circular outgrowth. We know this as the "potbelly," so common in many of the older men we grew up around. It is nature's way of storing energy against lean times. It's also common in younger (and sometimes very trim) young men. Many exercise regimens for middle-aged men such as jogging, hiking, and power-walking are geared toward pulling on that lower abdomen until muscle replaces fat.

A third type of male body surgery is on the gluteus maximus muscle, one's ass. Increasingly, this surgery is mostly on the lower portion of the muscles, in effect removing fatty deposits, and thus decreasing the size of and "raising up" the ass.

The fourth most common male surgery is the "lengthening of the penis," which is actually the removal of the lowest cartilage connection from the shaft of the penis to the scrotal sac, which makes the penis look longer, even though no real lengthening is done (see *Cock Size*). However, most doctors strongly discourage men from having the procedure for a number of reasons, not least of which is that while the cock gets hard afterward, it tends to hang down, not up. A number of "penis jobs" have been badly botched and cannot be corrected.

The benefits of cosmetic surgery are—or ought to be—immediately evident. The person's face, chest, abdomen, ass, looks better than before. In theory it's as simple as that. Yet, actually it's a bit more complex in that improved looks via plastic surgery can have a variety of mental effects. The first, and most obvious, is that it will increase self-esteem. You look better and thus feel better about yourself, and you more easily go to places you'd feared to go before, where you will be looked at and physically judged: the beach, bathhouses, pools, steam rooms, gyms, etc. Cosmetic surgery can totally revive your social, sexual, and romantic life.

Although it's not common, certain men have grown psychologically dependent on surgery, feeling that once one body part is fixed, another should be as well. Many psychologists see this small sector of "habitual" cosmetic surgery patients as emblematic of a larger problem. They call it *body dysmorphia*. It is a mental health condition characterized by continual dissatisfaction with parts of one's body. No matter how much surgery the man has, he is dissatisfied. He eventually becomes a "surgery junkie" and becomes obsessed about the "ugliness" of one or more body parts. These men provide good money for plastic surgeons, but their own lives are replete with unhappiness.

There are other drawbacks to cosmetic surgery. First, it's not cheap. A minor surgery around the eyes costs around $5,000. Most facial tucks and rhinoplasties cost double that. An entire face may come to $30,000. An entire face and body could run you $100,000. Health insurance plans do not pay for plastic surgery unless the need arises from an automobile accident or another injury. And only those people who can guarantee a certain number of personal and filmed appearances per year (e.g., major movie and television stars and athletes) can obtain a tax break of any kind, and then not a large one.

The procedures are by no means painless. In addition, medical complications, including infection, excessive scarring, and painful neuropathy as a result of nerves being severed, are, while not common, also not impossible. Some men have died after liposuction. At the least, you will look like hell—puffy, black-and-blue, beat-up—for days, possibly weeks, and with some procedures, even longer.

Couples

What is the origin of love? The Greek philosopher Plato answers this question in his *Symposium*. Plato has Aristophanes tell the following tale: In the beginning, there were three sexes: man, woman, and an androgynous man/woman. Each of the sexes was round, like a sphere, with a face and two arms and legs on either side. They would walk forward or backward, or tumble and roll on the ground. These three played and frolicked in the fields. But then they foolishly challenged the power of Zeus. For that, he punished them by splitting them in half so there were two of each. He also separated them so that they could never find their other half. What had been the double man (now two men), said Aristophanes, is the origin of gay male relationships; what had been the double woman (now two women) is the origin of lesbian relationships; what had been the man/woman, now split into a man and a woman, is the origin of heterosexual relationships. Plato said this of the man: "They who are a section of the male follow the male, and while they are young, being slices of the original man, they hang about men and embrace them, and they are themselves the best of boys and youth, because they have the most manly nature."

Aristophanes described the suffering of the three sexes after they were each split into two and separated. They felt as if their souls had been torn apart. Consequently, each spent all of its time searching for its other half, hoping to reunite. Each of the male halves was looking for his soul mate, and until he found it, he spent his days in sadness. Aristophanes said, "The pursuit of the other half of one's self is called love."

Today, we have the freedom to search for our soul mates, and with luck, we may find our "other half." Love between two men gives them the strength to ignore the scorn of a heterosexual world and immunizes them against a homophobic society. Gay love is a source of pride, courage, companionship, and security. Loving couples share more than their bodies; they share their souls.

There was a time when psychologists and psychiatrists claimed that gay men were incapable of real love, that their relationships were fated to break up because of emotional immaturity. There are probably still some professionals who maintain this biased belief despite all evidence to the contrary. Long-lasting gay relationships are common in our society, especially since World War II. It's not unusual to meet white-haired men whose relationship has lasted fifty years or more. It's always interesting to hear how they explain the success and longevity of their relationships. One such man said, "You each have to forgive and forget a lot." Another, more practical than the first, said, "I keep his stomach full and his balls empty."

Some gay lovers would like their unions legally recognized. Though some steps have been taken in that direction, legal marriage is not yet possible. Some states and municipalities now provide benefits for the spouses of their gay employees, as do a few private corporations (see *Domestic Partnerships; Civil Rights*). Perhaps the most significant advance in legitimating gay love relationships has taken place in the area of adoption. Thousands of gay men have quietly adopted children, and in many cities support groups for both fathers and children help sort out potential problems.

Many problems in relationships are due to differences in personality type between the lovers. One, let's say, spends his energies on his home, furnishing and decorating it with panache. Out of a strong sense of attachment to his lover, he's building a nest, and he believes that love should last a lifetime. To him, intimacy with his lover is the highest achievement, and sex between them represents love. He agrees completely with the Greek lesbian poet Sappho, who wrote about herself and her lover, "We came together like two drops of water."

A man with a different personality style, one who values autonomy and independence, is likely to be alarmed by the sentiment expressed in Sappho's quotation. The idea of losing his individuality or merging his personality with another man's is repugnant to him. While he enjoys a comfortable home, his life is not focused on domesticity. He likes excitement and novelty; he draws a distinction between lust and love.

The first personality described is characterized by what psychologists call attachment; the second, by what they call autonomy. The difference between these two

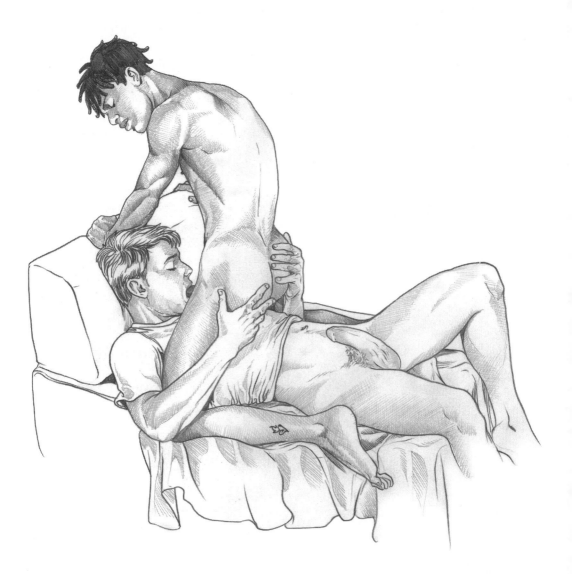

styles is at the root of many conflicts between lovers. It's not that one is good or the other bad; it's the mismatch that causes problems.

Two men who share the trait called attachment can make a happy couple, since their approaches to the relationship are similar. The same is true for two men who value autonomy in a relationship. Conflicts multiply when an attachment-motivated man sets up a relationship with someone autonomy-motivated. Neither kind of man loves more than the other; they feel and express their love differently.

No wonder sexual fidelity is the number one problem in gay relationships. Every couple faces the question of whether to maintain an exclusive sexual relationship (see *Fidelity and Monogamy*). Some lovers live together but have frequent sexual encounters outside the relationship. Sometimes these encounters are one-night stands; sometimes they involve steady partners. Many gay lovers who have been together for years seldom have sex with the other, yet remain deeply committed emotionally, as in heterosexual marriages in the more sophisticated parts of Europe. These unions are known as *mariages blancs*, literally "white marriages."

The problem of sex outside the relationship also faces gay couples who are still having sex with each other. One partner, for instance, may be content to be faithful; his need for security may outweigh his desire for novelty. The other partner, however, may feel a strong urge for sexual adventure. In every case, a solution to the conflict can be found if partners are willing to talk openly and honestly. Dishonesty is the chief enemy of good and enduring relationships. Partners who lie to each other are headed for disaster. Lying destroys trust, and if two men do not trust each other, the relationship is doomed.

Sex outside the relationship is particularly dangerous these days because of HIV disease (see *Safe Sex*). Each man has the responsibility to keep AIDS and other STDs out of the relationship (see *Sexually Transmitted Diseases*). Not surprisingly, many couples, regardless of their personality style, have agreed not to have outside sex because of their fear of disease. Other couples have outside affairs but insist that each man follow safe sex guidelines. Some couples use threesomes as a means of not cheating and ensuring that safe sex is practiced by all (see *Three-Ways*).

Another prerequisite for an ongoing, fruitful relationship is the realization that the relationship will change over time. When we find happiness with someone, we may feel that we have stumbled upon a timeless magic formula that must be preserved. Accordingly, we resist change, unwilling to recognize that all living things, including relationships, must change or fall apart. This problem is not necessarily a function of conflict between the men. It may be a gradual process in which they lose emotional contact with each other as the years go by.

Gay couples also suffer from external pressures. In many places, bigotry still persists, and if it's linked to economic discrimination, the couple may break apart under the strain. The parents of one or both of the gay lovers may also undermine the relationship. Some parents may attack the relationship openly; more often they take a subtle approach. They may pick a quarrel with the lover and manipulate their son to take sides. On the other hand, many parents want their sons to be happy and are supportive of their love relationships (see *Parents*).

Gay relationships commonly end because of personal conflicts. The primary psychological problem of our time is the fear of intimacy. Ironically, many couples break up because of their love for each other. One partner feels he is unworthy of love, and affection makes him frightened and suspicious ("He doesn't really love me, just his mistaken impression of me"). Another partner feels he is incapable of expressing love. Intimacy makes him feel guilty and inadequate ("He deserves someone better than me. I'm just a cold fish and I'm ruining his life").

More deeply, intimacy evokes feelings of vulnerability and loss of control. Because they have been disappointed in their childhood relationships with their parents, or because they have been hurt in earlier love affairs, gay men may be alarmed when they sense a growing closeness to another man. This fear seldom expresses itself openly. Often, it shows up in disguised forms, such as in an inclination to pick absurd arguments or to suspect a partner of sexual infidelity, or even in a frantic urge to trick with strangers and thereby disrupt the love relationship. Sometimes the only way to deal with these fears is by psychotherapy, often as a couple.

Jealousy is one of the most powerful and destructive impediments to a gay love relationship. It's a "red-hot" emotion that invariably consumes the waking (and sometimes the sleeping) life of the jealous partner (see *Jealousy, Envy, and Possessiveness*). The partner's every word, inflection of his voice, and body posture are interpreted and reinterpreted endlessly for signs of secret messages and "hiding the truth." That truth is deception, lying, and most of all the conviction that his lover is either tricking or, even worse, romancing another man.

Some jealous partners go to extraordinary lengths to "catch" their lovers in deception. Some actually follow their lovers at night to see if they are really going to dinner with friends. Others use the telephone as a weapon; they call his office at 8 or 9 P.M. to see if he's really working late. Better yet, when the jealous lover's on a business trip away from home, they call at 10 P.M. "Hi, honey," they say, but "Just checking to see you're in bed—alone" is what they mean.

Jealous lovers steam letters open and read them. They check their boyfriend's e-mail for sexual contact. They also snoop for their lover's computer password; especially astute snoopers may figure out that their lover has more than one password, one for family and one for potential tricks. They use these passwords to find their lover's profile on a gay sex site (see *Profiles*).

Sometimes it's true that the boyfriend has a profile and is on-line looking for tricks. But at other times, the jealous lover may mistakenly pick out the profile of someone who stimulates his own sexual fantasies, but accuses his boyfriend instead. Oh! Does the shit hit the fan then!

Still, with all the hazards of forming gay love relationships, we don't seem to be designed for going solo. The loving care given AIDS patients by their lovers is testimony to the deep sense of commitment that gay men feel toward their lover. It's just a matter of time until gay couples have full legal and civil rights in America. Hopefully this will become the model for gay rights throughout other parts of the world.

Cruising

Looking for sex is called cruising, and it can happen at any time, and at any place—over breakfast in a coffee shop, in line at the grocery store, at an exclusive reception, whether you're deliberately on the prowl or whether you're in the midst of errands and haphazardly find yourself in what seems to be an encounter. The most common time for cruising is at night, and the usual places are those streets, parks, bars, gyms, and clubs where gay men congregate. Most cities have an area or street that's been used for generations, such as Castro Street in San Francisco and Christopher Street in New York's Greenwich Village (although street cruising in New York City has now moved to Eighth Avenue in Chelsea).

There's an art to cruising, and its most important tools are timing and the eyes. The eyes first: You're walking down the street and you pass a man going in the opposite direction. Your eyes lock but you keep on moving. After a few paces you glance back and see that he has stopped in front of a store window, but is looking directly at you. If he's not your type, you'll probably register the compliment with a pleasant smile and leave. But if he does catch your fancy, you may go through the little charade of examining the shop window nearest you. After a bit, the frequency and intensity of exchanged glances will increase, and one of you will stroll over to the other.

There are a few safe, stock opening lines banal to the point of absurdity: "Have you got the time?" or "Got a light?" or "Where's Morales Street?" After these preliminaries, introduce yourself, ask his name, or suggest you have a beverage together.

That, at least, was how cruising usually worked in the past. Today in big cities men often wear a "uniform" so distinctively gay (at least when they've set out to cruise) that there's no doubt about their orientation (see *Uniforms*). Most people have become so open, casual, and fearless that the shop-window checking-out routine is skipped. You simply amble up to him and say, "Hi. Nice night, isn't it? You live around here?"

Once it's clear that one of you has an available space and both have the time and inclination, you're free to say, "Let's go!" Many men, especially those with narrow sexual tastes, may ask, "What do you do?" when you first meet—and they don't mean for a living. Some answer the question immediately, while others feel that part of the fun of discovering a new person is finding out what he does in bed. The very lack of certainty adds spice to the encounter.

On the other hand, many men don't like to move into sex without talking. It is not unusual to stop for a drink or a cup of coffee. The conversation will not necessarily be sexual but rather free-ranging, and exploratory. You're getting to know something about each other: your backgrounds, jobs, values, and other aspects of your lives.

There are some practical advantages in chatting for a while. Suppose you're attracted to him but you've heard disquieting stories about him. A talk will give you a chance to size him up more accurately. You might also feel there's something kinky, even dangerous about him. A talk will give you a chance to clarify your feelings about him.

Should your fears be confirmed, or if after talking with him you lose interest, *do not* go home with him simply out of timidity or politeness. *Never have sex* with anyone you're uncertain of, as this could lead to serious problems (see *Rape; Dangerous Sex*). Tradition has provided exit lines: "I had no idea it was getting so late; I've got to get home" or "I've got to meet a friend; give me your number and I'll call" or, more frankly, "I don't think it's going to work. Sorry." Exchanging phone numbers on the street isn't always a polite deception; sometimes one of you is actually in a rush and would genuinely like to get together later.

One recent and really very good (and necessary) use of a conversation during cruising is to find out what and how much your potential sex partner knows about HIV disease and safe sex. You can also inquire about his own parameters for safe sex and whether they jibe with your own. For example, it might be that he won't have anal sex at all, but will have unprotected oral sex. Or he may be so careful, he'll only indulge in voyeuristic masturbation from across the room.

Bar cruising is less matter-of-fact, more time-consuming, and often more frustrating. Everyone's reluctant to make the first move since he runs the risk of being rejected in full view of a room of other potential sex partners. As a result, the signals are as elaborate and subtle as the movements in Japanese Kabuki. He's interested in you, so he moves to your end of the bar and plants himself against the wall ten feet away and grazes you with occasional glances. Your interest mounts and you move— not next to him, since that would make it awkward for him to look you over more closely—to a position closer than before. At this point, if you stare, you may scare him away; but if you ignore him too long, he may think you've lost interest. This languid mating dance progresses until one of you ventures a smile and the other returns it. The conventional opening lines in bars such as "Come here often?" are often so familiar they're a joke. If the other guy has a sense of humor, he'll laugh good-naturedly.

One real problem in getting anyone's attention even long enough to spout a cliché in bars is that there are so many men to choose from that few are willing to zero in on an individual who, after an hour of chatting him up, may tell you he's got a lover.

Then, too, Mr. Right may be the next man to enter the door. Another peril is socializing; some people are there to see friends and have no interest in meeting anyone new. Finally, a few of those you see night after night propping up the bar want neither sex nor society; they're alcoholics and all they want is another drink (see *Booze and Highs*; *Drug Abuse*).

An extremely self-assured man can cut through the rigmarole of bar cruising, walk right up to someone, and say, "You look interesting. Want to talk? Couldn't we do something better than stand here?" This approach can result in failure; the object of your interest may be startled, too conformist, and simply walk off without a word. Then again, he may light up with pleasure. Everyone secretly dreams of approaching a man in a bar and saying "Wanna fuck?" but few have pulled off that particular fantasy.

If someone rejects you after enticing you, don't worry whether you said something wrong or ate too much garlic at dinner. He may simply not like your voice, or you may remind him of someone else, or he may not be wearing his contact lenses and so he has made a mistake. More likely, you will simply not be his type (see *Types*). Or he may be a cock-teaser. This annoying type haunts the bars and gets his kicks from turning people down; it's virtually a sexual thrill for him to say no, and after he's rejected three or four perfectly acceptable men, he'll go home alone, fully satisfied (see *Rejection*).

In one kind of cruising, a man who can keep a public phone in view from his home can dial the booth when he sees someone attractive. If the man on the street picks up, the caller propositions him.

Car cruising is a national sport with several variants. In small towns and rural areas, rest stops in parks or along highways are often the main place for meeting other gay men. After the pickup, the two men may have sex in the woods, in a car, or in any other available spot. Another variant is when you're driving and notice someone attractive behind the wheel of a neighboring car. There are many ways to attract his attention, the first being, of course, the kind of car you are driving. Some cars are considered "sexier" than others. Sports cars, European imports, and convertibles are high on the list; vans and campers with their family correlation are far less so (unless you're into daddies). Younger men are now being seen driving restored or long-garaged 1960s and 1970s gas-guzzlers, especially the glitzier chrome-embossed coupes and convertibles. West Coast gays prefer open-door Jeeps, the better to show off their bodies, especially in the summer when they wear nothing but shorts and sandals.

In cities with a great deal of car cruising, some of the more heavily cruised areas may have official signage discouraging it, with words like "More than once on the street in an hour is considered cruising." "Strip cruising" like that done on weekend nights on various main drags such as Los Angeles' Sunset Strip and Ventura Boulevard usually consists of slow driving in thick traffic in cars filled with people, who exchange greetings, conversations, and even passengers throughout the night. In a typical bout of car-to-car cruising, you pull up next to someone. His car or his face or something else catches your eye. You maybe nod. If he ignores you, it's all over. But if he nods or smiles back, you try to keep in eye contact at the next stoplight. Maybe one of you says something like "Going somewhere in a hurry?" Or some such. Sometimes at the point where you feel you have some but not complete interest, you might gesture with your hand as though masturbating in air; some guys prefer masturbating in air in front of their mouth, which of course conveys the idea of a blow job. Whether or not you do that, if you're both still interested by the fourth traffic light, one of you suggests you both pull to the side of the road. Do so only when and where it is safe and convenient. Get out of the car so you can size each other up physically, meet, and talk right there. If you're near one of your homes, you might suggest going there immediately, one following the other. Or, if that's impossible, you may exchange telephone numbers and/or e-mail addresses for a later date. Some car cruising, however, holds inherent dangers, besides the obvious ones of being distracted behind the wheel. Arrest through entrapment at rest stops and public toilets is common in small towns, especially around election time. And those who prey upon gays often use these spots to meet unwary men. Be careful!

Many gay men may go through shorter periods of intense cruising in their lives. They're bored with their work or their social set; they're in a new town, in a new neighborhood, in a mood to meet new people and try different things. Taken in the right spirit and with the proper precautions, cruising can be rewarding and fun. You're meeting new people, forming new friendships, and expanding your sexual repertoire. More than one satisfied gay couple met through cruising.

Daddy/Son Fantasies

The daddy/son scene has become more popular these days. It's difficult to say why. Is there a greater need for good parenting? Or has access to the Internet provided a boon to this special kind of relationship because of the new ease with which one can now find others who enjoy the fantasy?

The scene derives its power and interest from real-life psychological issues in many gay men's lives. There are an increasing number of books about the importance of fathers in the sexual development of their sons. As long ago as 1981, Charles Silverstein's *Man to Man: Gay Couples in America* (William Morrow) documented the sexual interest some gays have in their own fathers, including masturbation fantasies of being fucked by them. And clinicians tell us that some gay youths have attempted to seduce their fathers. Richard Isay's *Being Homosexual: Gay Men and Their Development* (Farrar, Straus and Giroux) discusses the importance of the erotic attachment of gay sons to their fathers.

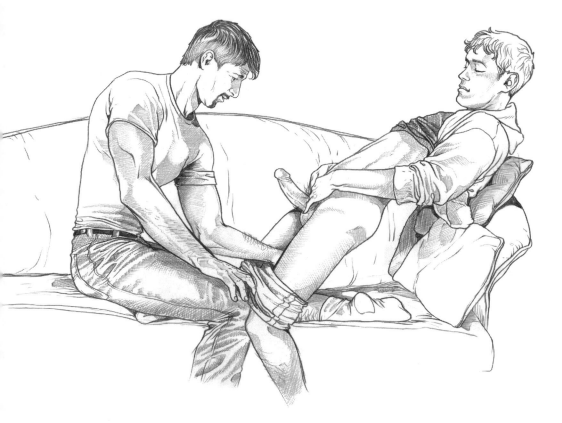

The primary goal of daddy/son scenes appears to be taking care of the son, helping him to grow within the context of a sexual scene. Occasionally the daddy/son relationship continues outside the bedroom as well.

In the gay scene, daddies tend to have certain physical characteristics: salt-and-pepper and sometimes thinning hair; facial and chest hair; faces that show maturity. Some sons prefer daddies with large hands (the better to spank them), but otherwise a daddy needn't necessarily be in the greatest physical shape. The actual age of the participants isn't fixed either: a son doesn't have to be much younger or even younger at all. He should, however, exude a boyish, even mischievous quality, and while he may not sport facial hair, either he or his daddy may prefer shaving off the son's body hair (see *Shaving*).

The daddy/son scenario is usually played out with the younger one being either a "good boy" or a "bad boy." Naturally, bad boys are punished, often by naked-ass-spanking over daddy's knees (see *Spanking*). Some, more deeply into the scene, may acquire and wear certain clothing coded to the fantasy: short pants for the son, a cardigan sweater and slippers for the dad. These accent the reality of the scene and heighten the sexual charge for the participants, as do the use of "authentic" belts and hairbrushes for the spanking. Obviously clothing isn't required: two naked men can play out the scene in bed perfectly well. As a rule, a son prefers to get fucked by the daddy and to follow the daddy's orders (but not too quickly). Many of these scenarios end with the "boy" being complimented for being "good"; the praise, we suspect, is the ultimate psychological goal of the scene. For gay men from unloving homes, the combination of being loved and being fucked by daddy may be nirvana (see *Bears*).

The entire sexual scene is filled with talk between the two men, with the daddy giving instructions to the son ("Show me how you can make Daddy proud"), and complimenting him for correct behavior. It's not unusual for the participants, particularly the son, to experience a rush of emotion after orgasm. Cradled by his daddy, the son may cry at the warmth and compassion he's experiencing, warmth he probably never experienced from his biological father.

One also finds "sugar daddies" in gay life, which may be a transformation of the daddy/son phenomenon. The sugar daddy is older, richer, and more powerful than the young man who becomes attached to him. While they don't call each other daddy or son, the older man takes on the role of protector and mentor, as well as being financially supportive of his charge—clearly the role of a father. Whether being cared for by an older man or being awash in his money is the primary motivation for the young man is unclear.

Dangerous Sex

Danger lurks everywhere in life, including gay life, where a simple walk down the wrong street can turn you into a statistic of gay bashing. While that may not be under your control, most other dangerous practices in gay life are. There are two main areas of potential danger: specific social behavior and specific sexual behavior. Both can be exciting—and both can turn deadly.

Some men only become aroused when there's a danger they'll be arrested or hurt while having sex, which generally means they only have sex outside or in public places. Why they deliberately court disaster is usually as puzzling to them as it is to others, and more anguishing. Perhaps their first truly satisfying sexual experience occurred in a public place, and that as well as the danger of discovery has become eroticized.

Another danger—one that in some cases has proved fatal—arises when a gay man is only turned on by encounters with straight (often teenage) hoodlums or with psychopathic homosexuals. If you're excited only when you go into a recognizably dangerous public park at night, a place haunted by muggers and brutal gangs, you better analyze your sexual tastes fast, before you are maimed or killed. Gay men *have* been murdered this way. Maybe you can be satisfied with the fantasy while jerking off, with a trusted fuck buddy or lover.

Another danger is the potential trick who tells you "I'm really straight. I go for pussy." This is a sure sign he hates his homosexuality—and *could* vent his anger on you.

The foolhardiness of gay men who put their lives in danger is not necessarily their characteristic way of dealing with the world. In business, with friends, in all other nonsexual contexts, they may be cautious and properly self-interested. But the sexual allure of danger—especially the erotic fantasies touched off by it—blinds these people and cripples their grip on reality. They should seek counseling or psychotherapy before it's too late.

Some men indulge in forms of sexual behavior that are potentially dangerous. The most blatant example is barebacking (see *Safe Sex*; *Barebacking*). Other unhealthy practices include not properly cleaning sex toys and not making certain that skin piercing is performed under sterile conditions (see *Body Decoration*; *Sex Toys*): these and other practices are potentially infectious (see *Scat*). Internal organs can also be damaged (see *Fisting*). Others involve breakable objects, such as glass rods inserted into the urethra (piss hole) (see *Kinky Sex*).

One unfortunate soldier was found with his dick snared up the tube of his bayonet sheath, while another man was rescued (one wonders by whom) when his dick was stuck up the bathtub faucet. One commonly finds men who insert dangerous objects up their butts, such as turkey basters, Coke bottles, and the like. That's what dildos are for (and a warm cock, for that matter). Social scientists know little about how these men developed such exotic ways to satisfy themselves. These behaviors are called paraphilias—which means "strange loves." While most of society regards them as disgusting, distasteful, or physically painful, to certain men they are charged with sexual excitement. But not all paraphilias are dangerous.

One paraphilia that is very dangerous is called *autoerotic asphyxiation*, sometimes known as *eroticized hanging*. It's a form of masturbation that can result in death. In one technique the masturbator literally hangs himself while jerking off (frequently while looking at porn). As he masturbates, he also progressively closes off his windpipe, aiming toward a mental-physical state in which mental awareness is supposedly increasingly limited and physical concentration is supposedly intensified, leading to an intense orgasm. The obvious problem is that he may not be able to release or loosen the noose around his neck after he comes, and he falls into unconsciousness, then death.

Professionals have no idea how this bizarre way to challenge the Reaper originated, nor do they know how to change it. It's evident the alleged delights have made this paraphilia popular among suburban and rural adolescents, who often do it while stoned on grass or alcohol and wearing headphones blaring out heavy-metal music. The bathroom is often used, and startled families find the nude or semiclad bodies of dead brothers or sons.

Good judgment is the best rule for avoiding danger. This includes making choices about tricks, lovers, and sexual practices. There are unquestionably some men who function effectively and safely in the world of the paraphilias, giving and receiving sexual pleasure. There are others, however, whose safety and judgment is in question. We hope that they will seek out friends or therapists with whom they can talk, and that ultimately they will either give up the behavior or learn to appreciate the excitement of sex that doesn't endanger their lives.

Depression

In most cases of depression you feel that no one in the whole world understands or cares for you. Or, conversely, that you don't care about anyone or anything in the world. It often occurs when you have no one around to praise you, or when you are unable to accept or to believe in the praise you receive. Depression can also follow a sudden and radical loss of status (either real or perceived)—conflict with one's family, say, the loss of a job, or losing one's home—and it is a particularly common consequence of hopeless love affairs or ending a relationship of long duration.

This kind of depression is different from sadness, what some people call feeling blue. Sadness is always a response to a real tragedy—say, the death of a loved one—the feeling of loss is appropriate. People who are sad may grieve for the loss of a friend, a family member, or even a job, but then, after grieving, move on (see *Letting Go*). When a person *cannot* let go of the sadness, however, he goes from feeling blue to being depressed, or moves, as some depressed people say, into blackness.

Psychoanalysts commonly say that depression is a repressed form of anger, a deflection of hostility away from its external object onto one's self. In other words, you are angry at the lover who abandoned you by dying, the boss who fired you, the landlord who evicted you. But either because the person is more powerful than you or the situation seems so hopeless, you turn your anger inward. Whether or not this theory is accurate, the appropriate, controlled venting of anger is often the best way to overcome this kind of depression, since expressing anger can reverse and banish some sense of powerlessness. When you assert yourself, you once again feel effective and worthwhile.

The psychoanalytic theory of repressed anger is probably too one-sided to explain the pervasiveness of depression in gay men. Clearly one cause of depression is the constant homophobia that gays are subjected to in our society: what's usually called *learned depression*. From childhood, gay men are taught that they have disappointed their parents by not being butch or conforming enough, or by not marrying and having children. Gay men are taught by their faith that they are sinners; are taught by the law that they are lawbreakers. One readily understands why many gay men have grown up feeling depressed about their homosexuality. A young man feeling rejected and unloved by parents, siblings, peers, and the community at large could hardly feel otherwise (see *Homophobia*).

An *acute depression* is caused by a specific event. An example is the loss of a lover or close friend through accident or disease. Gay men, especially those who were sexually active in the 1980s and 1990s, have watched the illnesses and deaths of their gay families, often remaining psychologically strong until the end, when the formerly repressed depression hits them hard (see *Gay Families*). They may need special help and counseling to move forward again. Several books have been written to help them; one of the best is *Gay Widowers*, edited by Michael Shernoff.

Chronic depression affects people over the course of their life. It is sometimes episodic, coming on without warning and lasting months or years at a time. For others, the depression begins in adolescence and never lets up. Chronic depression may also be either mild (a dull psychological pain) and always in the background, or severe, so painful that hopelessness colors a man's existence, potentially even prodding him toward self-destruction (see *Suicide*). Professionals believe that chronic depression is biochemical, probably inherited through the father's side of the family.

Other kinds of depression have different origins, although those causes remain unconfirmed at this time. Some men adopt a depressed attitude from a parent by *identification*. This means that the young boy internalizes his mother's and/or his father's low self-esteem and feelings of inadequacy.

Antidepressant medication is effective for either acute or chronic depression. The course of treatment in acute depression is usually short, while in chronic depression the drugs must be taken for significantly longer periods, sometimes for life. The Prozac class of drugs that also includes Paxil and Effexor are the most effective and most often prescribed. They also have the added advantage of helping people who suffer from obsessions and compulsions. Like all drugs, they have side effects as well. The most common is a sharp loss of libido accompanied with the inability to get a hard-on and/or the ability to come. The higher the dosage of the drug, the greater the effect you experience. Some men strenuously object to this side effect, while others do not because the depression has already reduced their sexual drive. Fortunately, other antidepressant medications can be substituted.

Psychotherapy is extremely valuable to gay men in an acute depression, with or without medication. Men in a chronic depression will be aided by psychotherapy, but medication is always required.

Any form of depression can be so damaging to one's self-esteem that suicidal ideas become common and, in some cases, are acted upon.

Some gay men treat their depression by turning to sex for comfort and relief. In most cases, sex does not provide the solace they seek. What this kind of depressed person really needs is affection and closeness. Someone who is depressed often isn't very good as a sexual partner. He is so compliant that he's inactive during sex, and this excessive passivity just isn't sexy. The depressed person sends out signals that baffle his partner. Disappointed after sex because he has not received the simple affection and affirmation he needs, a depressed person emits signs of his disappointment that confuse and wound his partner.

Yet touching is precisely what most depressed persons need most, though the form the contact takes may be holding instead of fucking, stroking instead of sucking. If you're depressed, ask someone to hold you. The person you ask will probably be a friend or lover, but, surprisingly, even a stranger may be moved and flattered by the request. Animal comfort, however, is not enough. If you're depressed, you need to be with people who like you, who value your opinions, who see things from your point of view. Being alone may seem like a Romantic pose, but when you're depressed, try to abandon it and be with supportive and loving friends. For deeply depressed men, this may not seem to work. But in time it can have a subtle and pervasive effect upon you, helping you gain needed self-esteem.

Many gay men become depressed when they are sexually rejected. If someone is already depressed, he can interpret the least sign of indifference as a rejection. A depressed or insecure man trying to make out in a bar, say, ensures his failure by going, with an unerring instinct for defeat, straight to the coldest strangers in the room. By contrast, someone in a buoyant frame of mind is relaxed, a bit choosy, and ready to admit that his appeal is not universal. He knows that this guy may go only for diminutive blonds, that one for overweight lawyers, and that one only for money (see *Types*). But a depressed person is frantic and quite often forgets the bewildering range of human sexual preferences. He never stops to say to himself, "But I may not be this fellow's type," or, "That guy may not want to go home with anyone if he has to get up early tomorrow for work." Rather, he makes nervous overtures in every direction and translates the first no into a total dismissal of his entire value as a human being.

A few gay men are depressed *after* sex, especially with a stranger. Sometimes your partner is a warm, affectionate person, but this very warmth can be threatening if you are depressed and afraid of intimacy. You get rid of the guy as quickly as possible—and then vaguely sense you've lost yet another opportunity to connect with another person and develop a rewarding relationship.

One way to feel productive again has come back into style: becoming a volunteer in some community or gay-based organization that helps other people. This has the double advantage of getting you out of your home where you would remain brooding and back among people, while at the same time it makes your own trouble relative.

Dirty Talk

Sex is not a simple agitation of the loins, a few squeals, a tussle, an ejaculation, and then the slow resumption of grazing on the meadow. Learning has shaped all human actions beyond a few (animalistic? bestial?) reflexes, and as a result, the same erotic combinations can be interpreted in hundreds of different ways, according to the value the imagination attaches to them.

That's where dirty talk comes in. Because we are creatures whose lives are caught in a net of words, naming the act we are performing heightens our excitement. Dirty talk can create sex as it describes it, for talk is one of the most potent means of changing straightforward sex into a defilement, a childhood prank, an obscenity, or a religious rite.

Dirty talk can be an occasional burst of four-letter words or the unwinding of an elaborate fantasy; it can be one-sided or a collaboration through which you instruct your partner in your sexual needs. For many men, going to bed with a guy with a really filthy mouth is the ultimate turn-on.

The Internet makes dirty talk all the more popular—and necessary (see *On-line Cruising*). So, too, does phone sex. Let's start with how you write your on-line profile (see *Profiles*). While some gay men use it merely to list their demographics, others also include dirty "talk" to hint at what they want to do in bed. How dirty can you be? That's up to you. While nastiness will get you nowhere, the careful unfolding of a sexual scene (even a rough one) may get you enough responses to keep you busy for months.

On-line chat rooms are a great place to talk dirty. It's common for gay men to jerk off together on-line (you'll need to type with one hand) while telling sex stories—usually what you fantasize doing to each other (see *Chat Rooms*).

Phone sex has long been the way to hook up both for jerking off and/or meeting men (see *Phone Sex*). Tissues handy, gay men draw verbal images of their favorite sex acts. Aficionados are highly skilled at providing a verbal environment reeking of sensuality and tuned in to what they sense is the other man's sexual needs—all created with words.

E-mail has also been a way for gay men to communicate. Lovers, hope-to-be lovers, and fuck buddies now communicate sexual fantasies via e-mail, and they are every bit as sexual as on the phone (see *Fuck Buddies*). It's not unusual for e-mails to end with "and when I come on your chest, I'm going to rub it all over your body. By the way, are you free for lunch tomorrow?" However, we advise you not to use your computer at work to talk dirty, as many employers are now checking employee e-mail. Wait until you get home.

We believe dirty talk is still an underutilized resource, far from its potential popularity. We believe that anything that heightens sexual excitement, and therefore pleasure, in consenting adults should become part of the sexual repertoire of gay life. Even ordinarily shy men have become wordsmiths on their computers and phones.

Talking dirty can also enhance your solo sex. Most men jerk off to videos, but a few talk out loud to the characters on the screen. Try this: If you identify with one of the characters, say what he's feeling toward the guy he's fucking—or to the man sucking his cock. If you're a bottom, say how you feel with his cock inside you and move your body as if it's happening to you. Or, if you like to be humiliated when getting fucked, yell out, "Shut up and take it, bitch!" as though you're him talking to you. This may look silly on the printed page, but it won't be when you're watching the video with one hand around your cock. Say gentle words if that's what you're feeling, or be powerful and controlling if that's your mood.

Words can be especially compelling if you're jerking off with a lover or buddy. While jerking off together, try telling him a dirty story. Lie next to him, your hand resting on his cock, then tell him a sexy story about having sex with another man. You'll know when you're hitting his fantasy because his cock will get harder. As you find what turns him on, keep the story going. Don't let him come too soon, even if you have to occasionally lift your hand away from his cock. At some point he will need to get off (and so will you), so either you finish him off or let him do it himself. But don't stop talking until he comes.

Talk about his orgasm. Talk about how strong it was, or comment on how thick his come is, or anything that makes him feel sexy and powerful. Obviously, this exercise has a lot of variations. Try them all.

Talking dirty can really help steam up a three-way (see *Three-Ways*). Start with a fantasy, but be a tease, and don't allow the others to start touching until after they have entered the fantasy you're constructing. Whisper in their ears (but loudly). We guarantee this will create a heightened passion when the physical sex begins. Don't be afraid to be aggressive about this; they'll thank you afterward.

Of course, some gay men hate anyone's talking while having sex. Instead of its turning them on, they find it a big turn-off. Some men won't even make a sound when they come. You should try to respect your partner's right to have sex his own way: silently or loudly. There's no evidence that "silent comers" are sexually inhibited. But what if you love to talk dirty and find yourself in bed with someone who doesn't? Don't be rude. If he's a nice guy, stay and finish having sex. Afterward try to discuss it with him. He might have a particular reason for not liking to talk during sex (say for years he overheard some family members shouting during sex while he tried to sleep). Or he may never have tried it. Discuss how the two of you can slowly work up to it. Try having sex that way. It might take a few sessions before he gets into it. Or he may never get into it, in which case you'll have to decide whether to see him again.

Domestic Partnerships

As a result of incessant gay activism, fifty cities and seven states now offer domestic partnership benefits to gay lovers (see *Gay Liberation*). Many universities, unions, and over two thousand private corporations also offer benefits to gay couples. When Hawaii almost legalized gay marriage, the idea so terrorized legislators from other states that they passed laws against gay marriage. Some European countries have been more generous by legalizing gay marriage.

Benefits (they vary from city to city and from state to state) usually include health/life insurance and retirement/survivor/bereavement benefits. But while these benefits apply to gay couples, they are usually not equal to those given to straight married couples.

Many governmental agencies and cities now also keep a registry of gay couples who receive a certificate noting their union. Most notable is the U.S. House of Representatives, where gay members and employees can receive this certificate. It is, however, more symbolic than real, since it offers few practical rights. It's best to keep up with these changes in benefits for gay people through the Lambda Legal Defense and Education Fund (see *Appendix*).

Until gay marriage is legalized (it's a state function) and recognized throughout the country, gay couples will have to protect themselves by consulting a sympathetic attorney who will advise them about property rights, health and retirement insurance, and the care of children (see *Insurance; Wills; Living Wills*).

Those who support the passage of domestic partnership bills claim they are as close to marriage as many gays will see in their lifetime. Heterosexuals, particularly the religious Right, who oppose these bills see them as endangering the institution of marriage. They do not explain how two gay men being in a domestic partnership can further harm the already catastrophic state of marriage in the United States, where divorce rates currently run over 50 percent and two-thirds of American children have three or more parents. Heterosexuals already appear hell-bent on destroying the institution without any outside help.

Some gay politicians and gay mainstreamers alike believe that obtaining domestic partnership rights in every state is the key to obtaining full gay rights (see *Gay Politics*). In Vermont, where a full domestic partnership bill recently passed, it has come at some cost to its adherents, whereas in California, where the rights have been legislated piecemeal, there has been far less vocal opposition. Either way, it suggests that the gay politicos are correct.

. . .

Domestic Violence

Lover battery is a form of domestic violence that is no different in its origins or effects than wife-beating and child-beating. Battery usually begins with an occasional slap or "loving" punch, often explained away as "not meant." Apologies and even lovemaking may immediately follow the abuse. As the batterer finds himself getting away with it, his lover finds the abuse increasing week after week, with the alleged reason for the slap or kick or punch becoming increasingly more trivial.

As the battering continues, the lover finds himself fearing punishment for any behavior not approved of by his battering partner. He finds himself doing virtually everything to please his lover and to avoid being hit. He also finds himself in the odd and humiliating position of making alibis for, lying about, and even excusing his lover's behavior to others who notice the bruises. He may even come to blame himself for his stupidity and his ineptitude, which is, after all, why his lover tells him he is being hit: a loving chastisement geared toward making him a better person, a more appropriate lover.

At last, the battered lover finds himself living in fear for life and limb, yet unable to tear himself away from the man who passionately kisses him one minute and severely punishes him the next.

What is really going on in such a relationship? Doubtless, some form of homophobia. For the batterer, probably it's self-hatred being passed on as hostility toward the partner. For the victim, it could be that his secret fear that he can never be worthy of anyone's love transforms him into a punching bag for someone else's fears and anxieties (read *Growing Up Gay in a Dysfunctional Family* by Rik Isensee).

Who can become a battered lover? Anyone. A national survey funded by the Centers for Disease Control and Prevention recently found that a greater number of men than one would think are physically abused by their intimate partners. So don't think it can't happen to you. You can be intelligent, cultured, rich, brilliant, or famous. Who can become a battering lover? Here the list is a bit shorter. The potential exists in many gay men, especially homophobic ones, and those who constantly harbor resentment and hostility toward others, blaming others for their own shortcomings. Alcohol and drugs are often contributing factors: the mix of liquor and hostility is a potent one for physical abuse.

Does your partner lose his temper easily? Does he hit objects or pets? Break things when angry? Does he verbally abuse you and others? Is he always right and never wrong? Has he become overly jealous and possessive of you? If this picture fits and he's begun hitting you (even if he cries afterward and begs your forgiveness), then it's time to get out of your relationship. And fast!

How do you escape? Get a trusted friend to help. You might also call a domestic-violence hot line. Do *not* tell your lover what you're planning. He'll only cry and apologize—once again—then harm you worse the next time he's angry, which will likely be soon.

Arrange with your trusted helper to get you away from your lover with as many of your belongings as possible. If you must, get out with nothing but the clothes on your back and your ATM card. Do not go to relatives or to people and places where he'd expect you to go. Find a new place. Make sure your battering lover does not know where you are, and that no one tells him where you are. People trying to make peace between you should be asked not to interfere and should *not* be told where you are staying.

Once you are gone, *stay away from him*. Accept no calls or letters. If you must see him to settle business matters, see him only in a public place, and with another person at your side, perhaps an attorney. Never see him alone. It may take a few meetings to persuade him—and yourself, too—that you want nothing to do with him. Remember, the rest of your life is at stake.

It is more than likely that this guy will move on and find himself a new person to abuse, and you may find yourself wondering whether to warn the new lover. Whatever your decision, remember where *you* were at this point in your relationship: The new lover will probably be as unwilling to accept your warning as you were unwilling to listen to your friends. By the way, once you've escaped, join a support group or get counseling so that maybe you can find out why you chose an abusive lover, so you don't make the same mistake twice. Often, both abusers and those who are abused come from families in which abuse was common. But remember, you *can* break the cycle of violence.

Gay (and straight) male victims of abuse can share their stories at a gay-friendly, new Web site, SAFE (Stop Abuse for Everyone): www.safe4all.org. It can help you identify, support, and properly refer male victims of domestic violence. It lists services as well as a number of highly qualified professionals ready to help and provide training to law enforcement, healthcare providers, social services, and crisis lines. SAFE also provides a brochure for male victims and their concerned family and friends that identifies typical reactions of abusers and specific advice on domestic violence. Send a self-addressed, stamped envelope to SAFE, Male Victims Brochure, P.O. Box 951, Tualatin, OR 97062.

Drug Abuse

There are two epidemics in the gay community. The first, obviously, is the AIDS epidemic; the second is the widespread use of a variety of "party drugs" that has caused irreparable harm to gay men. In contrast to AIDS education and treatment, the gay media pays little attention to drug and alcohol addiction; they treat it as a mildly serious problem. In a previous edition of this book, we took a cautionary stand on party drugs because scientific research on their effects was only in its infancy. In the past ten years, we've learned a great deal about them and the verdict isn't good for habitual drug users.

The common complaint by professionals against party drugs is that they are "disinhibitors." When we are under the influence of a drug (including alcohol), we drop our normal inhibitions and good judgment. Men who see themselves as shy, inhibited, or particularly sensitive to rejection like the feeling of "disinhibition" because it makes them feel alive and in tune with the crowd. We all have some kind of wall around us, but for most of us it's a permeable structure. Others have walls made out of concrete that restrain them from feeling alive. Disinhibition dissolves the walls, at least for a short time. So what's the problem?

Number one, disinhibition leads to taking other drugs. A few drinks of alcohol may provide a satisfying buzz in one person. Another might want to feel even "better," and that could lead to a few snorts of coke, a hit of ecstasy, and maybe a bit of crystal methedrine, a combination that spells trouble. The second problem is unsafe sex. Alcohol and drug abuse is the number one cause of unsafe sex today, including the lunatics out there who call themselves barebackers (see *Barebacking; Safe Sex*). While under the influence of drugs or alcohol, a man who would never normally allow someone to fuck him without a condom may end up getting fucked by one or more men who come in his ass.

Drug use can also lead men to participate in sexual activities that cause physical damage. Some party drugs are anesthetics, so men often aren't aware of serious damage done to their assholes, rectums, or other parts of the body by partners who are themselves oblivious to (and sometimes unconcerned about) the harm they're doing. Drug users might also participate in sexual scenes that make them feel exceedingly guilty in the morning—if they remember them at all (see *Fetish; Kinky Sex; Sleazy Sex*).

Drug use is not the only cause of disinhibition. The social environment is equally important. A common scenario is this: You're among friends and other gay men dancing at a dance club or circuit party. Shirts are off and the view is enticing. Everyone looks to be having a wonderful time. That's when friends suggest you take a hit of ecstasy or do some crystal. Why not? you think. You probably have no idea who produced the drug, what it contains, or how your body will react to it, and that's where disinhibition comes in. The combination of the social environment, the sexual vibes all around you, the peer pressure (everyone else is doing it), and the physiological effect of the drugs on your body often makes you unable to care, even though they may lead you to disease and/or addiction.

We don't want to be "nannies" and chastise you for having a good time. We simply want to give you the best information available about party drugs. The most common are listed below, with explanations of why men take them, their effects, and their dangers. As with all decisions about sex, it's your choice whether you use them at all, use them a little, or let them take over your life.

Ecstasy. Also known as X, technically called MDMA (methylenedioxymeth-amphetamine), ecstasy is a synthetic amphetamine, the type of drug that stimulates the central nervous system (what men call an upper). First patented in 1914 in Germany, it was used in animal experiments by the U.S. army in the 1950s. At the time, psychotherapists believed that the drug would enhance psychotherapy, and they used it for that purpose until the drug was declared illegal in 1985. Ecstasy has been popular among gay men as a party drug since the midseventies, when it had a slightly different formula, known as MDA (the "love drug"). In its most recent guise it has become immensely popular and it is probably now the most-often-taken drug at dance clubs.

Ecstasy is taken orally. The effect usually begins anywhere from twenty to forty minutes later, usually in the form of a sudden amphetamine-like rush, leading to a feeling of tremendous physical and mental well-being. Initially, there may also be an intense desire to defecate (known as the *disco dump*). It can remain at its height (plateau effect) for as long as three or four hours.

Ecstasy keeps men dancing all night. They feel a sense of relatedness to those around them, feel happier, and experience a pleasurable altered perception of time and the ability to perform mental tasks. Dancing relieves the agitation caused by the drug. Men also feel sexier on ecstasy, but the ability to get a hard-on or to come is much diminished. Therefore, it's thought of as a sensual rather than a sexual drug.

The drug works by stimulating the release of a neurotransmitter in your brain called serotonin. This jet flow of serotonin produces the high. When taken often, the high is diminished, while negative effects become more pronounced.

Ecstasy dehydrates the body significantly, and the drug taker should drink a lot of water or sports drinks during the evening. The problem is further complicated by alcohol, which also causes dehydration (see *Booze and Highs*). Dehydration can be dangerous, even deadly. How deadly was demonstrated in England at raves in 1992. Clubs decided to turn off their drinking fountains in an effort to sell bottled water. That year, dehydration left fifteen teenagers dead.

The release, then depletion, of serotonin can leave you feeling depressed afterward, or highly anxious. Ecstasy may interact with the Prozac class of drugs (SSRIs) and MAO inhibitors. There have also been reports of deaths when ecstasy was taken with protease inhibitors. If you are on any of these medications, discuss drug taking with your doctor.

The aftereffects of ecstasy usually last one to four days, as the body attempts to replenish lost serotonin. You may continue to feel depressed, lethargic, not hungry, and sleepy.

While research has shown that ecstasy causes *permanent brain damage* in laboratory animals, scientists haven't yet conclusively shown long-term brain damage in humans, but the belief is growing that repeated doses may lead to this. Ecstasy is not addictive.

Cocaine. Coke is probably the second most popular party drug in gay life. A stimulant as well as an anesthetic, it has been used for centuries to blot out physical pain. It is a product of the crystallization of the oils from the leaves of the coca plant, generally grown in a swath of Pacific Ocean mountainside terrain from Central America down through South America.

In the gay community, cocaine is most often found in powder form and snorted, but it can also be injected or smoked (crack). Some users inject a mixture of coke and heroin, called a speedball.

Cocaine enters the bloodstream, blocks nerves in the brain, and releases three neurotransmitters: dopamine, norepinephrine, and serotonin. You experience an initial rush of euphoria, confidence, and talkativeness. Like ecstasy, the drug taker feels highly sexual, without having any real ability to have sex. Many people who take the drug say they can't sleep, can't eat, and can't get hard or come. Constipation is a common side effect.

In higher or repeated doses over time, cocaine may cause irregular heartbeat, heart attacks, seizures, and strokes. Withdrawal lasts longer than the high. Over time, men who habitually snort cocaine will destroy their nasal passages. Some men (it may be dose-related) experience paranoia and hallucinations. Sometimes the hallucinations become tactile and you feel things all over your skin. This is called the *cocaine bugs*. While not a narcotic, cocaine is highly addictive, and kicking this habit can be extremely difficult. Narcotics Anonymous (NA) is the treatment of choice.

Methamphetamine. Commonly known as crystal or speed, this drug has become increasingly popular at dance clubs and circuit parties because, like ecstasy, it allows men to dance all night, producing a feeling of increased energy and a decreased need for sleep. Crystal (also called meth) can be snorted or injected. It heightens sensory awareness, self-esteem, confidence, verbosity, grandiosity, and euphoria, unlike opiates such as morphine and heroin, which usually promote social withdrawal. Crystal also elevates mood and sex drive, while decreasing feelings of anxiety and inhibitions. Crystal users feel more attractive and find it easier to cruise for sex. Crystal users are also more apt to indulge in kinkier sex, such as S/M or fisting (see *Sadomasochism; Fisting*). All this good feeling is caused by the sudden release of dopamine, an important neurotransmitter in the brain. Like ecstasy, crystal intensifies social interactions.

While sexual desire is heightened, sexual performance takes a nosedive. The user may not be able to get it up or come—hence the term *crystal dick*. Crystal users have a reputation—well supported in research—of getting fucked more often than they do without the drug (perhaps because of their temporary impotence?). Research has also found that two-thirds of men on crystal were getting fucked without condoms, and therefore, crystal users have a higher HIV transmission rate.

Other side effects are an inability to eat or sleep while the drug is in effect. Afterward, depression often sets in with a marked need for sleep. More significant aftereffects associated with long-term use include stroke, liver damage, high blood pressure, and in a few cases, psychosis. Crystal should not be combined with protease inhibitors.

Methamphetamine is highly addictive.

Poppers. Amyl butrate is sold as a liquid and produces fumes that are inhaled, a familiar rite in clubs. Poppers usually come in small vials. The drug is a vasodilator that produces its high by expanding your blood vessels so quickly that your blood pressure drops, you get dizzy, and the room seems to spin. The liquid may burn the skin if it makes contact. It is highly flammable. In the early years of the AIDS epidemic, poppers (then amyl nitrite) were mistakenly blamed for the disease, revealing both the level of misinformation at the time as well as the prevalence of the drug in the gay community. Some deaths have resulted from the combination of poppers and Viagra. Both drugs dilate blood vessels, and the combination can reduce blood pressure to a lethal level. Poppers should not be used by anyone with cardiovascular disease.

Ketamine. Known as Special K, or just K, ketamine is a derivative of an anesthetic used by veterinarians. It was first manufactured in 1965 and is still used for medical purposes. The drug produces a feeling of being detached and disconnected to people around you. The user is generally unaware of pain and may feel anesthetized and sedated. Many users say that it makes your brain feel disconnected from the rest of your body. Some men like that.

K is sold as a powder and is generally snorted. It may also be put on the tongue and taken with water. The intensity of the drug is dose dependent. At high doses it distorts perceptions of the body, the environment, and time. There may even be hallucinations and paranoid delusions. At "party"-dose levels it distorts sensory stimuli, producing illusions. The effect takes place about ten minutes after snorting. The peak effect is after thirty minutes, and then it gradually subsides. The trip is over in about an hour or so. The lethal dose is thirty times the party dose.

One scary possibility is that the user will go into what is known as a *K hole*. This is a catatonic state in which the drug taker stares blankly into space and is incapable of communication for hours. The man in the K hole usually comes out of it, but not before scaring the hell out of his friends.

K has a significant effect upon gay men's sex lives. Some bottoms view large, thick cocks as a personal challenge and use K for its anesthetic quality to allow getting fucked roughly by them for long periods. As with the use of other anesthetics, these men won't be aware of the physical damage until they wake up the next day. K is an addictive drug.

GHB (Gammahydroxybutyrate). Also known as "grievous bodily harm," GHB is found naturally in many mammalian cells. The manufactured variety of GHB was first produced in France over thirty years ago. In the 1980s, it was widely available over-the-counter in health food stores. Banned by the FDA since 1990, it is now used heavily in clubs and at circuit parties.

GHB is taken orally. It reaches its peak effect in twenty to sixty minutes. The high lasts for about ninety minutes. GHB induces a pleasant state of relaxation and tranquillity. The user feels placid and has a tendency to verbalize. Like ecstasy, GHB is a sensual but not sexual drug.

There are special dangers to this drug. The dosage can be confusing. There is little difference between a party dose and the dose needed to put you into a coma. Some men who have gone into comas have died, probably because they choked on their own vomit. Alcohol and GHB is a dangerous, perhaps lethal, combination. Other side effects include confusion, agitation, difficulty walking, and possible loss of bladder control. Seizure may occur when combining GHB with either crystal or coke. It also shouldn't be mixed with other depressants such as alcohol or Valium.

GHB is one of the "date rape drugs." The other date rape drug, less common in the gay community, is Rohypnol, known as roofies, or simply ro. It interferes with short-term memory and is commonly slipped into a person's drink. He or she doesn't remember what happened afterward. The drug is banned in the United States.

OxyContin. Oxycodone is the generic name of a medically approved opiate that doctors prescribe to control pain in cancer and orthopedic patients. OxyContin is the trade name of a sustained-release form of the drug that lasts for twenty-four hours. In the late 1990s, it was widely reported that teenagers were using the drug for its effect rather than for medical purposes, stealing the pills from their parents' medicine cabinets or from local pharmacies. The pills are crushed and snorted or injected for their heroin-like high. OxyContin abuse is now entering the adult gay population. It is highly addictive.

Anabolic Steroids. Steroids are used by muscle queens to add bulk to their body quickly. They're also used more productively by the medical establishment to combat body wasting in HIV patients. A particular kind of explosive temper called 'roid rage occurs in some men who use steroids; they should stop the drug immediately and get to a doctor. The side effects of synthetic testosterone include balding, pimples, reddish skin, and shrinking balls (because the testes stop making testosterone).

*　*　*

How any of these drugs affects you will obviously vary. Except for legally prescribed drugs, you have no way of knowing the degree of purity in the dose—whether the pill you take has any active ingredient in it at all, or too much of it. Each of us metabolizes a drug differently, so your body may, for instance, process the drug more quickly than your companion's. The faster the metabolism, the quicker and stronger the effect. And combining drugs increases the risk of harm. Your size and weight may also influence the effects of a drug. A dose of GHB, for instance, will have a greater effect on someone short and light than someone tall and heavier.

Depression is common afterward while your brain struggles to replenish vital chemicals—the neurotransmitters—that you lost when taking the drug. It can last for a day in one person, but days in someone else. Men who already suffer from depression may slide deeper into the hole, even to the point of physical pain.

Research shows that gay teens use more alcohol and party drugs than straight ones. Homosexuality in teens also increases the risk for health problems in general, suicide, victimization, and sexual risk taking. Teenagers (adults as well) may use drugs to combat feelings of depression and low self-esteem (see *Teenagers*; *Depression*). Psychotherapy is the treatment of choice.

Drugs and Sex

Alcohol and other drugs have always been used as a means of oiling social and sexual inhibitions. Shy gay men find that a few drinks make them bolder when cruising, and the fear of rejection can be tempered with a number of party drugs. Smoking pot before sex often stems fears of sexual performance, especially if a man suffers from a sexual dysfunction. Many party drugs have the reputation of producing a psychological state of sensuality and gregariousness.

If it were only that easy. While alcohol and some drugs appear to be safe in moderation, others are implicated in potential harm to the body, while still others interfere with, rather than stimulate, sexual functioning.

Going to bed with a drunk is like trying to have sex with a limp fish. He isn't sexy, lacks passion, and is not likely to remember it (or you) in the morning. He also won't be able to get an erection because too much alcohol is a brain depressant, not a stimulant. The brain (at least metaphorically) goes to sleep. That's why his dick (and the rest of him) is limp.

Pot appears to relax many men, so long as they smoke in moderation. Otherwise, they're likely to enjoy the marijuana buzz so much that they may forgo or even forget sex. Research suggests that the testes produce abnormal sperm cells while you are stoned, but that their functioning returns to normal the next day. In any event, not many gay men are likely to get upset about the condition of their sperm cells.

Viagra, the drug for men with impotence problems, is used by men who never had a problem getting hard. They take it to get harder, for a longer period. Tops like it because they can fuck like a horse, and rapacious bottoms are usually enchanted by their sex partner's staying power. Go-go boys and hustlers like staying hard with the drug because they can command higher rates and better tips. The same goes for male porn stars.

There are, as always, a few problems in this chemical heaven. Viagra is potentially harmful if taken too often within a short period, as it can cause a dangerous drop in blood pressure. The drug works by dilating the arteries, letting blood into your cock. Assuming you have a normal cock, the more blood that gets into it, the harder and more rigid it gets. But if the blood travels through wider arteries (Viagra opens all your arteries, not just those in your cock), the result is a reduction in blood pressure. That's why some gay men who take a high dose of Viagra find themselves getting dizzy, seeing stars, and walking into walls.

The blood pressure problem is life-threatening for some uninformed gay men. It should be obvious that if you take Viagra, under no circumstances should you ingest any other drug that may also dilate your arteries. Do not use poppers—their buzz is also an effect of dilation (see *Drug Abuse*). And do not, if you're using the injection for impotence, also take Viagra (see *Impotence*). If you are on any other medication, ask your doctor before using Viagra.

In a few recent cases, some idiotic gay men have operated under the principle that if a little is good, a lot more is better. They literally overdose on Viagra, doubling, tripling, and quadrupling the dose. It works! Their cocks get very, very hard—and they *never* go down. The condition is called priapism, named after a Greek and Roman god who had a huge and perpetual hard-on (and who ran after and fucked teenage boys). That's okay for a god, but not for you. If this happens, you'll have to go to the emergency room. They may be able to handle the problem with a blood thinner. If not, they will have to drain the blood in your cock (as you suffer the snickers of the emergency room staff) or the blood will turn viscous, harden, and cause scar tissue inside your penis, making future erections impossible—for life. Enough said.

We don't advise using Viagra all the time, unless you have a diagnosed impotence problem. Using it too often may cause you to lose confidence in your ability to have sex without it. That could be a psychological problem, to say nothing of the absurd expense of the pills.

If you decide to use Viagra, take the lowest dosage of those currently available, 25 milligrams, and see how well it works. If you're young and in good health, it should do the job adequately and safely. Don't take it again for at least twenty-four hours, preferably forty-eight hours.

You've probably already heard that Viagra is *not* a substitute for arousal. If you're not feeling sexual, taking the drug won't make you hard. If you're depressed and/or on antidepressants, the drug may not work. Be sure to check with your doctor about the safety of using your antidepressant and Viagra.

Virtually all the party drugs interfere with sexual performance. These include ecstasy, cocaine, crystal, and GHB, which have reputations of creating a feeling of sensuality and increasing social interaction while at the same time inhibiting getting hard and/or coming (see *Problems of Ejaculation*).

Early Abuse

The child is father to the man," said poet William Wordsworth, and we couldn't agree more that childhood experiences lay important foundations for adult sexuality. Unfortunately, some of us come from dysfunctional families where we experienced physical, verbal, or sexual abuse. Homosexual abuse (sexual or otherwise) is *not* more common than heterosexual abuse, despite what many homophobes would have us believe. In fact it's statistically far *less* frequent.

Children are abused for many reasons. Emotionally disturbed and alcohol- and drug-dependent parents often terrorize their children simply because they are the handiest objects. Some parents sexually exploit their children (see *Rape*). More subtle damage occurs when children are brought up in families where parents and children hide feelings from one another, performing only the mechanics of family life as though they were actors on a stage. No wonder children born into these families grow up with a well-honed mistrust and, in adulthood, become overcontrolled (sometimes overcontrol*ling*) in love and sex.

A few gay men blame their homosexuality on an abusive father, but this notion is merely an example of internalized homophobia. More often one finds gay men feeling guilty about their erotic life. Oddly, some men counter these feelings by an obsessive sexual feast composed of nameless men and blank faces, night after unsatisfying night. One such man said that for him it was "affection at any price." A few men resolve their conflicting sexual feelings through celibacy, others by carefully controlling what sexual acts they'll perform, usually a limited lot. But all these men suffer one limitation: They cannot feel intimate with another man. Control becomes their substitute for vulnerability, even when they are in the arms of a loving, caring partner. This overcontrol is understandable as they are compensating for the horrific lack of control they experienced when younger.

The problem is how to get them to separate early abuse from adult sexuality. A number of obstacles intervene. A man may choose lovers every bit as abusive as his father (see *Domestic Violence*). Friends sadly marvel at the phenomenon, seeing their best counsel ignored while their friend runs from one abusive lover to the next. But most men choose lovers more wisely. Even so, their sex life may be strained and rigid.

Ellen Ratner, editor of *The Other Side of the Family: A Book for Recovery from Abuse, Incest and Neglect*, tells us, "The instrument of pleasure to [the body] is also that which holds the pain." She means that the formerly abused man can't let go sexually because, by doing so, he'll reexperience the painful abusive childhood. It is as if his memory were contained within his muscles, rather than in his brain. Memories of being abused may return during sex with a lover, perhaps as a quick flashback or in reaction to smelling an article of clothing. Psychologists call these reminders triggers.

If you were abused in childhood, you should consider looking into psychotherapy and joining a support group. If your memory of that abuse is interfering with your sex life with your lover, ask him to be part of the therapeutic process. Otherwise, he'll have trouble understanding how you can be ashamed and uptight at the same time that you're aroused. You may understand that your discomfort isn't your partner's fault, but he may not.

In the meantime, you and your partner can do things to help bring more complete trust into the relationship. You might try Simon Says. You, the abused partner, say, "Touch my———." Depending on how it feels to you, continue or discontinue the touching. Do it clothed or naked, as you wish. Another technique is to outline a body on a piece of cardboard and to identify the body parts that feel good to you when touched, and those that don't. Color them differently, and change colors as you feel more comfortable sexually. Try taking your partner's hand and moving it along your body, telling him what kind of touch and which places on your body feel safe. Finally, develop trust by trying a "blind walk." Your lover blindfolds you, then leads you by the hand around your apartment, stopping from place to place to let you feel objects and guess what they are. If you live in a rural area, go outside and touch flowers or leaves. Then reverse roles by leading him in a blind walk.

Effeminacy

This has turned into an issue of growing complexity and importance as our society becomes aware of the large number of children born with unclear gender identity, as well as the various social, political, and even financial reasons why having a distinct gender seems to be required. No one is sure whether male children are born with or learn effeminate behavior. Growing scientific evidence suggests that some traditionally feminine characteristics are biologically determined in some gay men.

Whatever the genetic or physiological cause for those boys' feminine traits and interests, they are as natural to them as an interest in baseball is to the stereotypical boy. In school, these boys are taunted constantly and mocked as "sissies." They are often rejected by peers, teachers, and in some cases, their own parents. Repeatedly told to "act like a boy," they come to believe that there is nothing right about them. This effeminacy is part of their character and remains throughout life.

On the other hand, some young men come out who never expressed effeminate behavior in childhood but may do so in adolescence. These are usually teens who are trying to get even with parents who don't accept their homosexuality. In some cases, they can drive their parents insane. It's rare that such behavior lasts very long; usually it disappears as they become more at ease with their sexuality. If they find a group of other gay young men, they may overemphasize effeminate traits and vocalizations whenever they are together. This is often allied to camping, and they are sometimes known as "screamers" and "twinkies" when together (see *Camping*). Alone, they tend to be far less affected. In fact, when they are acting effeminate, they are actually socially bonding, consolidating their group identity for themselves, one another, and everyone else.

Effeminacy is by no means limited to gay men. One will also find effeminate straight boys who are taken for gay and discriminated against as fully as are gay boys. From grade school right through adult life, the effeminate male is perceived as different from other males and is bullied and beaten up. Regrettably, even adult gay men may discriminate against an effeminate man. "He's too femme," they say, to rationalize their ostracism. This attitude is based upon the traditional notion of a strong and impermeable barrier between male and female behavior. "Straight acting" is the most important facade in their lives, and they'll only date another like-minded gay man. If you find yourself uncomfortable in the company of men with feminine traits, don't blame it on them. Instead, ask yourself why you're afraid; it could be that it's an expression of your own unconscious homophobia (see *Homophobia*).

Etiquette

Manners, as we know them, began around the twelfth century in the area of France known as Anjou, under the influence of Eleanor of Aquitaine, who, we must assume, was tired of the boorish manners of people surrounding her. Within a few centuries, an Italian, Castiglione, had codified her teachings into *The Book of the Courtier*.

By the eighteenth century, manners were reserved for the aristocracy and the upper classes, and that's what set them apart from the hoi polloi. By the middle of the nineteenth century, one could tell a man or woman's exact social standing by how well he or she knew to behave in company, as well as by his or her accent. And by the first third of the twentieth century, manners continued to make class and financial distinctions that often seemed inflexible.

What role does etiquette have in gay life and particularly gay sex? Plenty, although perhaps not exactly in the way that Amy Vanderbilt would have suggested. Fortunately, her conservative approach has been amended by the gay-friendly Miss Manners.

Manners begin in public places. Say you're in a bar or restaurant or club and you're minding your business and enjoying the music and ambience. Someone comes along and asks you to dance. Do you take one look at him and, not at all liking what you see, reply, "I don't associate with trolls"? Or do you instead answer, "Thanks, but I'm enjoying myself fine alone"?

Both statements might be true. Truth is not the point here. What is the point is how you are going to behave in an uncomfortable situation. Etiquette is all about how to do that.

What is required is a bit of empathy. Recognize that "he" is as easily hurt as "you." A smile is in order, a "thank you," and then a face-saving (for him) white lie, such as "I'm here with a friend; he's just coming back from the bathroom."

Another example. You've gone home with someone you just met, and after a terrific beginning, the two of you have ended up having a less than spectacular sexual session. In fact it was downright terrible. Maybe your chemistry wasn't as strong as you thought, or maybe you got your signals crossed. But you've gotten off, and all you want to do is to forget about the experience. As your trick is getting dressed, he offers you his phone number and asks for yours, saying something like "Maybe next time, we'll really sizzle."

This is sweet and he means well. In fact, he's probably as disappointed and unhappy as you are. But you are certain you two will never have good sex. What do you do? Do you say, "It'll never work out. You're lousy sex"? Or do you obligingly exchange phone numbers and instead say something like "Sex isn't everything. If we find out we don't do that well together, maybe we can go out dancing (or to brunch or to a movie or shopping together)"?

The second is a sign of your ability to discern the truth and yet to stay open to possibilities: the possibility of his friendship to begin with, or at least his company in some nonsexual way.

Using good manners doesn't mean being prissy and prim and proper, although the word has been misconstrued as meaning this for decades. Using good manners says that you are calm, confident, manly, grown-up, and aware that not everything in life works as it ought to and that you are prepared to put as good a spin on whatever does happen as possible. It's a lovely characteristic. The ancient Chinese called it grace and said that it is how the superior man acts all the time, no matter where he is or among whom he finds himself.

Etiquette also means being physically clean for sexual encounters—unless, of course, you and your partner have agreed to "pig out" (see Sleazy Sex). It means being safe, and not forcing your partner to do something he's unsure of or doesn't want to do.

Exhibitionism and Voyeurism

One of the real surprises of the so-called sexual revolution was how many people unexpectedly revealed themselves to be exhibitionists. Among gay men, it turned out to be incredibly easy to find guys who were willing to striptease for others, to perform sex acts in public places, to throw sex parties and carry out sex acts of even the most extreme and kinky nature in front of their friends, tricks, and neighbors. Equally surprising was how many other men were eager to watch.

Of course, all sex involving two or more people consists to one degree or another of exhibitionism and of its natural corollary, voyeurism. Part of the turn-on is looking at your partner before sex, anticipating; during sex, enjoying; and afterward, fantasizing about the sex you've just had. These dynamics seem to be a given of the human condition. The earliest examples of world literature are filled with stories of men and women passionately interacting during moments of exhibitionism and voyeurism, from David and Bathsheba, to Susanna and the Elders, to Diana and Actaeon, to Apollo and Hyacinth, and so on. In recent studies of gay sex in rest rooms and other public places, sociologists have remarked on how few exhibitionists there usually are at any one time, and how many more voyeurs (as well as how easily voyeurs can turn into exhibitionists). If you've ever been at a sex party or gay bathhouse, sex club, or backroom bar, you'll probably agree. One reason for this is that most men are physiologically visually oriented when it comes to sexual relations (this is true for both straight and gay men); as opposed to women, who have more complex, usually emotion-oriented reactions. Another reason may be that most people are inherently shy, or modest, or simply unwilling to bare what others might consider physical flaws or shortcomings.

Perhaps it's less easy to understand how, with the right surroundings, men can so easily transform themselves into sexual displays for one another. Gay life encourages men to sexually show off for one another and to join with other gay men in watching sexual displays whether they be in gay bars, a Mr. Leather contest, or a gay pride parade.

We believe that exhibitionism and voyeurism in gay venues such as strip clubs are normal and healthy for gay men, unless a performer is being injured, exposed to unsafe sex, or exploited without his permission (see *Barebacking*; *Dangerous Sex*). In the privacy of your own home, exhibitionism and voyeurism can—and probably ought to be—used to stimulate or add spice to your sex together (see *Kinky Sex*; *Versatility*). Equally healthy, if you are without a partner, is accessing sexual Web sites on your computer, and using chat rooms and even Webcams to have "real time" mutual masturbatory sex (see *Chat Rooms*; *On-line Cruising*; *Webcams*). In fact, computers and the Internet have brought a new intimacy, immediacy, and sophistication to exhibitionism and voyeurism. Who knows where it will go? Perhaps one day virtual reality will bring an exhibitionist into *your* home.

Face-to-Face

Facing your partner while you fuck is the position preferred over all others by most gay men. You can look at each other, you can kiss, you can read each other's face for cues or just for the visible signs of pleasure given and received. For some men, face-to-face is also the position that enables the deepest possible penetration.

Some men find the penetration too deep (see *First Time*). Others dislike getting fucked in this position because they feel passive or feminized, while for others, the passivity is a turn-on. Some object to face-to-face fucking on more practical grounds. Their legs become cramped. If sex goes on for a long time, the man on the bottom may get tired of having his legs up, hooked over his partner's shoulders, and his knees pressed to his own chest.

If you're doing the fucking, when you are both fully aroused and at ease, stimulate and relax your partner's anus with your finger, and insert a lubricant into his asshole. Then, after you've put on a condom, he's ready to be fucked (see *Condoms*). Formerly, many men liked to rim the asshole, since tongue stimulation is highly pleasurable to both parties. The saliva also serves as a good lubricant. Unfortunately it also increases the chance of transmitting parasites and other STDs (see *Rimming and Felching; Sexually Transmitted Diseases; Sit on My Face*). Kneel between his legs, lift his ankles, and place them on your shoulders. He may prefer his right foot hooked over your shoulder, his left foot below, wrapped around your back; this position gives more flexibility, and it places his asshole at a slightly different angle in relation to your cock, which may ease entry.

While fucking face-to-face can be the most exciting of sexual acts between men, getting inside in this position is where most problems occur. Guys of different sizes, shapes, and weights can often encounter problems. With a little patience, and a will to succeed, no problem is insuperable. You may be really raring to go, but you should calm down and be tolerant of your partner's comfort: You'll both enjoy it better. Entry should be slow and gentle, allowing his sphincter muscles to relax to accommodate your cock (see *Anus*). Once you are all the way in and he feels comfortable, you can bend over and kiss or tongue any part of his upper body. And if you both are comfy, you may also be ready to try hard-thrust fucking. Some men really like that and shout and slap each other's buttocks to increase the excitement as they get closer to climax (see *Spanking*).

If you're both agile and your bodies fit together in a particular way, it may also be possible to fuck and suck him at the same time. Sit back on your heels, simultaneously pulling your partner up onto your lap; he should wrap his legs around your waist. Then lower his legs; the more direct the pressure against his prostate gland,

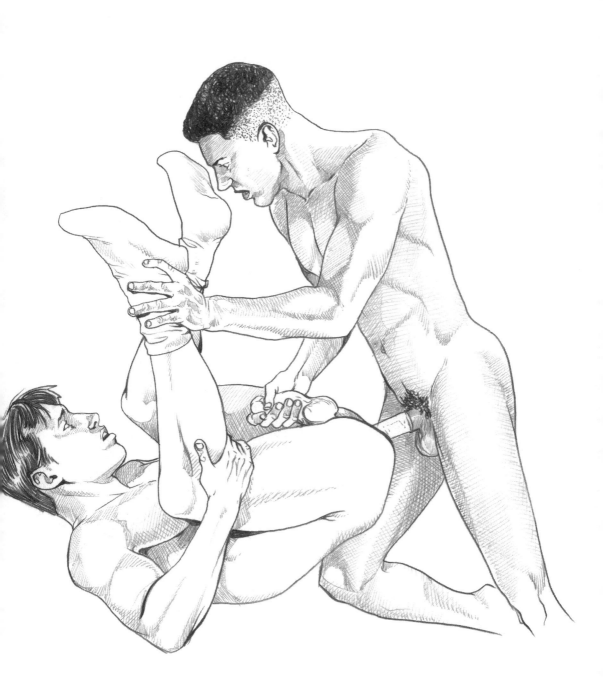

the more pressure (and thus pleasure) he feels. He should not try to sit up to fold his arms around your neck (that's another position, with its own merits), but should continue to lie on his back on the mattress, with his pelvic area propped up on your thighs.

If you now bend your head down to his crotch, you should be able to suck his cock. You may have to angle his cock down, or you may have to use your other hand to form an extension to your mouth (see *Blow Job*). You won't be able to deep-thrust in this position, but you can get some movement. Try this: As you pull out your cock, go down on him. As you push back in, lift your mouth away. Or you can jerk him off as you fuck. For deep fucking, bend him back until his knees nearly touch his shoulders. His weight will rest on his spine and neck, and his ass will stick straight up. Go up on your toes and fingertips, as though doing push-ups. Grasp his ankles and open his legs wide without forcing. You may have to balance yourself by shifting your weight from your toes to your knees.

Another position: Stand or half-crouch on the floor beside the bed (you may want to elevate your partner slightly by placing a pillow under him). His back will rest on the mattress but his legs will be straight up against your chest. To avoid losing your balance, lean over and steady yourself against the wall. An alternative is for you to grab his ankles and open his legs as wide as possible, relying on the resistance of his body to keep you from falling over on top of him. If you're strong, you can even lift your partner off the bed and carry him around while still inside him.

If you are the one getting fucked, be sure to communicate what you are feeling to your partner. Say your legs or back begin to ache. Don't grin and bear it: Tell him you want to rest or to try some other position. If your partner is masturbating you and you sense you're about to come, gently move his hand away and jerk yourself off. This will help you achieve an orgasm simultaneous with his. No matter what your scene, being fucked takes getting used to. If you have lower-back problems, or some other disability, you may want to avoid face-to-face fucking altogether or warm up to it slowly. Remember to tell your partner what feels good. If need be, adjust your position to find the most pleasurable angle, and if that's not working for you, suggest changing your position to side by side or doggy style (see *Side by Side; Rear Entry*).

Face-to-face admits variability of sexual and emotional expression, and partners can move from gentle, cherishing tenderness to athletic roughness.

• • •

Feet

Most people think of their feet as a functional but not very attractive part of their body. Fashion models earn a living by exhibiting their faces, chests, or butts, but only specialized foot models ever show their feet, even in beach scenes. To some men, however, feet are as sexually stimulating as a cute ass or a big dick is to men with more traditional tastes. And while odors from the feet are repugnant to some, they are the ambrosia of smells to others—especially after a long, hot day at the office.

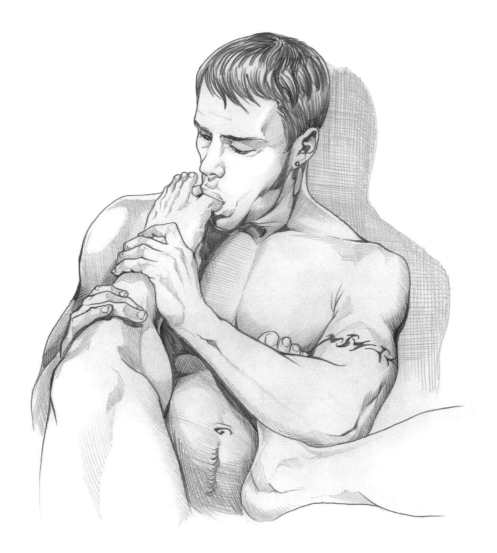

We have the impression that sexual adoration of the feet has increased in popularity over the past decade. An alternative explanation is that foot fetishists have come out of the closet, encouraged by the spread of foot-fetish clubs on both the Internet and in specialized bars.

As in almost all forms of sexuality, foot fetishists come in many varieties. There are tops and bottoms, for instance, those who want their feet adored, caressed, and licked, and their counterparts who want to do the adoring, caressing, and licking. Cleanliness is also a variable. Some men prefer spick-and-span feet straight from the bath, while others prefer musky odors and a patina of sweat.

As a side dish to a larger entrée of sex, playing with feet adds spice to the menu, and we believe should be part of every gay man's sexual repertoire. It treats the feet (clean or otherwise) as part of, and connected to, the rest of the body.

Foot fetishists psychologically isolate feet, making them equivalent to the cock as the symbolic locus of pleasure. Some foot fetishists choose not to participate in genital activities altogether, such as sucking cock and fucking ass. Their main activity is jerking themselves off while adoring another man's feet. Or in some cases, jerking off into the shoes (especially sneakers) of their idol.

The greatest problem for lovers of feet is finding another man to love, since their fetish has reduced the number of potential available partners. While most gay men are willing participants in harmless fun with their feet, they usually expect to move farther north—where they can get off.

Fetish

Professional descriptions of fetish activities go back to the work of Krafft-Ebing, a famous nineteenth-century medical researcher of pathological sexuality, who wrote about straight men jerking off into women's panties and bras. To him, and to the medical authorities that followed, a fetish was defined as a man's sexual arousal by nonliving objects. Modern sex researchers are more informed about the subject, mainly because they have attempted to objectively understand the relationship between sex and fetish objects, rather than, like Krafft-Ebing, categorizing them as normal or abnormal.

Gay men feast on an enormous number of fetish objects. They can be divided into two categories: part of another man's body, such as his hair or cock, or something the man wears, such as leather or a jock (see *Bears; Cock Size*). When concentrating upon part of another man's body, in an extreme form you look only for men who possess a particular hair/eye color, facial features, height, or appearance—one man, for example, said, "I go only for troglodytes" (see *Types*). We all have our types; it becomes a fetish only when one part of the other man takes center stage and virtually *all* other physical characteristics are ignored. Psychologists sometimes call this *fractionalization,* meaning that the visual turn-on is wholly dependent upon just one physical characteristic. The rest of the body and personality is ignored.

Wearing apparel is the most common nonhuman fetish. A gay man, for instance, who's "into" underwear wants to jerk off watching the other man wearing his underwear, or wearing a jockstrap (especially after a sweaty workout at the gym), or clad in tight-fitting Speedos. These undergarments emphasize and concentrate the watcher's eyes on the prize, the other guy's cock.

There's no end to the list of wearing apparel that turns us on. It includes popular items such as leather boots and clothing (the smell of leather turns men on). Leather (and other wearing apparel) helps create a mood congruent with a sexual "scene" (see *Sadomasochism; Role Playing*). More recently, rubber and vinyl have become popular, best for those without the income to afford a full leather outfit. Less popular with gay men than straights are other fetishes such as diapers (called *infantilism*) and silk.

Body parts (besides the cock) are also favorite fetish objects with gay men. Feet are very popular (see *Feet*). Big hands are desired by aficionados of fist fucking (see *Fisting*). Gay men who love ass (are there any who don't?) prefer one shape over another and adore watching men wearing jocks—more for the view from the rear than from the front. Hairstyle, ears, the shape of the nose, and more lately, six-pack abdomens all have their admirers. The list of fetishes, like styles in general, changes over time. Johnny-come-latelies include men smoking cigars and men wearing business suits (often with their cock out of the pants, or the shirt open to expose one nipple). You'll find a cornucopia of fetishes (no matter how obscure) available on-line and through chat rooms (see *On-line Cruising; Chat Rooms*). There you'll find other like-minded men.

Are there psychological problems connected to focusing upon a fetish? As a rule, they are no more psychologically hazardous than other sexual situations. A fetish *can be* a problem if it's the only thing that gets you sexually excited. Say you like to jerk off looking at photos or videos of men wearing Calvin Klein briefs—and that's the limit of your sex life. Then you've probably got a problem. But it's not the fetish that's the problem; it's your inability to bring other sexual behavior into your life, especially behavior that might create emotional attachment between you and a partner.

Perhaps you can make a "scene" out of your fetish. Your sex partner, for instance, might frustrate you for a while by taking off his clothing slowly (see *Seduction*). He might prevent you from touching your cock while he fondles his own through his underwear. He might "force" you to lick his boots or feet (see *Licking; Bondage and Discipline*). He might "make you" suck his cock or his asshole (see *Rimming*). He might leave on his Calvins and fuck you, have you fuck him with them on, or even get you to wear them. The object of these exercises is to reconnect your fetish with the person you're with.

Fidelity and Monogamy

They are not necessarily the same. Fidelity between lovers excludes the possibility of having sex with a third person, while monogamy means that two people have declared themselves lovers, an intimate emotional and sexual relationship, but one that does not exclude the possibility of tricking outside the relationship. Not surprisingly, some couples, especially since the AIDS health crisis began, insist the terms are synonymous: no sex outside the relationship.

Arguments about fidelity are the commonest reason that couples break up (see *Couples*). Gay men are subject to the same emotional ideology as straights, which means they often maintain mistaken notions of possession of the partner, just as in some forms of marriage where the husband has direct rights of ownership over the wife (see *Jealousy, Envy, and Possessiveness*). Movies, books, and poems all bolster the idea that love is possession, and this confusion between them often underlies disputes about infidelity.

If you suspect your lover of infidelity, sort out your feelings. Jealousy can be the product not only of possessiveness but also of a lack of confidence in yourself. What you really fear is that if your lover has sex with others, he may find someone more exciting than you. Jealousy may be a mask for envy; perhaps you believe he is more attractive than you and is having more success.

Relationships inevitably go through changes and difficult patches over the years. The most problematic times for gay men seem to be around two and seven years into the relationship. Generally, if you can get past those problem epochs, you can sustain a lifelong relationship. These two benchmarks are important times for couples to address issues of monogamy. Some gay men, especially those who have had no or few previous relationships, may become bored with only one sexual partner, and one sexual menu. They may provoke a decision whether to "open up" the relationship to others, to continue it (unhappily for one of them), or to end it altogether (see *Open Relationships*). As many European and some American heterosexuals have discovered, often the longest and best relationships are those in which the decision was made to have sex outside the marriage under specific rules.

If you plan to go this route, you need to be explicit in devising rules to suit each other's needs and vulnerabilities. That requires honest (not cruel), possibly lengthy (not tedious) conversation; in a love relationship there are responsibilities as well as opportunities.

It's always complicated for lovers to set up rules about having outside sex, since each of them may fear abandonment. That's all the more reason why they should agree on the parameters. Sometimes a settled couple will set up a rule that if they go out together for an evening, they will always return home with each other. If one meets someone he likes, he may take the person's phone number or e-mail address and make arrangements for getting together, but he may not desert his lover during their night out. Some partners have a rule that they will have sex with outsiders only in threesomes that include the other lover (see *Three-Ways*); other couples will trick out only when one of them is out of town. Some couples designate nights off (one night per month, every two weeks, etc.) in which they are free to pursue outside sex. Such rules can and should change as the relationship evolves, as it is bound to do, and as the lovers discover and come to accommodate each other.

One should also note that some gay couples have always insisted on both fidelity and monogamy, adhering to the belief that gay relationships, like heterosexual marriages, exclude outside sex. Though many find it hard to believe, there are numerous cases of sexual fidelity in gay relationships.

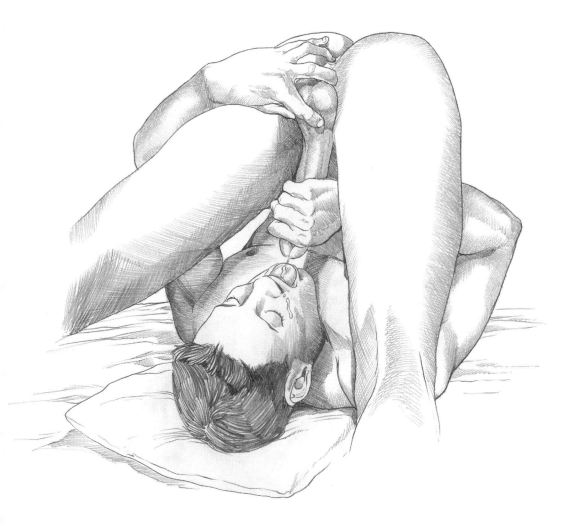

To a different set of men, tricking out represents such enormous health dangers that even raising the subject is painful. They fear the HIV may be introduced into their relationship by a third party, and they've sworn off tricking "for the duration" of the epidemic (now more than twenty years).

Remember, lovers have a primary responsibility to each other, and not to the standards of either the gay community or to society at large.

Finding a Physician

Gay men have special health problems that can be understood properly only by a doctor who has worked with and is sympathetic to gay patients. Many gay men insist on consulting with a gay physician because so many straight doctors are both ignorant of gay medicine and actively hostile to gay patients. But straight doctors, especially because of their experience in the AIDS epidemic, have become far more sensitive to what we might call gay medicine. What you want is a gay-friendly physician.

Some gay men have two doctors, one for their ordinary health problems and one for sexually transmitted diseases. This is irrational. Our bodies are not cordoned off into gay and straight zones. So-called gay health problems such as hepatitis, parasites, and venereal diseases may produce symptoms that will damage parts of your body not originally infected. It's best to have one doctor to keep track of all your health needs, and if you cannot come out to him or her and discuss your sex life and lifestyle, you need a different doctor, or you need to cure your own homophobia (see *Homophobia*; *Sexually Transmitted Diseases*).

How do you find a doctor sympathetic to the health needs of gay people? Gay service organizations usually have a list of local gay-friendly physicians. Some doctors even have health clinics with which they are associated. Friends will recommend doctors who have treated them competently. Gay health centers are listed in the *Gayellow Pages*, available in bookstores, and gay magazines and newspapers usually contain ads by gay physicians. The Internet also has a number of gay referral sources. Gayhealth.com is currently the best of the lot. In many cities, you can be treated at low-cost gay health clinics. (See the Appendix for a list.)

If you should find yourself in a strange city (or country) and be unable to locate a gay-friendly physician, you need to be able to tell a straight physician what you think may be wrong—especially if it's a sexual condition. Say it up front and without ambiguity. If you need a swab up your butt to check for the clap, for instance, or down your throat, say so. Don't be intimidated by the doctor.

If any doctor refuses to treat you, threaten to make a formal complaint against him or her with the local medical association. Of course you may not carry out the threat if you feel you must keep your homosexuality secret, but if you're already open about it, make the complaint. You're doing it for yourself and for other gay men who need proper treatment. A bit of gay militancy is in order when dealing with hostile straight doctors. For too long the health problems of gays have been neglected by irresponsible physicians.

Demanding your medical rights is extremely important if you or your lover is HIV-positive or symptomatic for AIDS. Although it is changing rapidly, some physicians and nurses will still treat you like a leper if you have the HIV. One hospitalized AIDS patient, for example, was visited by a house physician wearing work gloves and a paper bag over his head with eyehole slits. The doctor spoke to his patient from the threshold of the room. Needless to say, the patient recognized that he had a fool for a physician and complained to the hospital administrator. Within an hour a new and competent physician was at his bedside. The moral? Don't take shit from a homophobe, with or without a medical degree.

First Time

Throughout history men have fucked one another and relished the experience. Etruscan tombs in Italy, for instance, have paintings of men fucking other men. Sex between men has persisted despite the persecution by clergymen, judges, and doctors. This persistence in the face of harsh penalties such as hanging, burning, castration, imprisonment, and commitment to mental hospitals indicates that fucking and getting fucked is a great and enduring pleasure.

To get fucked and enjoy it, you may have to overcome some negative attitudes about your asshole (see *Anus*). The best preparation for getting fucked is to explore your anus and some of the sensations it can provide. Some men like to do the following exercises in the bathtub. The warm water helps you to relax, and the bathroom provides some privacy for gay men who still live with their family.

Wash your anus, including just inside, with soap and water. Lubricate your finger with your preferred lubricant and insert it into your asshole (see *Lubricants*). As you feel increasingly relaxed, apply more lubricant and push deeper. You'll feel the sphincter muscles at this point; these need to relax for you to get fucked. Deliberately tighten them. You'll be surprised how strong they are. Relax them. Grip and relax these muscles several times.

Now move your finger in deeper. You'll find the sphincter muscles are more extensive than you thought, and they open and relax of their own accord around your exploring finger. If they don't, stop and relax for a minute or two.

Once your finger gets beyond the inner sphincter, it enters the rectum, a wider space. You'll notice the change in texture. Move your finger in and out a couple of inches at a time. If you've been fearful about anal penetration until now, you'll be amazed how easy this is.

Remove your finger, breathe deeply, and relax. Tell yourself out loud that you're coming along beautifully. Complimenting yourself may seem absurdly narcissistic, but in fact it's a useful reinforcement, well known to behavioral psychologists. If, after this break, you insert your finger again, you'll notice how much more easily it goes in—but don't rush. Ironically, going slowly gets you in faster.

After several exploratory sessions, try two fingers. If you feel the sphincter muscles closing, return to the tightening and relaxing exercises. You may now use a dildo if the idea appeals to you. Make sure it's reasonably sized, and not one of those monsters that stunt artists absorb (see *Sex Toys*).

Two other exercises may be of value. First, if you have a fuck buddy or lover, ask him to explore your asshole with his fingers. Then put your finger in his anus. The second exercise is to jerk off with one hand while you insert one or two fingers of the other hand into your anus. As you masturbate, move your fingers rhythmically in and out. Again, you may want to invite your partner into the bathtub to perform these exercises with you (and if you have a large enough tub). Given the close quarters, the session may end up both instructive and hilarious.

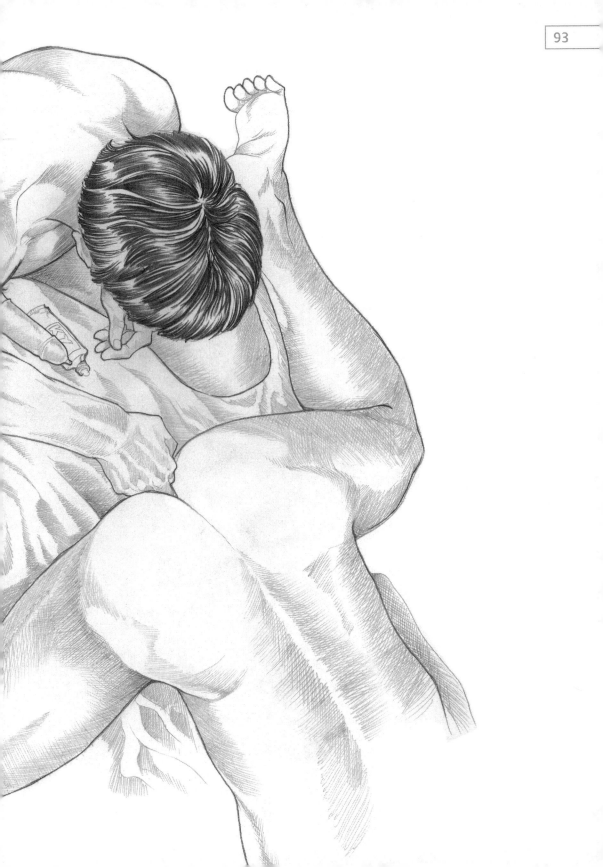

One note of caution. Fingers, dildos, and cocks can be pleasurable and safe. Never put anything else up your ass. No glass bottles, sweet potatoes, or other exotic objects. They may elude your grasp, get lost in your colon, and require major surgery.

You should prepare in a number of ways for getting fucked the first time. Physically, all you need to do is to clean yourself out with a small enema. Some men find that a squirt from an ear syringe does the job well enough. You should also have condoms ready, and always insist that your partner use them. We strongly advise you not to drink alcohol heavily or to use mind-altering drugs at this time (see *Drug Abuse*). They may interfere with good judgment about safe sex (see *Booze and Highs*). Choose whatever lubricant you generally use to jack off (see *Lubricants*). Lubricate your asshole and the outside of your partner's condoms liberally. You can also use your favorite jerk-off lubricant to work on your own dick while getting fucked (see *Condoms*; *Safe Sex*).

There are two good positions to start out with. In the easier one, both you and your partner lie on your side, pitcher's front to catcher's back. However, sometimes a novice will prefer to be on top so he can control the situation. In this position you face your partner, who is on his back, and you sit on his cock (see *Sitting on It*). Being on top will relieve what may be one of the main anxieties: that he will enter too quickly. If you are on top, you can control the rate of penetration yourself, but remember that the average man can accommodate quite a large penis with no great difficulty. If problems about size occur, it may be because your partner's cock is unusually thick. When his cock is about a third of the way in, you may feel pain. Pull away gently and rest before trying again. The interval will give the sphincter time to relax and open.

On the second attempt, everything should go well. You should be able to accommodate the whole cock—in fact, you may be surprised how easily it goes in. If it doesn't, simply repeat the process, trying to relax. Make sure you're breathing; when you get anxious, you tend to hold your breath.

The first few times you get fucked you may have the uncomfortable sensation that you are about to defecate. Only after several experiences will you learn to tell the two sensations apart.

Suppose you're at home with an attractive man, and you're both undressed. Suddenly he announces that he's never been fucked before but wants to learn. Your reaction is crucial. Do you want to take on a novice? You may not be interested—or, on the other hand, you may be flattered. If you're not willing to take the time to do it right, skip it. Initiating a neophyte must be done patiently and carefully.

Your job is to get him to trust you. You must teach him to relax, guide him through clear, unambiguous instruction, reassure him that he's doing well—and never rush. Tense people are seldom aware that their bodies are rigid because their muscles have contracted. Point out to him where on his body he tenses up. Rub the spots, massage them a little. You don't have to be a professional to help him to feel good and relax (see *Massage*).

Enter him gently with one finger. After he's adjusted to one finger, enter with two—but not too quickly. Once you've got both fingers in his anus, masturbate him with your other hand. The familiar pleasure of masturbation, which he's known since puberty, is now linked with the new sensation of anal penetration. You could masturbate or suck him almost to the point of coming, but don't. Frustrate him a bit; make him wait for his climax.

You might want to have him do the same to you, and even reverse roles, taking turns jerking or sucking each other, until he's comfortable and hot.

Now you're ready to fuck him. Let's say he's on his back with his legs around your shoulders. While massaging his cock with your hand, explore his anus with the fingers of your other hand, then with the head of your cock. Ask how he feels, and when he seems eager and fully relaxed, put the head of your cock in, but not entirely. Let him get used to the sensation before continuing.

The first entry should be slow and gentle. Partial entry is par for the course; don't try to force your way in. If he tenses up, withdraw and use your fingers to massage his anus again. If he begins to panic, stop what you're doing. If you're partly or completely inside him, ask if he wants you to pull out. Say it calmly. Even begin to retract a little. It's his body being invaded; let him guide you. Sometimes knowing that you can be trusted is enough to relax him.

Let him know what you're feeling—how exciting it is to be inside him, and how sexy and handsome he is. Continue to jerk him off, but not to the point of climax. Get him to vocalize what he's feeling: Vocalizing it will help him feel more pleasure (see *Dirty Talk*).

Thrust slowly and gently. From time to time let him initiate the movement; vary his position until your penis massages his prostate—a sure site of pleasure. Finally, after you both come, kiss him, hold him, and tell him how good it felt to be inside him.

Fisting

Fisting—also called fist fucking—is the insertion of the whole hand through the rectum and into the colon. It is dangerous and could result in complications that lead to death. A sharp fingernail can leave a deep, painful cut in the rectum that could take weeks to heal. A fist ramming the sigmoid colon—the part of the intestine eight inches up from the anus—could be fatal.

The tissue lining the sigmoid colon has the consistency of wet paper towels. In some cases it can expand to accommodate a closed fist, but internal bleeding can result, as can infection of the peritoneum (the membrane lining the abdomen), causing peritonitis. Since the bleeding is internal, it produces no visible blood. Some men have recognized the symptoms (stomach cramps, chills, and fever) and rushed to a surgeon. A colostomy, rerouting the intestine to a sack on the side of the body, saved their lives.

The harm done in fisting comes about because the intestines lack pain receptors. The person being fist fucked can't tell what's going on inside him. Since a lot of fist fucking occurs while people are drugged, physical sensitivity is reduced. Drugs may also interfere with good judgment (see *Booze and Highs*; *Drug Abuse*; *Drugs and Sex*).

Many gay men may consider this description unnecessarily alarmist. Despite these obvious dangers, fisting was quite popular in the past, mostly among sadomasochists, and some of the best-selling porn films of the pre-AIDS era—*L.A. Tool & Die*, *Fists of Fury*—dealt with it in a most erotic manner. The Fistfuckers of America (FFA) assures us that there are numerous cases of men taking a fist with no apparent damage. Not all fisting depends upon pain and dominance. To take a whole hand requires such total relaxation that after getting fisted a man might feel great tranquillity.

Often the person getting fisted has already been fucked for a while by his partner's cock, and his rectal muscles are relaxed. The fister should coat his hand and forearm with a thick layer of lubricant (Crisco is often used) and should apply more lubricant throughout the process (see *Lubricants*). The fister ought to have previously removed rings and bracelets from his hand and wrist, trimmed his fingernails, sanding down rough edges. If the person to be fisted notices that his partner's nails are

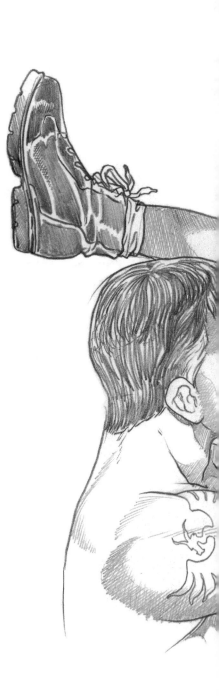

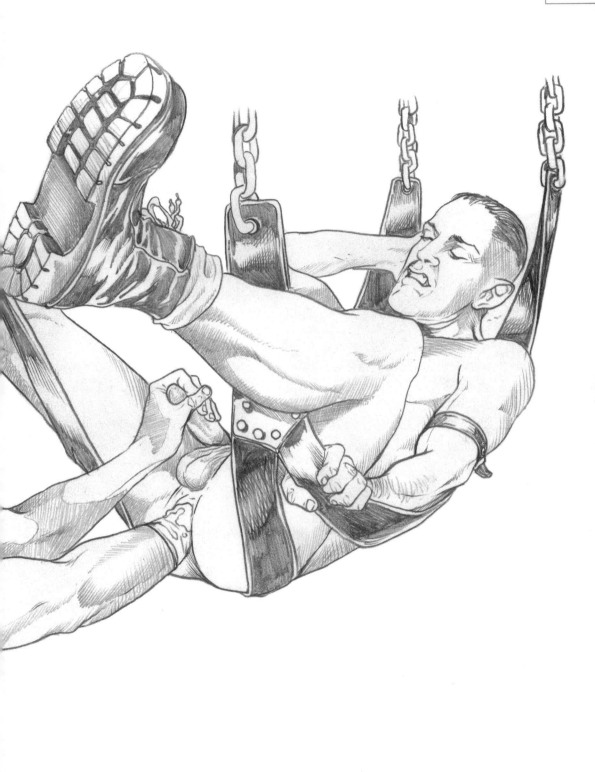

long or sharp, he should insist they be trimmed there and then. Many men report having had potential tricks take their hands and check their nails upon meeting, and long before any discussion of potential sex: He's checking to see if you keep your nails short and are open to this kind of sex.

For most people, fisting occurs experimentally and seldom goes beyond the insertion of several fingers deep into the rectum. Less often, fisting is the final experience of an intense session of sex when neither man is able to sustain an erection. While they seemingly have done everything else with each other's body, they still want to remain sexually intimate and active.

Fisting should begin with a cleansing. Enema bags of various kinds are available at your local pharmacy. Buy one, read the directions, and make sure that you are completely clean before beginning. Fisting begins with the insertion of one or two fingers to loosen up the muscles; three or four fingers follow. The fister then pulls out his hand, folds his thumb against his palm, and wriggles his entire hand back in. The difficult part is getting the hand past the sphincter. The man getting fucked will take whatever position facilitates entry. Some lie on their back with their feet in the air, others crouch on all fours. Perhaps the best position is standing and slowly sitting on a vertical forearm. To achieve climax while fisting, some men masturbate. Sometimes the fist is removed and fucking with a cock is resumed.

A new problem has arisen with fisting—AIDS. Most researchers believe that the HIV and illness-producing bacteria are easily transmitted through the blood-rich system of the anus, rectum, and colon. Any practice that causes trauma (damage) to any part of this area is therefore deemed an unsafe sexual practice. Some fisters try to minimize this danger by wearing a latex glove during fisting, condoms when fucking, and by never ejaculating in the bottom's asshole. Still, fisting remains a questionable practice, one that demands both skill and concern for one's partner. Needless to say, you should never insert any dangerous object into your ass (see *Dangerous Sex; Sex Toys*).

Foreskin

In the days of the Roman Empire, having the foreskin on your cock was cosmetically important, since the penis was perceived as a mark of beauty and a symbol of a man's masculinity. Athletic games required competitors to have a foreskin that completely covered the glans penis (the head of the cock). But some athletes came from North Africa and the eastern Mediterranean, where circumcision was common. These athletes underwent an operation in which a new foreskin was surgically formed so that they could compete, although we have little evidence about the success of the procedure. In any event, with the fall of Rome, foreskin restoration stopped.

Circumcision originated among the ancient Hebrews as a way to mark their separation from the gentiles. It was also a way to prevent male Jews from hiding among gentiles, much as the Christian Copts of Egypt today still tattoo a cross on the wrist of a newborn child. Circumcision is still practiced in the Jewish and Muslim religions, and throughout the United States by most gentiles. Sir Richard Burton, the nineteenth-century English explorer, noted that some physicians believed circumcision discouraged masturbation, then called *onanism*, after the biblical story of Onan, who wasted his "seed" by allowing it to fall to the ground instead of impregnating a woman. The belief was another example of the anti-jerk-off crusade of the time (see *Masturbation and Fantasy*).

Circumcision became routine in the United States in the nineteenth century, some say for health reasons, others to prevent masturbation. Today it serves no practical purpose (it certainly doesn't prevent masturbation), though it is frequently justified as a hygienic measure. A circumcised cock may be a bit easier to keep clean, but the uncircumcised need spend only a few seconds more to be perfectly tidy.

Uncircumcised men occasionally claim that circumcision removes some sensitivity during sex, but one wonders how they know this. When erect, circumcised and uncircumcised cocks look and feel much the same.

Many gay men register strong preferences for "cut" or "uncut" meat; in fact, personal ads in gay publications often specify which is desired (see *Profiles; Sex Ads*). For these men, the *appearance* of the partner's cock is probably an important factor in their fantasy life, though it limits the reservoir of potential partners. It's sad to think that men are rejected as sex partners or lovers because of a piece of skin.

We've met a few men who say that a foreskin is required for "docking": You place the head of your dick against the head of your partner's dick (face-to-face, so to speak). Then you pull his foreskin over both his dick head and yours—and you are docked. You masturbate yourself as your partner masturbates himself, all the time rubbing your two cock heads together until you come (see *Mutual Masturbation*). We also note that some men like to place jewelry on their foreskins, often connecting a Prince Albert to a chain, but it's hard to leave the house that way (see *Body Decoration*).

Sometimes medical circumcision is required on an adult man because the prepuce is too tight and prevents a full erection (this condition is called *phimosis*), or because of recurring infections. Circumcision of an adult can be serious and painful and should not be undertaken for purely cosmetic reasons. Occasionally, men attempt to restore their own foreskins or circumcise themselves without medical assistance. Don't do it, and don't let a friend do it. This can result in mutilation and serious infection.

We have little sympathy for circumcised men who seek foreskin restoration for cosmetic reasons, or for the uncircumcised who want to be cut in order to fit in. We believe the underlying problem has nothing to do with cocks, cut or uncut. It's probably what shrinks call *body dysmorphia*, a mental condition in which a man has an obsession about the inadequacy of some part (or parts) of his body and chooses surgery as the means for changing it. Since he's usually never satisfied anyway, we believe that a better treatment is psychotherapy, medication, or both.

We have a different solution for gay men who will only have sex with a cut or an uncut man. Grow up.

Friendship

Friendship means more to most gay men than it does to straights, and gays learn how to value and cultivate it. Both straight and gay teenagers know the intimacy and ardor of friendship, but all too many straights "grow out of" those fierce involvements and pour all their emotional energies into their husband or wife and children.

Parents of gays often puzzle over how their children can endure the loneliness of single life. Since the parents are usually rooted in their marriage and often receive little real sustenance from friends, they would naturally have difficulty understanding a lifestyle in which friendship is central. Typically, a gay man will have two or three close friends, male and female, with whom he shares his hopes and doubts about his job, his health, his emotional and spiritual growth, and his personal goals.

Exceptions abound; some married straights maintain intense one-to-one friendships, and conversely, gay couples may socialize only with other couples. Nevertheless, experience suggests that gays, especially those without lovers or between affairs, enjoy friendships that are active, supportive, candid, and nurturing.

Contrarily, some parents of gays cannot seem to fathom—even after many explanations—the difference between a gay man's closest friend and his lover. Because gays often travel together, room together, and spend so much of their time together with close friends, they're always having to explain, "No, Joe isn't my lover, Mother. He's"—big chorus here—"just a friend!"

It's that *just* that helps the problem along. Friendship is by no means a makeshift or a substitute for love; it is its own province, one that some philosophers have considered a higher affection than love—higher because, at its best, friendship is free from the need to dominate, to possess, or to use. Because friendship is so crucial to the happiness of most gays, they should take pains. Nothing is more irritating (and self-defeating) than the gay man who drops his friends and goes into hibernation the moment he finds a new lover. Especially if, as often happens, a few weeks or months later, after the romance has cooled, he sails back into his friends' lives, needing to discuss in endless detail what went wrong, trying to pretend he was there all the while. Gay friends can and should be able to tell each other everything, including what they need and really want—say, a birthday party thrown for one of them, or a movie matinee at an animated or trashy film, or even a vacation on a cruise ship neither can really afford. Many men who've had strong partnerships and equally strong friendships find it difficult to assess which has been more important in their life. And when you are older, often friendships step in to fill the gap tricking and partying no longer can fill (see *Growing Older*).

Compared with the glamour of a new passion, friendship may seem a mild pleasure, but it's a pleasure that endures and ripens. Friends should not be taken for granted. They should be selected with care and their feelings regarded with sensitivity.

Frottage

Rubbing against someone (while clothed or naked) to the point of climax is called frottage. Unpleasant, beady-eyed straight men—and not bad-looking gay men, too—practice it standing up in crowded elevators, in rush-hour subways and buses, or waiting on line in front of theaters. Teenagers in the fifties and sixties did it to excess in the backseats of jalopies; it was called heavy petting by the media. It's also something two naked men can do together at home. Some even prefer it these days, because there is no exchange of bodily fluids and so it is considered safe. In the wrong circumstances, however, it can be quite dangerous.

Some gay men rub against men in crowded subways and buses, sometimes even reaching around and fondling the cock of unconsenting straight men. This can obviously lead to a punch in the face at best, and getting beaten up and arrested at worst. Still, we have heard of gay men who get off this way (even coming in their pants), and while it obviously provides a heightened sense of excitement and danger, it seems to us to be indicative of serious emotional problems probably arising around issues of masculinity.

Sometimes frottage is called belly-fucking, or more pejoratively, the Princeton rub. One lubricates one's partner's stomach or one's own cock, climbs on top, and pumps away. If one's ass is out of commission for some reason, belly-fucking can be a good substitute, though it has appeals of its own and need not be considered a makeshift. Some men also like the feeling of rubbing their genitals against those of their partner until they come. If he's smooth-skinned between his legs, you can lie behind him and fuck the space between his thighs, just below his crotch (inter-

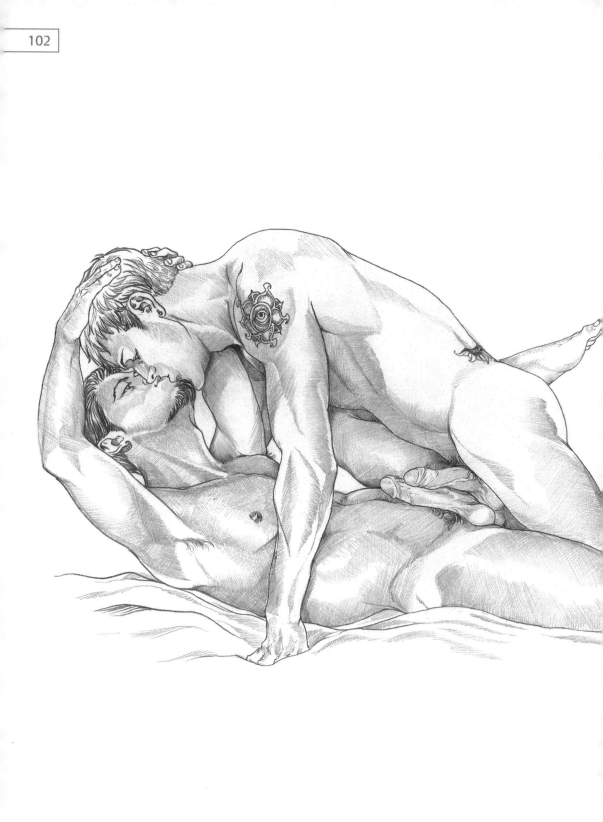

femoral fucking, as it's called). Armpits, the gully between the pecs, the crevice between the buns, and the space between the clavicle and chin when the head is tilted to one side are all similarly available. If you're wrestling, you can both rub against each other to the point of climax. You can even masturbate a cock with the soft soles of your feet.

Fuck Buddies

Let's say you meet someone and go home with him, and the sex is so successful that the next time you meet in a club or bar you go home again. After that, you bump into each other on the street, flirt, talk dirty, and end up having sex again. You exchange phone numbers and call each other up and arrange more sex. You're seeing each other regularly, having hot, satisfying sex, and you've come to look forward to these encounters. Yet the two of you have not become lovers, and intuitively you both know you never will. Also, while you talk before and after your hot sex sessions, you intuit that you two don't share enough in common to ever really become intimate friends. No problem, there's a perfectly good name and acceptable relationship in gay life for you—you're fuck buddies.

Fuck buddies allegedly also exist among heterosexuals. During the sexually liberated sixties and seventies, playwrights and filmmakers especially presented scenarios of men and women having repeated sex without emotional complications—*Same Time, Next Year*; *Darling*; and other films showed such relationships. However, it never really caught on among straights the way it did among gays.

Having a fuck buddy means you can have successful sex without entangling alliances, without the emotional turmoil of a romance. Of course finding a compatible fuck buddy is as difficult as finding a lover—looking for one doesn't work: He either comes along or he doesn't. A good fuck buddy is naturally, wonderfully useful if you have no interest in having a more intimate relationship, particularly if you already have a lover (see *Couples*).

Use your fuck buddy to perfect your technical skills and to expand your sexual repertoire. It's not unusual for someone to integrate new sexual skills discovered with a fuck buddy into his relationship with a lover. In this way, the relationship with the fuck buddy can help the relationship between two lovers.

Tops who want to be bottoms for a day, or vice versa; men who want to experiment with all the different kinds of fucking and sucking that are found in this book; and guys who are interested in trying out kinkier stuff can do so freely as long as their fuck

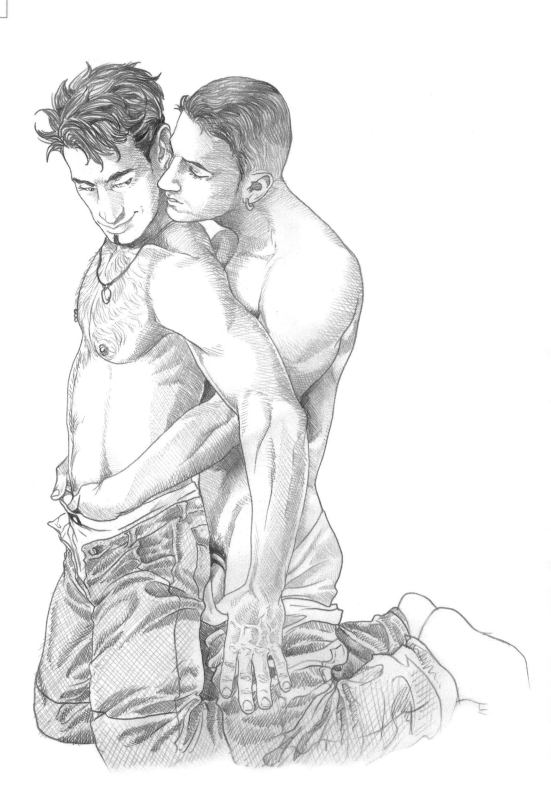

buddy agrees (see *Kinky Sex; Sleazy Sex*). But the best use of a fuck buddy is simply to have sex in safe surroundings.

The mutual pleasure of the fuck buddies is the quid pro quo of the relationship, with the implicit understanding that the relationship can be ended at any time by either party with no hard feelings.

Gay Families

For many gay men, one of the greatest downsides of coming out is that it sometimes means having to give up their natal family. It's sad but true that, for many families, there is no tolerance for gay children. For every mother who embraces her gay son after he's come out, there's another who curses him and tells him never to call or come back home. Even worse, it's not always that simple or that black-and-white: Many families, whether for religious or other reasons, don't outright disown and ban their gay sons. Instead they try to change them, ignore their lifestyle, or insist that, when they are at home, they follow the family's antigay rules. It can be stressful, and needless to say, as gay men grow older, their natural desire to have more to do with their family becomes deeply frustrated. Instead of coming closer, they find themselves forced to draw further apart.

No wonder that gays form their own "families" and that increasingly they come to live within those fabricated families more intensely and fully than they would ever have done with their natal family.

What is a gay family and who can belong to it? A gay family is any group of individuals a lesbian or gay man draws around herself or himself as (s)he begins to settle down into life. Some of these families are similar to those friendship groups among younger gays, teens especially, first coming out. Often those early groups contain more mature and less developed members, brothers and "sisters" as well as a "parent" who may actually be someone's parent or sibling, or may be a teacher or coach or local social worker, or pastor, or even local CD-store or video-rental-shop owner where the kids hang out. These groups often form with apparent ease and almost unconsciously. They exist to give young gays support and a sense of belonging, to air problems and provide solutions, sometimes just to blow off steam and whine about life. And of course they offer protection from a hostile outside world.

Gay families among adults are no different. Who can belong? Anyone, regardless of sexual orientation. Mostly, however, a gay family consists of a gay man and his closest two or three friends, as well as one or more former tricks, a partner, or an ex-boyfriend. Like the teen's gay family, generally one person is deemed the youngest and treated by the others as the "child"—one gay family actually referred to theirs as "David, Our Problem Child." Someone else—it could be anyone of any age—often becomes the parent. "Yes, Mother," one gay man will say to someone in his gay family. And although he's joking, he may also be telling the truth: that friend or ex has become his substitute parent, one more loving than the first.

Straight friends, especially straight women, are often drawn into gay families, and they often find considerable strength and privilege in their newfound status. In fact, for some women who are interested in playing the field and/or following their career and not getting married, being a member of a gay family is one sure way to always have a date or escort, as well as to try out and develop facets of her personality she may find are now holding her back from forming her family. Straight men, especially younger ones, often from broken homes or in better need of parenting than nature has provided, often fit themselves into stable older gay families, and they, too, can benefit greatly. Occasionally a natal brother or sister of a gay who's also out of step with his or her relatives for other reasons than sexuality may seek membership in a gay family.

Some gay families consist entirely of lovers, past and present. It's often quite intriguing (sometimes painful) watching a new boyfriend enter such a ménage of former partners (see *Couples*). The rest of the family is made up of close friends, both gay and straight.

What can having a gay family do for you? You always have a shoulder to cry on or someone to share your achievements. You always have somewhere to go on the holidays when natal families are celebrating. One of the authors and his gay family celebrated the Hanukkah/Christmas holidays extensively, attracting large numbers of people to dinners and gift-opening breakfasts, including straight couples and their children. Over the years, the big holidays continued, and even when parents separated and divorced or moved away or died, their children still had somewhere to go when they most needed a home, a family, love, stability, and a sense of belonging. The other author gives large New Year's Day parties for his gay family, complete with amateur theatricals of growing complexity.

A gay family can provide you with worldly things, too: contacts and connections, advice, legal help, money, employment, health care, a place to live as well as a sure place to be appreciated for who you are, without any sense of feeling different or discriminated against. One of the real tragedies of the AIDS epidemic was that entire gay families were wiped out, or most of a gay family. A gay man who may have existed for years within his carefully cultivated environment of love was suddenly isolated and without the support network he'd relied on, at exactly the time he most needed it. Pulling together a new gay family can be a daunting, nearly impossible project later in life. Still, it's worth trying to accomplish.

• • •

Gay Liberation

The homosexual civil rights movement began in 1869 in Germany when a Hungarian physician, Karoly Maria Benkert, published an open letter to the Prussian minister of justice protesting legislation penalizing homosexuals. Benkert coined the word *homosexual* and used it for the first time in the letter. He also coined the word *heterosexual*. Before that, the medical profession used *contrary sexual desire* as a diagnosis, while other physicians hospitalized gay men for *moral insanity*. The law referred to gay sex as perversion, sodomy, or buggery, while the educated homosexual population of Europe called themselves *congenital inverts*, a term first used by the German neurologist Krafft-Ebing.

The word *congenital* was important to gays because it implied that their sexual orientation was biological in origin, and therefore, they were not responsible for it. The alternative belief was that sexual behavior was subject to "free will," meaning that it was under voluntary control. The rapidly changing nomenclature indicated two factors: society's confusion about how to deal with homosexual men and women, and the political struggle between biological and social-learning explanations for the origin of sexual orientation. This argument is as lively today as it was 150 years ago (see *Mythic Beginnings*).

A decade earlier, the German scientist Karl Heinrich Ulrichs popularized the theory that male homosexuals made up a "third sex," endowed with male bodies and female brains. His descriptive term for homosexuality was *Urning*, which comes from a speech by Pausanias in Plato's *Symposium*, in which a group of men discuss the nature of love around the dinner table (see *Couples*). Ulrichs was probably the first nineteenth-century writer to argue that homosexuality was biologically determined or, as he put it, "congenital." In 1889, Magnus Hirschfeld, a German physician who had been profoundly influenced by Ulrichs's third-sex theory, founded the first journal devoted to the study of homosexuality. In 1911 he founded the Institute for Sexual Science, a repository for biological, anthropological, and statistical research relating to sexuality. (Christopher Isherwood, who visited the institute while living in Berlin, describes it in *Christopher and His Kind*.) The Nazis destroyed Hirschfeld's center and all of his research papers when they came to power.

The First Congress of the World League for Sexual Reform was held in Berlin in 1921. It was an extraordinary event because it brought together leaders in the struggle for gay rights throughout the Western world. A year later, twenty-five branches of the homosexual rights movement were scattered throughout Germany. The tyranny of the Nazis, however, destroyed this movement, and during World War II many homosexuals were interned, forced to wear the infamous pink triangle, put to slave labor, and exterminated. *The Pink Triangle* by Richard Plant is an excellent history of this period.

In England in the 1880s, the poet Edward Carpenter (who was not gay) and poet J.A. Symonds (who was gay) openly campaigned for gay rights and made some progress in public opinion. But just before the turn of the century, the extraordinary public scandal surrounding the writer Oscar Wilde's two trials changed all that, causing homosexuality instead to be openly condemned. Not until 1959 was *The Wolfenden Report*, commissioned by the British government, released, recommending dropping all criminal penalties against homosexuality in Great Britain. Yet it took many years after the report before homosexuality was fully decriminalized in Britain, and in parts of the British Commonwealth it's still illegal.

In the Soviet Union, homosexuality was decriminalized after the 1917 Communist revolution, but it became a punishable offense again during the 1920s following Lenin's death, when the homicidal dictator Joseph Stalin took control. After World War II, the entire Eastern Bloc treated homosexuality as harshly as the Russians did. Now that the Cold War has ended, social changes in Eastern Europe have brought with them a new era of acceptability toward gay life in all of these once Communist countries, with Romania and Bulgaria leading their way, and even Russia now has a vibrant gay life.

In the United States, gay liberation took its first steps with an organization modeled on the German gay movement and founded in Chicago in 1924. A precursor group without much lasting influence, it was called the Society for Human Rights. Its goal was to educate the public about homosexuality and to repeal sodomy laws. This organization was hounded by the police and the press and was soon driven out of existence. It was ahead of its time.

The sexual climate in the United States was extremely difficult for homosexuals right up to and throughout World War II. Those self-aware enough and bold enough to live openly were subject to arrest, police entrapment, imprisonment, psychiatric and medical mistreatment, and legal castration. Read *Becoming Gay: The Journey to Self-Acceptance* by Richard Isay, and *Cures* by Martin Duberman. Even so, gays and lesbians came to wield great power in the theater and strongly influenced the American film industry, with some of Hollywood's biggest stars of the day—Greta Garbo, Cary Grant, and Marlene Dietrich included—living openly gay or bisexual lives. The censorious Hollywood Hayes Office forced these stars and their public personas back into the closet in 1938. Read *We Can Always Call Them Bulgarians* by Kaier Curtin.

Many sociologists and historians consider World War II the key event responsible for bringing out American lesbians and gay men. Huge numbers of young people were drafted or enlisted, taken off the farms and out of the factories, thrown together in boot camps, on ships, in barracks, and allowed to socialize. Many gay servicemen joined entertainment groups putting on camp shows (no pun intended) for our troops in both the United States and overseas. For excellent coverage on this topic, read

Coming Out Under Fire: The History of Gay Men and Women in World War Two by Allan Bérube.

The publication of the first Kinsey report about male sexual behavior to a startled public in 1948 confirmed what many already knew: the widespread extent of male homosexuality at all levels of American society. Groups of gays began to meet, notably Harry Hay's pathbreaking Mattachine Society in Los Angeles in 1950, which published the first homosexual magazine, *ONE*. In 1955, the Daughters of Bilitis, a lesbian organization, was founded in San Francisco; its publication was *The Ladder*. When the United States Postal Service banned the distribution of *ONE* and pronounced any mention of homosexuality in mailed-out printed matter to be obscene, the ban was appealed. This was an extraordinary act of public bravery in a society that still imprisoned "sodomites." The Supreme Court decided in favor of the publication and against the post office—an important legal victory for gays. For more details, read *Making Gay History: The Half-Century Fight for Lesbian and Gay Equal Rights* by Eric Marcus, and *Out for Good: The Struggle to Build a Gay Rights Movement in America* by Dudley Clendinen and Adam Nagourney.

Even so, by 1969 there were still only about fifty gay organizations in the whole United States, none influential. In that year a significant, spontaneous upsurge of gay militancy occurred. On June 28, 1969, the New York City police raided and attempted to close a gay bar in Greenwich Village called the Stonewall Inn. Although the bar had been raided often, on this night, for the first time, the gay clientele, composed mainly of lower-class street hustlers and transvestites, actively resisted the police. Several cops were bludgeoned to the ground by the purses and high heels of the transvestites in the bar (see *Transgender*). The fracas became so fierce that police were compelled to lock themselves inside the bar until reinforcements arrived.

On this early summer night, a day after the funeral of the singer-actress Judy Garland, the neighborhood was already filled with gay residents—many upset by the death of the premier gay icon—who quickly joined the melee, turning it into a riot. The surrounding area in Greenwich Village was cordoned off and the riot squad brought in. The next afternoon, a protest rally was held at Sheridan Square. Seemingly overnight, a new spirit was born, one patterned to a great extent on the black and feminist civil rights movements.

Two major organizations were founded out of that protest against New York Police Department policies: first, the Gay Liberation Front (GLF), and after that organization failed, the longer-lasting, more successful Gay Activists Alliance (GAA). The GAA, though committed to nonviolence, confronted discrimination at the risk of arrest. They originated the "zap," a public demonstration using humor to highlight prejudice against gay people and to draw media attention, and to reduce gay bashing by the police. In one zap they brought two wedding cakes to the New York City Marriage License Bureau, which had previously refused marriage licenses to two gay men and two gay women. Atop the cakes were the customary images of brides and grooms, except that two grooms were on one cake and two brides on the other. While officials frantically phoned the police, gays from the GAA cut the cakes and handed slices to the office staff together with coffee to wash the cake down. There were no arrests, but lots of newspaper publicity, which was, after all, the objective. In another action, a member of the city council was holding up passage of a gay rights bill. One Saturday at 3 A.M. about a thousand gay men, just out from a nearby GAA dance, marched to the councilman's apartment house and demonstrated in the streets, keeping him (and his neighbors) up for hours. Thereafter, gay militancy became the order of the day, and activist groups were formed in many American cities, all devoted to achieving civil rights for gay people.

The radical gay groups of the 1970s were a far cry from those that had come before in the 1950s and 1960s. (Although, of course, all groups stand on the shoulders of those who came before.) The earlier groups, such as the Mattachine, advocated a politics of "fitting into" society, as part of an attempt to prove that gays and lesbians were participating and productive members of society deserving equal rights. When Mattachine members demonstrated, for instance, the men wore suits and ties and carried attaché cases, and the women wore dresses. Seventies gay radicals, by contrast, came from the ranks of the anti–Vietnam War activists. They knew radical politics by their experiences fighting the federal government against the war. Their goal was to change society, not to assimilate into it. While nonviolent, they had no reservations about civil disobedience, nor about breaking up antigay meetings of politicians or psychiatrists.

Today, radical gay groups exist, especially on many college campuses, but they are a much smaller and less visible part of the gay movement. This is understandable. ACT UP, which fought government inaction on AIDS research and treatment, was probably the last major radical group. It reflected a renewed activism among a younger generation of gay men who had not had to fight for gay rights themselves, but who drove the AIDS epidemic to the front page. Gay men diagnosed with the virus were deeply frustrated by what they saw as bureaucratic inaction. The diagnosis was, after all, a death sentence at the time. To bring their plight to the public's attention, and feeling that they had nothing to lose, they organized large sit-ins and hit-and-run demonstrations against governmental agencies and health officials across the United States. During the 1980s and early 1990s, ACT UP achieved levels of sophisticated nonviolent protests involving a manipulation of the media that had never before been seen in any civil rights movement.

In contrast were groups such as the Gay Men's Health Crisis (GMHC) and other gay AIDS service organizations that became mainstream advocates for men infected with the virus. GMHC is the oldest and still the best funded of them. These less radical groups, working with state and federal legislators, governmental health agencies, and the media, have had a phenomenal effect in making the lives of those with AIDS and the HIV more livable. Disability insurance for AIDS patients, and the ADAPT (in

New York State) program that pays for patient medication, are two examples of their effectiveness. The movement from radical to moderate gay politics is an understandable evolutionary change. The gay rights movement may no longer need radical gay politics to secure our civil rights. Moderate gay groups— those that work *with* power brokers instead of *against* them—now carry the ball to end discrimination against us.

As a result of both radical and moderate gay activism, gay service organizations now exist throughout the country. They include health services such as New York's Callen-Lorde Community Health Center and Washington, D.C.'s Whitman-Walker Clinic; self-help groups such as the People with AIDS Coalition (PWAC) and the Gay and Lesbian Alliance Against Defamation (GLAAD); and gay counseling centers such as New York's Institute for Human Identity. Virtually every major city in Europe and the United States has its own lesbigay community center, in addition to gay political clubs, legal services, and gay caucuses in most professional associations. Many work to reverse discriminatory statutes, to educate the straight public about gay life, and to provide badly needed services to a changing community, one that is both aging and newly youthful. See the appendix for a list of these groups.

Gay Politics

Gay politics arose out of the Stonewall riots in Greenwich Village in 1969 (see *Gay Liberation*). A number of militant gay liberation organizations were formed soon after the riots. These included the radical Gay Liberation Front, Gay Activists Alliance, and the more moderate National Gay Task Force. They had four clearly defined goals. First, to secure freedom from harassment and arrest for gays who gathered in bars, restaurants, clubs, or on the streets. Second, to repeal all local, state, and federal legislation that criminalized homosexual acts between consenting adults. Third, to end the media's misrepresentation of all gays as effeminate, perverted, child molesting, violent, and murderous. Their final goal was to change the psychiatric profession's diagnosis of gays from mentally ill to normal.

To a greater extent than anyone thought possible, these goals have been met— only partially, true, and only in selected cities and states, and always against a background of unceasing antigay prejudice and antigay activity by right-wing religious and political groups. Even so, in a short time—other groups such as women and African-Americans have been fighting a century or longer for equality—we gays have done well. The freedom of gays to associate is now a constitutional right upheld even where prejudice is strongest. Sodomy laws have been repealed in thirty-seven states, and there is constant lobbying and legislative activity to repeal them in the other thirteen. To be sure, there have been civil rights setbacks, such as Colorado's state referendum in 1999 rejecting equal rights protections for gays and lesbians. But these are atavistic calls to turn back the clock, and they will ultimately fail. Virtually every large city in the country has passed gay rights ordinances. Today even counties and non-urban population centers are eliminating outdated antigay laws. And in southern California, the community of West Hollywood broke away from the surrounding city of Los Angeles to become the first independent city in the United States with a majority of gay and lesbian residents, and with a gay government.

Unfortunately, the Supreme Court in 1986 upheld Georgia's sodomy law, even though a previous Georgia attorney general spoke out against it and asked for its abolition. The case, *Bowers v. Hardwick*, was brought by Bowers, the then attorney general. It involved a local policeman who walked into the bedroom of a gay man's apartment and found its occupant having sex with another man. The occupant, Mr. Hardwick, was arrested on the charge of sodomy. (You can find this decision and other court decisions important to gays on the Lambda Legal Defense Web site — www.lambdalegal.org).

The much publicized murder of Matthew Shepard in a small Wyoming town in 1998, and the murders of other gays and lesbians in the past few years, are a barometer of how much hatred still exists against gays in the country.

Much of the real work of today's gay politics is done behind the scenes, in political party headquarters, in city hall corridors, in statehouse offices, and in legislative committee rooms. It's there that laws are drafted, rules are changed, and politicians are persuaded to make gay rights part of their legislative agenda. Gay politicians are campaigning and winning seats on municipal councils, and being elected to state and federal chambers.

While it has been a struggle, the media have made great strides toward eliminating outright lies, slanders, and misrepresentations of gays in their pages and on the airwaves. An entire new generation of media workers is sensitized to gay images and issues. Of course the media always had their share of gay people, but now these workers are more open about their homosexuality. Hollywood and TV, which once ignored gay issues or presented them only in stereotyped terms, have now taken the lead in presenting gay people in a sympathetic light.

AIDS has been one of the most important issues to gay men for the past twenty years. Gay activists, the Gay Men's Health Crisis, and other AIDS organizations have worked tirelessly to gain access to life-extending drugs, as well as medical, legal, and financial protection, even the protection of wills from antigay relatives (see *Insurance*; *Living Wills*; *Wills*). The effectiveness of their work has been nothing less than astonishing. ACT UP took gay politics back to the militant, radical days of the seventies, participating in scandalous demonstrations that galvanized public attention and, as often, polarized both gay and nongay people.

In the eighties and early nineties, "outing" was one of the most controversial practices. Those who out others do so because they believe the closeted individual, who may be a public figure or leader in government, entertainment, or the arts, has hurt the gay community through his or her hypocrisy and homophobia. Clergy who condemn homosexuality from the pulpit by day, but practice it by night, are a good example. Outing the closeted person reveals this hypocrisy and self-hatred and reduces his ability to do further harm. Many who out public figures stop there, but some go further, outing people who may never have done harm to gays. The reason given to support this kind of outing is that every gay is needed to help the movement, or that every gay must stand up to show our strength and numbers.

Many gays oppose outing, calling it an invasion of privacy and an unnecessary threat to a person's reputation and employment. This is true, although in the United States public figures have limited rights of privacy, and most public figures accept this as a by-product of fame. Gay political leaders prefer that admired gay public figures come out so as to provide good role models to gay youth. Given our homophobic culture, outing is always a risky venture with unpredictable results.

There has been a significant change in the gay rights agenda in the past few years. The civil rights agenda has given way to what has been called the assimilationist agenda. Many gay people are demanding the same "family" rights that straight people have. Gays are insisting on the legal right to marry and to adopt children, to a reaction of sheer fright from heterosexual legislators. Terrified more states may make gay marriage legal, other states have rushed laws through their legislatures making gay marriage illegal.

Growing Older

At the beginning of the new millennium, in the "first world" nations, the fastest-growing population is not newborns, but older people. Thanks to advances in medicine and social care, the mortality rate of adults has dropped incredibly during the past century, and men and women can now expect to reach well into their dotage before death. For many, living into the mideighties and even midnineties is not unheard of, and the centenarians club has grown considerably. We're all getting older, and that includes gay men.

Obviously *where* they live when they reach retirement age influences the mental and physical well-being of gay men. Senior citizens who live in well-organized gay areas tend to live the longest, have the best mental and physical health, and be the most content with their lives. We suspect that the freedom to live an openly gay life contributes to longevity. This was confirmed by studies reported in *The Journal of Gerontology* that found that the following factors affected longevity:

1. How many friends you have.

2. Whether you live with someone.

3. How much contact you have with a former spouse or grown children.

4. Whether you're out to your support group.

Internalized homophobia and low self-esteem are among the surest signs of a troubled and unhealthy life. Alcoholism, depression, and suicidal tendencies are the most extreme manifestations of homophobia among senior gays as well as among younger ones—to no one's real surprise (see *Homophobia*).

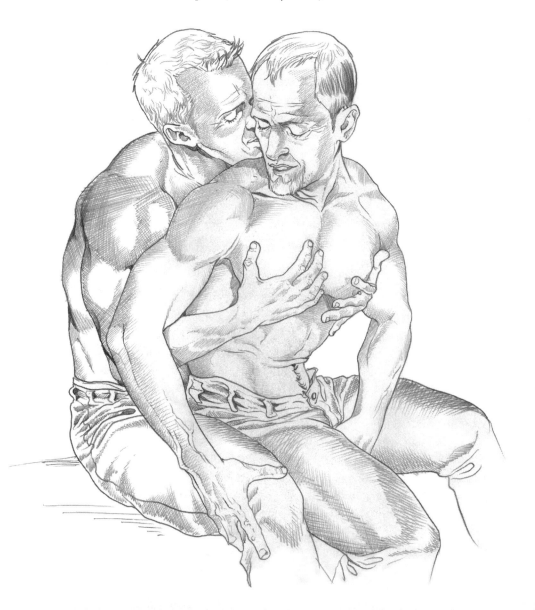

What was surprising in the research findings was how widely and deeply most older gay men constructed their support systems. The average network for gay men stretched from six to ten people, compared to half that size for heterosexual seniors. These included partners, old lovers, previous spouses, children, siblings, parents, and many younger people. Another surprising fact is that the average age of most people in the support system is ten years younger. Being "young at heart" seems to help you lead a rich life later on, too.

For many gay men, sex and romance *can* begin at sixty. Or at retirement. Many older gays alive today were closeted or married for much of their lives. Some waited until their children were married before divorce or separation; others waited until their wives died before coming out. For them, gay life is new and exciting.

At the same time, scores of gay partnerships have survived the AIDS epidemic. These older gay couples lead fulfilling lives, both emotionally and sexually. In fact, many older gays have found that despite some losses in their sexual abilities with increased age, in other ways their sex is better. Over time, and with repetition, sexual skills usually get better, and many older gay men are sought after for their technique and for their interest in satisfying their partners.

Among the biggest problems facing older gay men is finding sex partners. If you are over fifty and single for whatever reason—your partner died, you were too busy with your career to find a lover, you were married and raising a family—it can be difficult to find companionship. Companionship, rather than sex, may turn out to be your goal at this time anyway. A friend or sex buddy or sometime trick may satisfy your sexual needs; but finding someone you can have dinner with regularly, talk with on the phone often, or go to the movies with weekly may be what you need even more. As we get older, we tend to routinize our lives. Spending all morning in bed playing with a lover may not be as satisfying at seventy as doing exercises, reading the paper, talking to pals by e-mail, and working in the garden.

Other problems in growing old when you're gay include age discrimination, both in the straight and the gay world. Our society doesn't value maturity as, for instance, many Asian or European societies do. Instead our young people are taught to be vain about their youth and young bodies, and phobic about wrinkles. From a sociological point of view, an increasing generation gap exists among gay men (greater than among lesbians), and in the United States it is almost entirely a result of the loss of gay men due to the AIDS epidemic (see *HIV Disease*). In the past, going to a gay bar or gay party meant being in the midst of several generations of gay men. Younger gays came to rely upon older ones for information, financial and social aid, and advice to advance their careers. Often there was dating across generations, so that twenty-year-olds dated thirty-year-olds, some of whom dated forty-year-olds, some of whom dated sixty-year-olds. In the past, the gay community gained considerable strength from all of its generations working together, but today many gay bars and clubs admit to playing earsplitting music specifically to keep senior gays out. Older gay men who go into bars, clubs, and restaurants frequented by younger gay men report being ignored by bartenders and waiters. Those few places where senior gays do gather are given derogatory names like Dragonwyck and Jurassic Park by younger gays. It's not known how much age discrimination takes place in gay-owned businesses and housing, although studies are under way to find out.

Other problems faced by older gay men concern the inevitable decline in health. A multitude of diseases gain entrance to our bodies, and as the years pass, concern over disease and its treatment absorbs more and more of our time. Age (and disease) also take their effect on our sexual abilities (see *Impotence*; *Problems of Ejaculation*). We can't get it up as often (or as hard), can't come many times in a week, but most of all, don't feel as driven sexually as we did when we were young. The last is not necessarily a liability. Most senior gay men make better choices in sex mates than they did during their young years when any hole (or dick) would do. Sexual contact takes on a balanced tone, mixing friendly social contact with sexuality. There's always Viagra to help in the physical department (see *Drugs and Sex*).

However, the Internet has become a haven for young and old wishing to meet, whether in chat rooms or via bulletin boards.

Another upside are membership organizations devoted to the needs of older gay people. Organized in 1976, Senior Action in a Gay Environment (SAGE) in New York City is now America's oldest and largest organization for senior gay people. While there's no required minimum age, most members (male and female) are over fifty. SAGE also has affiliates in at least a dozen cities in the country. Call them for information about an affiliate in your state (212-741-2247), or check out their Web site (www.sageusa.org). SAGE's activities are vast. Clinical services include individual and group therapy, and a Friendly Visitor program for homebound elderly gays. Their educational and advocacy programs include an annual national conference and liaison with other senior-citizen organizations, such as AARP, and fighting against age discrimination. They've just begun a community organization program in which they go out into the community to provide local activities and meetings in New York City. SAGE has become the model of how to provide advocacy and needed services to gay seniors.

As influential in California is the Coachella Desert area club known as Prime Timers, a large social group for senior gay men. Its membership commands considerable local economic and political power, and invitations to its parties are among the most sought after in the area.

The first retirement communities specifically built for gays and lesbians have opened, one in the Midwest, one in Palm Springs, California, another in Florida. If the current trend of gay age segregation continues, we can envision that senior gays will live in closed communities where people under fifty-five years old aren't allowed and will tend to their own concerns with their substantial experience and income, ignoring the problems of younger gay men; while younger gays will have no one to help them get through the often difficult middle years before they reach retirement age. It's a situation that needs addressing on a national scale.

If you are a older gay or about to be one, don't get caught in any of the traps of how you *ought* to live your senior gay life, whom you can date, and how much fun and satisfaction you can get out of life. For many older gays with some financial stability, new hobbies, vocations, volunteer work, and especially travel can become important and fulfilling activities. For others, a daily "mall walk" or trail hike and weekly bridge game is enough. You've earned your free time—enjoy it.

Guilt

Guilt is a deep and persistent problem for homosexuals, and overcoming it is a long but fulfilling and liberating experience. Like the devil, as described by the Puritans, guilt insinuates itself into the most private corners of the heart and comes dressed in many clever disguises. Most of us feel that we are far too intelligent and sophisticated to be plagued by anything as old-fashioned as guilt. But it's precisely the intelligent, sophisticated person who has the most difficulty in clearly labeling the guilt that haunts so much of his behavior.

Some gay men so disapprove of their own homosexuality that they hate themselves not just for what they do but also for who they are. Often this sense of guilt is not experienced directly but masquerades as chronic depression. A person suffering from profound guilt believes he should be punished for . . . well, not for his wrongdoing but for his wrong-being. Accordingly, he does nothing to stand up for his civil rights (see *Depression*). Extreme forms of guilt can become so incapacitating that they lead to suicide attempts (see *Suicide*).

Many gay men, however, from time to time suffer from less severe forms of guilt. They feel guilty not for being, but for doing specifically "bad" things, which can range from cheating on a lover to experimenting with S/M and liking it. Or they may feel guilty about being gay—but only intermittently, when they read a condemnation of homosexuality in the press or when their parents look hurt and disappointed.

Guilt may be either conscious or unconscious, the latter being particularly hard to root out. It can manifest itself in excessive cleanliness, in excessive politeness, in a compulsion to work too hard. Unhappily, many gay men who suffer from internalized homophobia transfer their feelings of guilt to other gays and despise them as a substitute for hating themselves. Your guilty feelings may also be motivated by a desire to please your parents (see *Homophobia*; *Parents*).

Analyzing your guilt feelings, you may learn that lying just below your guilt about being gay is a more general guilt about sex of any sort. Some children are brought up in families where sex is bad, no matter what form it takes. The relationship between the parents is so poor that it leaves children with a sense of despair about all love relationships (see *Sex Phobia*).

Guilt manifests itself in other aspects of gay life—endless cruising, inability to succeed in business, romantic fascination with straight men, an exclusive taste for quickie sex, or a penchant for "hopeless" love affairs with unavailable partners (see *Sex with Straight Men*). Guilt breeds a fear of intimacy and the self-contempt and longing for punishment that underlie so many of these behaviors. A more elusive expression of guilt is a desire to do endless favors for other people, to woo them in hundreds of little daily acts, to be a professional nice guy (see *Pleasure Trap*). This compulsion to please, usually linked to an inability to say no, often arises from the need to demonstrate that one is likable in spite of the terrible fact of one's being homosexual. Self-contempt endows the individual with an inexhaustible trust fund of guilt that can be drawn upon by anyone and on any occasion.

How can you overcome your guilty feelings about being gay? We suggest participating in gay organizations. The more conservative-minded person might work as a volunteer in an AIDS service organization or join a gay athletic group such as Front Runners in New York City. Being part of a group will help you develop greater self-esteem and allow you to socialize. By joining civil rights organizations, you can actively fight against the institutions that are to blame for your guilt (see *Civil Rights*; *Gay Liberation*). When a person is isolated from the gay community, he has a much reduced chance of dealing with his guilt feelings.

Gyms

Given the great emphasis Americans place on health and fitness, and the increasing pressure upon younger men to conform to more muscular and masculine body images, gyms have become increasingly popular. In fact, gyms have become to our time what bars and clubs were in previous decades: a basic, central location where gay men can meet and socialize. While gyms aren't necessarily sexual hangouts, they certainly can be, especially in showers, steamrooms, and saunas.

Before the 1970s, most gyms were straight-owned and straight-operated, functional spaces with wall-to-wall carpeting, low ceilings, and walls of mirrors. As a rule, they were located in urban downtowns or within ethnic middle-class enclaves and catered to off-duty policemen, firemen, the occasional boxer, and a few die-hard bodybuilders. During the 1970s, especially following the success of the film *Pumping Iron*, which introduced Arnold Schwarzenegger to the public, bodybuilding became more respectable. The most famous straight gyms were the Mid-City, in Manhattan, and Gold's Gym, in Venice Beach ("Muscle Beach"), California. Gold's subsequently opened branches all over the country.

By contrast, the earliest known gay gyms were small and attached to private homes or businesses in resorts such as Fire Island Pines, Fort Lauderdale, and Laguna Beach. Spots such as Merrill's and the slightly more public Botel Gym at the Pines became crowded social gathering places on Saturday afternoons. Before every sizable party, some men pumped up to maximum visual effect. Naturally, that was in the PNE, Pre-Nautilus Era. Movable weights, not solid machines, formed the full selection of equipment, and it wasn't unusual to see someone step off the Sayville ferry at Fire Island with luggage consisting entirely of a ton of dumbbells, barbells, weights, and a small paper bag containing a fresh T-shirt and a Speedo.

Nowadays, with a minimum of one gym per gay neighborhood, you can find guys working out to get or keep in shape, or merely to socialize, see, and be seen, or to catch up on the latest gossip, while trying to achieve that elusive "muscle queen" or "gym bunny" perfect look. On weekend afternoons the clientele can be as hurried and impolite as a rush-hour crowd on the Hollywood Freeway or the Lexington Avenue subway line as members angle to get at those Nautilus machines, which promise lats and deltoids to die for.

While most men rely only on physical exercise to increase the size of their muscles, others look to augment or shortcut the tedious process by using health supplements. Most gyms and health food stores offer a full range of supplements that are both safe and legal, from protein shakes to performance-enhancing soft drinks, to creatine. While these are mostly considered safe, the jury is still out pending further testing, and you should exercise caution. On the other hand, anabolic steroids are also sought out by gay men. These steroids are illegal in amateur and professional sports for several good reasons. The main effect of steroids, which are androgens (male hormones), is to increase body bulk. In high doses, they may cause high blood pressure and bring on and exacerbate liver damage, and they have been implicated in testicular cancer and some melanomas. They also shrink the testicles. This occurs because the testes don't need to produce androgens after they are artificially introduced into the body. So, if you find yourself in bed with a man with big tits and small balls, you've taken home a steroid user. Tell him that the practice is medically unsound.

Naturally, many gays not only prefer a more natural look but also argue that gyms exacerbate the problem of gay men tending to look like one another in order to attract those similar, not opposite. Are gay men really afraid of looking too different? Or have they been browbeaten by what writer Michelangelo Signorile has called the "body fascism" of gay magazines and movies (see *Body Image*).

Hair

Who can forget the long, overcombed, oiled hair of young men in the 1950s with their DA (duck's ass) backs and single falling curl over the forehead, iconized by singers like Elvis Presley and the Everly Brothers? Or, the flat-top crew cut, with every bristle stiffened by hair gel? In the 1960s the hippie look provided men with hair galore, from stylish pageboys to powder-puff Afros, with everything in between. In the 1970s that look was shortened and cleaned up somewhat, and men's hair most often resembled those sitters in paintings from the Middle Ages through the Renaissance. Mustaches and beards were common, complex, and lavish.

We are not living in an epoch where men's hair is especially erotic or eroticized. And—with the exception of the goatee—facial hair, too, seems to have become passé in the last few decades.

Of course, short hair has its charms as well, for though a buzz cut makes you look like a clipped cadet, to a lover it feels like a luxurious sable brush as you burrow your head in his armpit or crotch. And baldness is a forceful, masculine feature, especially to those who think it results from an excess of male hormones. Virtually every hairstyle can have its own erotic appeal, at least when viewed from a distance. Up close, however, hair bristle with excessive gel or mousse can be unappetizing. If you've lost your hair, polish your dome and let it catch every light. If you can't bear to be bald, then have those expensive and painful transplants. Please don't wear a toupee or comb long strands across your barren desert—you're fooling no one.

Body hair also has its admirers. Some men have plenty of it (see *Bears*). A sure sign of a heavy pelt of fur is a tuft of hair showing at the collar or on the wrist.

Nothing is more versatile than hair. A full beard lends a saturnine (even satanic) look to the face, especially if the beard is precisely trimmed. Shaggier beards run the gamut from looking windswept and philosophical (old hermit in a mountain cave) to seeming robust and outdoorsy (lumberjack in town for a day to raise some hell). A droopy mustache can be poetic and deepen the eyes to spiritual pools; a neater, sharper mustache can turn you into an Edwardian roué. Some men insist upon a mustache on their partner; others recoil from facial hair as being unhygienic. Older men especially find that as their facial features soften with age, by adding a mustache or beard, they can become remasculinized (see *Growing Older*). Gray-haired gays often discover new life (and new dating partners) once they've put on a new mustache or beard.

In a perfect world you should be free to experiment to find what style you like best and how you may attract a new class of admirers. Playing around with your facial hair is the main way you can modify the image you project. A pretty boy bored with a world of doting daddies who consider him cute can transform himself into a tough punk by growing his beard for three days, cutting his long locks, or shaving his head almost to the skin. A middle-aged hunk with a beard, a bald head, and a leather jacket, weary of having tricks ask him to piss on them or burn their chest, can attract respectable types by shaving and dressing in a jacket and tie (see *Shaving; Types*). While this would seem to be ideal, the current reality is far more boring and predictable.

Hands

Since the hands are our most sensitive nongenital equipment, precisely coordinated and packed with nerve endings, they can be used to perform the most delicate work. They can be feathery, making just noticeable contact with the down on another man's body—especially the tiny hairs above the tailbone, along the nape, around the nipples, on the insides of his thighs, and on his balls. To

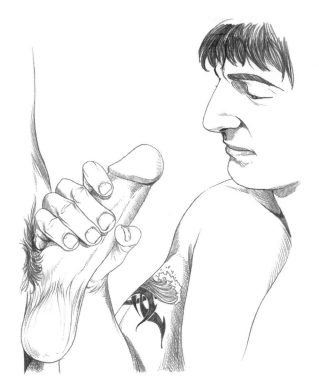

appreciate the pleasure hands can provide, lie beside your partner and kiss him, but don't let any other parts of your bodies come into contact. As he becomes more excited, trail your fingertips over the sensitive flesh of his stomach. Pull back more from the kiss and lightly trace the outlines of his mouth with your finger. Explore the inside of his mouth with your fingers, especially the front of the gums and the roof. Reach down and slowly trigger the hair on his balls. Wet your hands with your saliva and draw two lines on his stomach beside his penis (without touching it). Then graze his cock with your hand.

Hands can also stimulate other parts of his body, playing with his asshole, stroking his thighs and the backs of his legs, rubbing the bottoms of his feet, or pinching his nipples. Remember, as your partner becomes more excited, he can tolerate and will enjoy slightly rougher touching. When he gets sweaty and comes close to a climax, stop for a breather. As he calms down, blow a cooling stream of air over his sweaty body and follow this jet trail with light motions of your fingertips. While you're sucking him, you can stick a finger up his butt to give him an extra sensation he will find exquisite. (He'll have a stronger climax, too.) Or you can reach under and grab his balls while he's fucking you; some guys like their balls to be pulled hard. In rough sex, hands can make a vital contribution. You can pin your partner's wrists to the mattress as you fuck his face. You can squeeze his tits hard or slap his ass. And when all is done, you two can just lie there, exhausted, bodies too sore or overstimulated to touch, with hands intertwined.

From the moment you first connect and your hands meet and begin to know each other at a bar, on a beach, or across a candlelit table, to the end of lovemaking, hands communicate and elaborate the language of love (see *Touching and Holding*).

HIV Disease

Before 1995, AIDS (acquired immune deficiency syndrome) was the number one killer of gay men (especially young men) in America. Today the virus continues to kill gay men, albeit at a lower rate than before. In third world countries it promises to exterminate huge numbers of people who are too poor to afford the expensive regimen of drugs required to keep the virus at bay. Intravenous drug users now constitute the largest number of new infections in the United States.

Many of the young gay men coming out today seem to be unaware of the incapacitating illnesses and drawn-out deaths of gay men from the early 1980s until 1995. Watching friends and lovers waste away to skin and bones is just not in their experience, as it is for gay men of an older generation.

In those days, one could search the horizon of the AIDS landscape and see nothing there, no treatment whose efficacy was assured. Infected men went biweekly to their physician's office to sit before a vaporizing machine and inhale aerosol pentamidine, the contemporary prophylaxis for PCP (Pneumocystis carinii pneumonia), much as the elderly go to health spas to inhale gases from the ground to cure real or imaginary diseases. It was considered a medical advance when HIV-positive men could buy their own aerosol machines and breathe pentamidine at home. Some men sarcastically called it "getting pasteurized."

The darkness of the landscape, medicine's ineffective treatments, and the hysteria and fear in the gay community laid down the perfect soil for charlatans, who emerged from the mud to prey upon men desperate to buy strange concoctions that offered no relief. The authors know far too many men who volunteered for bizarre treatments, such as the friend who went to Russia to be treated by "electromagnetic energy" captured from the earth by a doctor who also claimed to have found a cure for cancer. The friend died soon thereafter.

Everything changed in 1995 with the advent of HAART, or highly active anti-retrovirus therapy, which has changed the AIDS landscape from a sentence of death to one of hope. Most gay people just call it the cocktail. Today, newly diagnosed gay men are usually given this cocktail, a combination of three or more different antiviral drugs. The gay community has watched this metamorphosis with wonder. After taking the cocktail, men whose flesh had evaporated, leaving behind a skin-covered skeleton, suddenly gained weight and muscle mass. Hollowed eye cavities filled out, and cheeks regained the rosier color lost years before. Energy surged through their bodies like electricity waking up a set of simple dormant pleasures, such as eating out or going to the movies or the gym. Their testicles swelled with hormones as lust reawakened from its long-term hibernation. It was, and is, a picture of a body rejuvenated, alive once again—a person who, for the first time in years, thinks about the future, instead of planning his memorial service or struggling to find the courage to end his life.

But HAART is not a cure. For many people infected with the HIV, the cocktail provides longer life, but at the cost of being ill some or much of the time because of the toxicity of the drugs. Some recent research also informs us that some people are already resistant to antiviral drugs. Fortunately, tests can identify the resistance so that the person can be switched to other, effective drugs.

The following pages represent the minimum you should know about HIV disease. There are books and newsletters written to help you understand the disease and your part in either containing or spreading it. Web sites like gayhealth, GMHC, the CDC, and Johns Hopkins are particularly useful sources of information about new research in the diagnosis and treatment of the disease. But as we have made clear in this book, where your head is at is even more important than the information you have in it. Information serves no purpose if you don't think you have to be careful. Since research and treatment are progressing rapidly, some information contained herein may become out-of-date. It is your responsibility to keep abreast.

What Causes AIDS?

HIV stands for "human immunodeficiency virus." Medical authorities have proven that this virus or a group of closely related viruses causes the disease, and that this HIV is transmitted mainly by blood and semen. Some strains of the virus are more virulent (aggressive) than others, and this is called the virus factor. But three "host factors" are also important. Some of us have a genetic makeup that slows down (or speeds up) reproduction of the virus. Concurrent illnesses are a second host factor. They include sexually transmitted diseases, e.g., herpes simplex virus and syphilis (see *Sexually Transmitted Diseases*). Getting infected by the virus while suffering from these diseases accelerates growth of the disease. Finally, malnutrition makes you more susceptible to other infections that lower the effectiveness of your immune system, allowing the virus to reproduce even more quickly.

No one knows with certainty how the HIV originated, or where. Some people believe it is a new disease, while others believe that it remained confined to one geographically inaccessible area until modern transportation gave it the opportunity to spread.

How Is It Transmitted?

Intravenous drug users are at greatest risk because they both share needles that contain the virus and have poor general health. Bottoms who get fucked are in the next category of risk, followed by tops who fuck (see *Bottom; Top*). Participating in blow jobs is relatively low (but not no) risk (see *Blow Job*). Deep kissing has never been implicated in transmitting the virus (see *Kissing*). Kinky sex and even fisting are not implicated unless blood is drawn and there is no barrier (such as a condom) to prevent transmission of the virus (see *Kinky Sex; Sleazy Sex; Fisting*). Rimming, although a route for many STDs, is not implicated in HIV (see *Rimming*). The number of sex partners you have *is* highly correlated with becoming HIV-positive. That makes sense and is confirmed by virtually every research study. Finally, the use of alcohol and drugs is a significant risk factor since you are more likely to have unprotected sex when you're high (see *Drugs and Sex; Booze and Highs; Drug Abuse*).

It is impossible to know for sure the HIV status of every man you have sex with. In many cases, your lover or sex partner may be infected and not even know it. Virtually all gay and AIDS groups recommend that you assume that your sex partner is positive (and if he has any brains in his head, he'll assume the same about you) and that you act accordingly, which means having safe sex (see *Safe Sex*). When fucking, condoms are absolutely required (see *Condoms*). Some medical authorities also recommend a condom when giving a blow job. Advocates of barebacking, or fucking without a condom, are only keeping the epidemic alive (see *Barebacking; Saying No*). It is nothing less than self-destructive behavior.

Should I Be Tested?

Only nuns and other celibates don't need to be tested. Assuming you are not professionally celibate, and your sexual activities go beyond mutual masturbation, you should be tested regularly. How often you are tested depends upon how many sex partners you have and what you do sexually. Bottoms should be tested regularly, especially if they get fucked often, but tops should also be tested periodically. However, counseling should be included in the testing so you can be aided both medically and emotionally should your test turn out positive. Also, the very act of getting tested can be upsetting to some people.

The first test is merely to establish whether there are HIV antibodies in your blood. If there are, then you have HIV disease—but not AIDS. Your doctor will then probably do at least two other tests. The first is to check for *viral load*. That is a measure of how much of the virus is circulating in your body. The higher your viral load, the more rapidly the disease will progress. If your viral load goes over 55,000, your doctor may recommend HAART. The goal of HAART is to end up having undetectable viral loads. The second test is to measure your *CD4 helper cells* (also called T cells). The CD4 is one type of white blood cell necessary to fight infections. It gives a snapshot of how well your immune system is doing in fighting disease. A normal T-cell count runs anywhere from 600 to over 1000. However, the count can temporarily go down whenever you are ill or fighting off a bug of some kind, and it may also vary widely during the day. Even the common cold can temporarily affect T cells. It's therefore best to get T-cell testing when you are well rather than acutely ill. As the number of CD4 cells declines, the risk of getting sick increases. HAART is often started when the CD4 cells decline to less than 350. If the CD4 measure gets below 200 (or you get an opportunistic infection), you will be diagnosed with AIDS.

If you've read the last paragraph carefully, you'll understand that there is an inverse relationship between viral load and CD4 helper cells. The higher your viral load, the lower your CD4 helper cells.

The question of how often you should be tested remains one only you and your doctor can answer. Naturally, if you believe that you have symptoms of the disease, or if any of your sex partners have developed the illness, you should be tested. It's been suggested you be tested within three months after you've been exposed to the virus. By that time, your body will have had enough time to develop antibodies. But wait for at least one month, as difficult as that may be. The actual test results are usually available within a day or two.

What Happens to This Information?

The answer to this question depends upon state law. We'll use New York State as an example. By law, everyone who tests positive must be reported by name and birth date to the Department of Health. It's similar to the law about reporting venereal disease. However, there are laws to protect the confidentiality of this information, and while the state is supposed to inform your sex partners of your infection, this provision of the law is not enforced. Counting HIV infections is required for epidemiological purposes; states receive funds from the Ryan White legislation based upon infection rates. There is no evidence that the confidentiality of this list has been broken. Employers and insurance companies, for instance, cannot gain access to it. But remember, if you sign a medical release for your health-care insurance company that goes to your doctor, you've given up your right to confidentiality and he can release any and all of your records to the insurance company.

Many municipalities provide anonymous testing through local clinics. Gay and AIDS service organizations usually have a list of these sites. They will not report your name (since they don't have it) to the Department of Health. But if you test positive, you will need treatment, and your doctor is required to report it to the Department of Health.

What's the Difference between HIV Disease and AIDS?

The diagnosis of HIV disease means only that you are infected with the virus, while a diagnosis of AIDS means that your T cells have declined to less than 200 or you have developed an AIDS-associated opportunistic infection. In other words, a diagnosis of AIDS usually means your immune system is significantly damaged. In the "old days," virtually everyone who was seropositive moved on to one or more "opportunistic" illnesses, and eventually to death. The progress might take years, with repeated hospitalizations. Nowadays HAART is usually so effective in curbing the HIV that few HIV-positive men suffer from opportunistic illnesses. The only exception is gay men who were already ill at the time they began HAART treatment. But even these men, although occasionally subject to various opportunistic infections, manage to enjoy functional lives. Without HAART, they would likely be dead.

What Were the Opportunistic Illnesses in AIDS Patients?

Before HAART, a number of opportunistic illnesses led up to a diagnosis of AIDS and continued for years. Death from AIDS was marked by the appearance of one opportunistic illness after another.

It would start with swollen (but not painful) lymph nodes and severe night sweats that soaked your sheets. Thrush, a yeast infection (like women get in the vagina), would appear in your mouth and eventually move down your throat. Hairy leukoplakia, raised discolorations, appeared under your tongue, making eating difficult. Shingles, a herpes-type virus, caused a painful blistering on your legs or back. Other symptoms were a dermatitis (scaly rash) on your eyebrows, scalp, and sides of your nose, and unexplained weight loss and fevers—which gave HIV the name "slim disease" in Africa.

The major opportunistic diseases caused by a suppressed immune system were awesome. They included PCP (Pneumocystis carinii pneumonia), which was the major cause of death in AIDS patients, and KS (Kaposi's sarcoma), deep brown, purple, or black-colored cancerous spots that covered the body and internal organs. Other major illnesses that led to death were toxoplasmosis (a protozoan infection of the brain), cryptococcal meningitis (an infection of the membranes that cover the spinal cord), and dementia (deterioration of the brain), one of the late signs of the disease.

Who's Getting Infected with HIV Today?

We have a good deal of consistent research about gay men and infection. There is no question that the younger you are, the more you're at risk. For the past decade, newly diagnosed gay men have been overwhelmingly younger, and therefore, less experienced both sexually and in life in general than older gay men. Younger gays have considerably more sexual partners and are more likely to fuck without a condom, proving the truth of the Yiddish proverb "When the penis is hard, the brains are soft."

All of the above is obvious, but there is another reason why young gay men head the list of the newly diagnosed. Doctors are certain that most men who become infected with the virus get it from other men *who are only recently infected themselves*. In the first few weeks after infection, the viral load is sky-high. That's because the body hasn't had time to recognize and fight the HIV. After it does, the viral load takes a nosedive (but will go up again if not treated). So in that short period, the likelihood of transmission is that much greater because you are carrying an unusually large quantity of HIV.

This is one of the most important reasons why the epidemic of HIV disease stays alive. If we add to it alcohol and drugs leading to unsafe sex, we end up with a nasty epidemiological problem. Several books have addressed these problems, among them *Sexual Ecology* by Gabriel Rotello, and *Life Outside* by Michelangelo Signorile.

Why Is HAART More Effective for Some Men Than Others?

Gay men who were infected with the virus ten or more years ago may still suffer from one or more opportunistic illnesses. They may also have more trouble tolerating some antiviral medications. It's not unusual for these men to suffer from frequent diarrhea, debilitating headaches, and other complaints. Their doctors are usually able to switch them to other effective antivirals, which may have fewer side effects. At last count, about twenty drugs were approved by the FDA. There is a sound principle here: *It's easier to keep a healthy person well than to cure a sick person.*

The medical term *adherence* is also one of the factors that influence the effectiveness of HAART. This means sticking faithfully to the time schedule for taking your medication. If you miss more than one out of twenty doses of your antiviral cocktail, your body may become resistant to the antiviral therapy, making HAART much less effective. The mentally ill, significantly depressed men, and those who are alcoholic and/or drug abusers are at greater risk for missing doses, and therefore screwing up their treatment.

Ninety percent of diagnosed men who adhere to drug therapy do extraordinarily well. The other 10 percent usually do better when they are switched to a different cocktail. The often-reported debilitating side effects of the cocktail are less common for most newly diagnosed men, although your doctor may need time to fine-tune your meds. Until he finds the right antiviral, you may experience a number of minor, but uncomfortable, problems.

Because of HAART, the death rate from AIDS in the United States has declined by 95 percent, but that means a small number of men have *not* been helped. Fortunately, more antiretroviral medications are being tested and may become suitable for these men.

When Will Vaccines Be Available?

Two kinds of HIV vaccines are being tested. The first is a therapeutic vaccine meant to slow the progression of the disease for those already infected. When available, it will probably cut down on, not eliminate, the need for HAART. The second vaccine is the traditional kind, using a dead virus meant to create immunity in uninfected people. Estimates are that both vaccines will be available within a decade. Even then, the long-term effects of the vaccines remain unknown. It's best to keep track of them via gay Internet sites and the gay media.

Herpes Viruses and HIV Disease

Herpes is a family of viruses that cause a number of illnesses from cold sores (herpes simplex) to shingles (herpes zoster). The herpes virus group also includes cytomegalovirus (CMV) and Epstein-Barr virus (EBV). None of these causes HIV disease. However, if you have the HIV, any dormant herpes viruses already in your body may be activated, and CMV and EBV may break out, weakening an already compromised immune system. The symptoms are variable; there may be none, or the infected person may suffer flulike illnesses. Of course, not everyone has been exposed to the different herpes viruses, and therefore not everyone with HIV disease will have complications because of them. Herpes-type viruses are usually easy to diagnose, and a variety of treatments are available.

In addition to herpes, a number of common illnesses become harder to treat in the presence of HIV disease, such as cryptosporidosis and venereal warts. But the most important of those is syphilis. This is yet another reason to practice safe sex (see *Sexually Transmitted Diseases*).

What Are the Social Consequences of HIV Disease?

All HIV-positive men will inevitably face the question of whom to tell about their HIV status. Each gay man must decide whether to tell his family, friends, former lovers, and tricks. Telling each of them presents different problems. For instance, you may not yet be out to your parents (see *Coming Out; Parents*). Or, you may be afraid of an excessive concern by your friends. But what seems to worry gay men most is how to handle the situation when tricking or dating.

When tricking, most gay men believe that divulging one's HIV status is unnecessary as long as you *always* follow safe sex guidelines. That's the easy answer.

More difficult is how to handle the situation if you've begun dating someone. The inevitable question is *when* to tell him. The obvious fear is that your potential lover may flee for fear of contracting the disease himself. Unfortunately this happens all too often—many men just aren't mature enough to handle their fear. But if there is to be any future in your relationship, you cannot keep the secret for long, even if you are rigorously safe in your sex together. Your lover will feel that you lied to or betrayed him, and that can create a deep crevasse in the development of trust between you. "If I can't trust you about this," he'll think, "how can I trust you about anything?"

The longer you put off telling him your HIV status, the more difficult it will become to have the conversation. Our advice is to have the discussion sooner rather than later. If he's going to dump you, it's probably better to find out now, instead of after months of dating.

Coming clean about your HIV status is a first step, but even the healthiest of relationships can be strained when one lover is positive and the other negative (see *Mixed HIV Couples*).

A great deal of potential psychological molasses can be produced in this situation. Sex can often become baffling because each lover is trying to be supportive, but the conflicting feelings of fear and responsibility contaminate the air. Couple counseling may be necessary to help the couple talk about their fears.

.   .   .

Homophobia

Why have homosexuals been persecuted and despised for centuries? What is the basis of homophobia (the fear of homosexuality)? On the most obvious, surface level, a major explanation is that the dominant Western religions, Christianity, Judaism, and Islam, have condemned homosexuality and those who practice it. For centuries gay people have been persecuted and sometimes executed for practicing their love. The Catholic Church and fundamentalist Protestant groups have been aggressive and self-righteous, and until recently no one would stand up against them on the issue of homophobia. While this is slowly changing in our society, the effect of such teaching within towns, schools, and families often remains intemperate. More than one gay Christian, Jewish, Muslim, or Mormon child has been irrevocably drummed out of his home and school because of unyielding religious beliefs. Evidently, other beliefs about love and tolerance, which make those religions otherwise attractive, are not efficacious enough to counterbalance the intolerance. It is equally evident that in parts of the world where religions hold sway that do not condemn homosexuality—Buddhism, Shintoism, Taoism, Hinduism—bigotry is by no means as overwhelming or as lethal to gays, although it does still exist to some extent.

There are several theories as to why these religious theories have taken hold so strongly among people who may not otherwise be very religious. One belief is that society is sexually repressed and that homophobia is only one aspect of a more general condemnation of sexuality (see *Sex Phobia*). While most people would agree that Western society is repressive, the theory does not really explain why gays have been singled out with such particular animosity.

Another theory, derived from Freud, holds that we are all born bisexual, with the capacity to respond erotically to members of either sex. The homophobe, according to this theory, is the person who has not come to grips with his own latent homosexuality, who has neither adequately repressed nor accepted it. Instead of hating himself, the homophobe turns his anger against other homosexuals—a classic case of "projection."

A third theory is more recent. Research by social psychologists suggests that homophobia crops up in a society that maintains a strict distinction between male and female roles, especially one that assigns power and high status to men and dependence and low status to women. Gay people are feared and hated because they are perceived to be challenging this distinction, muddying the otherwise pure, clear waters of gender-linked behavior. A gay man who could enjoy all the privileges of masculinity (respect, a good job, legal and economic superiority) is seen as willfully and perversely throwing away these advantages and embracing the lower status of a woman. Conversely, lesbians are seen as wanting to usurp male privileges. All the stereotypes invented by the straight world to punish gay people (the sissy faggot; the mannish lesbian) are designed to protect against a breakdown of gender identity and of the unequal and unfair world of power, status, and wealth that identity represents. We can call this the *gender theory of homophobia*, because it says that homosexuality as a social role, rather than as a sexual practice, is what upsets some straights.

It's ironic that society should define homosexuality as deficient masculinity. History is replete with examples of gay (or bisexual) military leaders who were every bit as capable as straight generals in the supposedly masculine arena of brutality and conquest. Julius Caesar, Alexander the Great, General Gordon of Khartoum, Lawrence of Arabia, and Lord Kitchener all had male lovers or gay experiences.

At one time, gay liberationists were sensitive to questions about the masculinity of gay men. We used to say that gender identity (our feeling of maleness or femaleness) was independent of our sexual identity (being gay or straight). Like the society around us, we didn't want to be identified as deficient men—or to put it another way, be perceived as being like women. Although we didn't know it then, we were still identifying with society's concept of masculinity, and we chastised effeminate gay men for not being masculine enough.

Many gay men feel comfortable that their personalities contain both masculine and feminine components (see *Versatility*). Some gay men feel their feminine side is stronger and go out of their way to nurture it. One also finds androgynous gay men expressing maleness or femaleness according to the occasion. Deprecating any of them is homophobic, whether the put-down comes from another gay man or from someone straight (see *Effeminacy*).

We believe that the gender theory of homophobia outlined above also helps to explain internalized homophobia. The self-hating homosexual hates himself because he feels deficient as a man, and his self-hate is projected upon all other gay men. He can have anonymous sex or admire the masculinity of straight men, but he will be incapable of establishing an intimate relationship because it will mirror his hatred for himself (see *Guilt*).

Self-hating homosexuals are in emotional conflict. Guilt plunges them into what psychologists call an approach-avoidance pattern. As they approach a lover and get to know him, they are happy and hopeful. But once the affair looks as though it might work, they back away and avoid the beloved because intimacy upsets them. As they withdraw, they breathe a sigh of relief, glad to be rid of this latest entanglement, but they are once again alone and miserable. Loneliness drives them to attempt a new affair, with the same disastrous results. These dynamics are seldom expressed at the conscious level of a person's life. Instead, there's always something wrong with a new lover: He's lousy in bed; he's too young or too old; too extroverted or too introverted. But the real reason such a man rejects his lover is self-hate for not being the man his parents (and society) demanded that he be.

What cannot be denied is that, whatever its underlying causes, homophobia is a daily affront to gay men and lesbians and exerts an unseen yet unceasing burden on gay people's actions and behaviors every day. Until homophobia is recognized as the societal disease it is and then eradicated, no homosexual can be fully safe or entirely sane.

Hustlers

Male prostitutes in the gay world are called hustlers. In politically correct circles they're called male sex workers. Some make hustling a full-time profession, while others do it part-time, only on nights and weekends, to supplement their income. Some work the streets and hustler bars; others meet clients through escort services or advertise in gay publications and on the Web. Hustlers hired off the street are potentially the most dangerous, whereas those hired through a service are generally the most reliable (also often the most attractive and expensive). All prostitution—male or female—is, of course, illegal in the United States.

Why do people hire hustlers? Sometimes they're in search of a particularly kinky and hard-to-arrange scene (rubber, or the enactment of a highly detailed fantasy). If the scene is particularly elaborate or off-the-wall, hustlers will charge more. Others hire hustlers because they want a specific type (a small blond with a small cock, say, or a hairy man with a big cock), or they want to perform specific sexual acts (the small-cocked blond must fuck them, say). The point of hustlers is that one can fulfill a fantasy. A tall, masculine-appearing man may have a secret yearning to be thoroughly dominated by someone, but in bars he is typecast as a "stud." By hiring a hustler he escapes others' projections and satisfies his desires. Hustlers are also employed by people too busy or too famous to cruise, as well as by tourists, businessmen at meetings and conventions, and married or bisexual men looking for some excitement. And then there are those johns (as men who hire hustlers are called) who are more turned on by paying for sex than by getting it free.

Many johns strike defensive postures (usually after they come). A john might insult the hustler overtly or covertly; tell him he has never hired a "whore" before; attempt to impress with his superior wealth, intelligence, and connections. Hustlers are familiar with these stratagems. An encounter with a hustler can be pleasurable and civilized if each partner recognizes what can be gained from the experience—and what cannot: The john can forget love and companionship, and the hustler shouldn't expect a lifelong patron or an all-understanding father.

Hustling isn't easy. It takes mental and physical stamina to be able to deliver the sexual goods night after night. Many hustlers, especially those from the streets, are addicted to alcohol and/or drugs (see *Booze and Highs; Drug Abuse*). Others, especially those who begin hustling as young teens, can be left with deep psychological scars: alienation from their own body and distrust of affection. The work can also be physically dangerous.

Gay liberation changed the sales pitch of hustlers. Instead of presenting themselves as straight, most hustlers admit they're gay and do anything (well, almost) the client likes. They are also up-front about hustling as a career. Several recent books about how to hustle professionally have recently been published. A recent witty, practical, and shrewd one written by out hustler Aaron Lawrence is *The Male Escort's Handbook*. After reading it, you'll be able to better calculate if it's the occupation—or avocation—for you. Lawrence and other hustlers also have Web sites. Other self-confessed hustlers seeking celebrity have been nude models for magazines such as *Playgirl, Men,* or *Freshmen,* a fact they'll considerably play up in their newspaper and magazine ads. The benefit there is you may already know (to the quarter inch) exactly what you're getting.

Think twice before hiring a hustler. While most of them are ordinary guys with good looks or extra equipment, who may be oversexed and looking to make a few dollars, a few are angry, desperate, even psychotic; every year gays are robbed, burglarized, scammed, beaten, or killed by hustlers, though the numbers are probably no greater than those for murders occurring as a result of having sex with strangers. As you might expect, some hustlers are HIV-positive or suffering from AIDS, yet won't divulge this information because they need the money. If you must use a hustler, find someone reputable: Hire him through people you know or, better yet, call an escort service. Their business depends upon your safety—and pleasure.

When hiring a hustler, either through a service or directly, in person or by phone, you'll have to discuss the type of man you're looking for, any special fantasy or kinky acts you'd like included, and whether it's "in" (on their turf—usually cheaper) or "out" (they come to you—usually more expensive). Don't be embarrassed to engage in this step, as it is a business transaction to the hustler—a verbal contract, in fact—and should be a business transaction to you, no matter how kinky or fetishistic the activities may end up being.

Many big-city hustlers advertise themselves as masseurs, in the massage column of gay periodicals. Even though they may promise "total release" or "full satisfaction guaranteed," before setting up a date with them it's a good idea to discuss exactly what the masseur will do and what his (ordinarily sliding) rate is for each step along the way. A few may be bargained with. And once at the scene, a masseur who told you on the phone he'd only give you "full manual satisfaction" (a hand job) may end up doing a great deal more for the same amount of money, especially if he's horny or turned on by you.

Some men are aroused by the fantasy of being a hustler and play it out with sex partners. This seems like harmless fun to us. And more than one gay man who thought he was having consensual sex with a stranger awakened the next morning to find a $50 bill in the soap dish or on the bed table. He might ask himself if he acted "like a whore," whatever that may mean. But the truth is usually that as some men must receive money to have gay sex, and thus to assuage their shame, guilt, or other uncomfortable feeling, so others must pay money to have sex with another man, for approximately the same reasons. While it may be guilt money to him, for you it's a meal out or a CD or item of clothing—so enjoy!

Impotence

We men have a special sensitivity about our cocks (see *Cock Size*). How it looks and performs is our measure of being a man, and it's difficult for us to escape that early socialization.

Every man has a problem with impotence from time to time. Perhaps the worst part of the problem is our embarrassment discussing it. We hide it the best we can.

Of course, impotence can't be hidden in the bedroom. When the clothes come off, the failure to raise and maintain a hard-on becomes painfully obvious. That's when men start looking for reasons. They blame alcohol, drugs, something they ate, fatigue, even their partner (see *Booze and Highs; Drug Abuse; Drugs and Sex*). Although there may be truth to some of these explanations, by and large they are excuses employed to alleviate feelings of humiliation. These are examples of situational, not chronic, impotence.

Before you decide you have a problem with impotence, ask yourself a few questions. Does this happen often or only occasionally? If it's the latter, don't worry. Everyone experiences variations in sexual performance, and an isolated bout with an uncooperative dick may mean nothing more than that you weren't really turned on to your partner, that you had too many other things on your mind, or that you're coming down with a cold. Too much alcohol and drug use almost always affects sexual functioning and may also cause temporary impotence.

Repeated episodes of erectile failure are another matter. To begin with, repeated failures increase the tension surrounding sexual activities. "Am I going to get it up?" becomes so anxiety-producing that you may avoid any sexual contact. Humiliation turns to hopelessness.

Psychoanalysis used to be the treatment of choice for impotence because analysts believed that impotence was a psychological problem stemming from unresolved conflicts about one's parents or family. It was usually ineffective.

With the rise of sex therapy in the 1970s, direct behavioral intervention became the preferred treatment. Sex therapists believed erectile dysfunctions developed because of poor habits or attitudes about sex. They (like the analysts before them) claimed that 80 percent of impotence was caused by psychological factors, only 20 percent by physical ones. Sex therapists were no more successful than psychoanalysts.

How does a cock get hard? The brain sends a signal through the nerves that arouse you. Blood rushes into your cock through the penile artery. The blood stays there because veins leading out of the cock shut tight. The fluid pressure created by blood rushing in and not being able to get out makes your dick hard.

Four problems can occur in this process. First, nerve conduction by the brain to the peripheral organs. Your cock doesn't hear the message to get hard. Diabetes is the most frequent culprit. Unfortunately, many physicians don't discuss impotence when diagnosing diabetes because they're uncomfortable talking about sex. Second, arterial deficiencies. Your penile artery or its branches may be clogged with cholesterol and the effects of smoking. Ultrasound tests can measure the ability of these blood vessels to expand and deliver blood. Leaking veins in the cock could be a third possibility. To identify leakage, doctors inject a dye into an artery in your cock and use X rays to check the progress of the dye.

Side effects of medication are a fourth reason for a limp dick. Prozac and other SSRIs are notorious for reducing sexual desire, causing impotence or the inability to come (see *Depression; Problems of Ejaculation*). Changing or stopping use of this medication brings erections back. Blood pressure medications may also be a culprit. Some HIV-positive and AIDS patients have significantly reduced testosterone levels, either as a result of the disease itself or a side effect of medications. It makes thoughts of sex as appetizing as eating bugs. A testosterone patch or gel might help. If you're HIV-positive, speak to your doctor about how to maintain your sexual desire.

Today, our best guess is that 80 percent of impotence has a physical origin, and only 20 percent is psychological. Diagnostic procedures are used to distinguish between physical and psychological problems.

A few hospitals have clinics—usually in their urology department—that take down your sex history, give you a physical, and check your hormone levels. Special tests are administered, using highly sophisticated equipment. You're given a computerized gadget to take home and put around your cock when you go to sleep. It's like a cock ring, and it measures the number of hard-ons you have while you sleep and how rigid your cock gets with each one. This is the best test to distinguish between physical and psychological impotence. If it's a physical problem, you'll have fewer, less rigid erections, and a second test will be performed, a pharmacological screening. A drug injected into the cock produces a roaring hard-on. How long it takes to get hard, how hard it gets, and how long it stays hard gives the doctor a good idea of whether the problem is arterial or venous in character.

In the last few years, there's been a revolution in the treatment of physiologically based impotence. Here are some of the choices:

1. Viagra is the current "wonder drug" for impotence and is being administered across the world in extraordinary quantities, with former U.S. presidential nominees singing its praises. We've discussed the use of Viagra in our entry *Drugs and Sex*, so we won't repeat it here. We will merely mention two dangers: It should not be used with any other drug that lowers blood pressure (it could kill you), and an overdose could bring on priapism, in which the blood in your cock must be drained.

2. The only currently used noninvasive treatment for impotence is a vacuum-restricting device. It's a scientifically designed cock ring; it can help some patients.

3. Of the more invasive treatments, the mildest is self-administered. Just before sex, you inject a prescription drug through the shaft of your cock and into the corpus cavernosum. It produces a hard-on. The greater the quantity you inject, the longer the hard-on lasts. Some men can stay hard for up to ninety minutes. The sexual sensations are normal. Some men get upset with having to inject themselves, but it works. Porn stars use this drug for long photo shoots as well as for keeping hard-ons during those video sessions where they won't necessarily have to produce an orgasm on camera. But for those who are playing around with the drug, it can be quite dangerous. One acquaintance of the authors found himself not only still erect and rock-hard six hours after a photo shoot, but also reddening, swelling, and even running a fever. After repeated ice baths failed to bring down the swelling and fever, mild convulsions began and he had to be rushed to the emergency room.

   If, however, you are using this injectable drug for a bona fide problem, use a bit of imagination. Your urologist will give you specific instructions. Follow them. Perhaps you and your lover can play doctor!

4. Surgical procedures available today are more invasive. Many urologists recommend a prosthesis: a surgical implant inserted into the cock. These have been used for over a decade, with mixed results. The newest consists of a self-contained pump and reservoir. The pump is in the head of the cock; when you squeeze it, fluid is forced into the shaft and produces an erection. The release valve is also in the head of your cock. In another "fully inflatable" design, the pump is placed in your balls and the reservoir of fluid in the abdomen. You get a hard-on by squeezing your balls. Other operations are being developed, such as microsurgeries to tie off leaky veins and to open blocked arteries. But all these procedures are still in early stages of development. Always start your treatment with the least physically invasive procedures, because they are reversible. If an implant doesn't work, you cannot reverse the damage done to your cock by the surgery.

We recommend you have an evaluation and take the "cock ring" test that measures hard-ons during sleep. That will give you a good idea of how much of your problem is physical and how much psychological. If the test shows that the problem is psychological, try therapy with a professional who respects gay sexual life.

If the problem turns out to be physical, don't jump into surgery, no matter what any surgeon says. See other professionals before choosing invasive procedures. Consult with your personal physician. If you can't talk to him or her about sexual problems, get another doctor. You may also need a competent psychotherapist with whom you can discuss your feelings about sex. It's important that your therapist maintain a good working relationship with both your personal physician and the sex clinic. The therapist should be someone to stand by you after surgery and guide your progress.

Counseling, before and after surgery, serves an important function. Some men blame all their social and romantic problems on not being able to get a hard-on. They sometimes fantasize that when they're restored to full sexual functioning, their life will be magically transformed, with idyllic love relationships and marital bliss. But there's no magic in treating sexual dysfunction. Even after surgery, it's hard work establishing and maintaining a love relationship.

Of course all men want to perform well in bed. It's every bit as valid to want to overcome one's impotence so as to enjoy a good fuck as it is to want a long-lasting love relationship. Sometimes sex is about passion. At other times it's lust and excitement we crave. We should be able to function well in either situation.

Insurance

Learning about insurance may seem such a bore, especially for those gay men fortunate enough to be automatically insured by their employer. However, some of us are required to buy our own insurance because our employer doesn't provide it, or because we're self-employed, or because we've been laid off from a job. Gay men who are HIV-positive obviously have special needs and interests in the matter. So what's a bore today could be critically important tomorrow.

There are three kinds of insurance to discuss. The first is medical and dental insurance, which pays doctor and hospital bills; it may also cover office visits, home visits, or surgery. The second type is disability insurance, which pays a monthly stipend if you are temporarily or permanently unable to work. Finally, there is life insurance, which upon your death pays a specified sum of money to your beneficiary.

When you are first applying for any of these policies, most insurance companies ask questions about your past and current health and seek permission to obtain further information from your physician. You may also be required to undergo a medical examination conducted by one of the insurance company's physicians or be asked to take a blood test, which may include a test for HIV.

Insurance companies don't like to insure what they call preexisting conditions. That means any illness or medical condition you suffered from before your application or are still suffering from. Sometimes they will refuse to cover a particular illness altogether. For instance, virtually all insurance companies refuse to insure anyone who tests HIV-positive, while some others will not insure people with cancer or heart disease. Other companies may require a "waiting period," during which you cannot have coverage for a preexisting illness, but after which you will be covered. Furthermore, some insurers won't pay for medicine and treatments that are "experimental" (including needed organ transplants), even if the treatment is the only one that may save your life. If you work for a large employer, the group policy may stipulate that all preexisting conditions will be covered immediately. You really have to read the insurance booklet provided by the employer to see what applies to your case.

People always wonder whether they should lie about their medical history. "How is it their business?" some gay men ask. This is a complicated question for a number of reasons. Obviously, we can't recommend that you lie on insurance forms, since it's against the law. If you lie about your medical condition on the insurance application, then make a claim for a doctor or hospital payments—and the insurer finds out you lied to them—they can claim fraud and refuse to pay. The company may even cancel your insurance. The problem of coverage for preexisting conditions is delicate. You need to have a good relationship with your personal physician and take an active part in your treatment by discussing the medical diagnoses he writes on insurance forms. It's also advisable to seek the counsel of a sympathetic insurance agent who can advise you.

One factor that makes discussing insurance so complicated is the variation in state laws governing such policies. Federal statutes govern some insurance, as well. It's important to search out a local gay or AIDS service organization and inquire about the laws in your state. They can probably recommend insurance agents and/or attorneys who specialize in getting insurance for gay people. Listen to what they have to tell you because the laws controlling insurance change frequently.

A few municipalities have recognized domestic partnerships, cities such as New York, San Francisco, Boston, and West Hollywood. A few states have done the same, such as Vermont, and to a lesser degree Massachusetts, Hawaii, and California. A few private companies have done the same, with Walt Disney–ABC, Microsoft, and IBM leading the way. Employees and their lovers of these municipalities, states, and companies may be provided with some (or all) of the benefits, including insurance, usually provided only to married couples. If you work for a city government, inquire at a gay service organization to see if any benefits are provided for your lover.

Should you have to leave your job because of illness or because you've been laid off, a federal law protects your insurance. It's called COBRA, and it covers all private companies with twenty or more employees. Under this law, and regardless of your medical condition, you can continue your group coverage for up to eighteen months by paying the group rate. If you stopped working because you are legally disabled (say for example, if you have been diagnosed with AIDS), your coverage continues for an additional eleven months, a total of twenty-nine months.

The COBRA law even helps get around the waiting period for preexisting conditions. Let's say you leave one employer to work for another, but the medical insurance of the new employer has a waiting period of one year. You have the option of continuing the COBRA coverage you received through your old employer (which covers the previous medical condition) until the one-year waiting period is up. You then drop the old coverage.

In light of the AIDS epidemic, there are a few facts you should know about life insurance. The company can claim fraud on your application for only two years from the date you applied. Most policies pay for suicide after the policy has been in force for two years, but not before. Many gay men are surprised to learn that you can't necessarily name anyone you want as your beneficiary. This is due to the stuffy, prudish morality of insurance companies. (Unmarried straights can't name their lover as beneficiary, either.) Unless you want to pursue a civil rights case, there's no point in arguing with them or they may refuse to insure you. The usual tactic is to name either a relative or your estate as your life insurance beneficiary, and then, once the policy is in force, to change the beneficiary to a lover or a friend (see *Wills*). In many states, group life insurance can be converted to an individual policy, regardless of your health.

Some entrepreneurs have recently offered "viaticals"—in short, they "buy" the life insurance of AIDS patients, but at a substantial discount. You've probably seen their ads in gay magazines. They argue that this provides money at a time when it is needed. And indeed, when HIV-positive status was a death sentence, this was true, but it is less true today. While viaticals may be attractive as a source of quick cash, you should be very careful about "selling" your life insurance. Getting advice from a lawyer is crucial because you might be required to pay taxes on the proceeds and/or become ineligible for Medicaid or other forms of public assistance available to those with AIDS.

Finally, let's note that many state laws are changing in ways that help the consumer. It is no longer possible for an employer to fire an employee because he's HIV-positive or has AIDS. One can even appeal the rejection of a claim by an insurance company because they contend the treatment is "experimental" or too costly. Your employer's benefit book will explain how to do this. What is important for us gay people is to demand our insurance rights as often and as vocally as possible. This is usually accomplished through pressure on state insurance departments and via state laws. Those who work to lobby for favorable insurance laws have made and continue to make some of the more important advances in gay rights.

Jealousy, Envy, and Possessiveness

Jealousy is as rampant among homosexuals as among heterosexuals. Because homosexuality provides so many more opportunities for quick, concealed sexual adventures, it can be an even worse torture for the jealous gay man. The problem, as Marcel Proust pointed out, is that "jealousy, which wears a bandage over its eyes, is not merely powerless to discover anything in the darkness that enshrouds it, it is also one of those torments where the task must be incessantly repeated."

Proust's novel *In Search of Lost Time* can be said to be a three-thousand-page dissection of this most destructive of all passions. Proust suggests that not only can jealousy never discover the truth about infidelity but it can never be brought to a conclusion.

Jealousy is such an overwhelming emotion that it seems to be both natural and ineradicable. The truth is different. Jealousy is a learned emotion, often patterned after that of one's parents, and it exists in some societies far more violently than in others. Since it is a learned response, it can also be unlearned. Jealousy is often based on the belief that sex is the sole foundation of love. The jealous lover feels his only hold over his partner is erotic, and once his physical hold is broken, his lover will leave him. In other words, jealousy is a mask for your fear that your lover will abandon you (see *Fidelity and Monogamy*).

In other cases, jealousy is a "projection" of one's guilt about one's own lapses. A jealous man may have sex on the sly with dozens of other men, but each time he "cheats," he will redouble his interrogation and suspicion of his lover. The fact is, he cannot face his own adventures; instead he attributes his own philandering to his lover, who may be quite faithful. In today's world, one finds this jealous lover checking the e-mails on his boyfriend's computer or scrolling through personal ads on a gay cruising site to see if his boyfriend has a profile posted.

For other gay men, jealousy isn't felt, but is something he thinks he ought to feel. If, for instance, he was brought up in a heterosexual culture that places great emphasis on feminine chastity, such as Mediterranean, Latin, or Arabic cultures, a gay man may be as jealous of his lover as the straight men in his family are of their wives. Jealousy is actually but one aspect of an entire macho complex, one where his role, in his mind (if not in reality, nor in bed), is always that of the male, his lover's role always that of the female. A gay man from such a background may be especially impassioned because he feels guilty about being gay and needs to constantly prove his "masculinity," which he sees as already diminished by being gay (see *Homophobia*).

In other cases, jealousy is a smoke screen for envy. If you were really honest with yourself, you'd admit you're not plagued by jealousy over infidelity but rather by your envy of your lover's success. If you felt you could attract men as easily, you would give up being the jealous lover. Even though you may not acknowledge it, you are secretly competing with your lover over who is more sexually desirable (or so you believe), and you fear you may come up a poor second. Unfortunately, your low self-esteem will probably keep this mental process unconscious, a guarantee of constant bickering (if not outright abuse); it's bound to result in a broken relationship (see *Couples*).

Most jealousy is built upon possessiveness. A man believes and acts on the belief that his lover is his property, something he owns, and every time the lover flirts with outsiders, the jealous man feels that he's been robbed. In virtually all cases, the immediate problem that brings on the intense rage felt by so many jealous men is a sudden, strongly felt lack of self-worth. Therefore, jealousy isn't really between two people, but completely self-generated.

If you suffer from jealousy and are striving to overcome it, you must first begin by admitting that it's *not okay*, it's an emotion unworthy of you, one that is spoiling your relationship and may well ruin all future ones. As long as you believe jealousy is normal and justified, you will never beat it. Stop quizzing your lover; stop trying to catch him out in lies and phony alibis. Do not read his diary, letters, or phone bills or try to sniff out his computer profile. Every time you feel jealous, forget your lover's actions; instead, examine your own emotions. What feelings underlie this frenzy? Are you feeling guilty about being gay? Are you guilty about your own dating around? Are you envious of him? Are you unsure whether your partner really loves you? Once you are honestly able to locate the deep disorder beneath your jealousy, articulate it to yourself and then to your lover.

If your partner suffers from jealousy and it's getting worse, you may be in real trouble. Jealousy can often lead directly to physical abuse (see *Domestic Violence*). If you cannot get your lover to look at the problem realistically, you may need couples counseling or psychotherapy. If that doesn't seem to be working, you may have to end the relationship before it becomes physically dangerous. But keep in mind that, for many couples, while only one partner is expressing jealousy, both may be contributing to it. Sometimes one lover is consciously or unconsciously feeding his partner's jealousy. Why would anyone do that? To keep him in suspense—to keep him fascinated (nothing is as blinding as jealousy, at least when it's under control—the jealous lover never thinks of anything except his partner). If this is your case and you admit that you're equally to blame, you better find out why. Are you afraid of being abandoned? Do you expect jealousy for a relationship to feel real? If your relationship is being held together by this constant anguish, it's time to get into psychotherapy.

J.O. Buddies

Jerk-off buddies can be partners in fantasy. They may talk dirty; wear provocative costumes such as jockstraps, leather jackets, and chaps; and while they keep up a sex rap, masturbate themselves and each other (see *Dirty Talk; Masturbation and Fantasy; Mutual Masturbation*). Some J.O. buddies operate long-distance, jerking off while talking on the phone. They describe themselves in erotic detail, talk about their cocks and sexual desires, and fantasize having sex together (see *Phone Sex*). Still other J.O. buddies exchange letters, photographs, or audiotapes and videos of themselves. Sometimes they send each other their semen-stained underwear. Of course the Internet has opened up new possibilities of finding a J.O. buddy, as long as you can type with one hand (see *On-line Cruising*).

Jerking off with someone else is the preferred, sometimes the only, sexual outlet for some men (see *J.O. Clubs*). For others, it may be a form of foreplay or an exciting alternative to the more usual repertoire of sucking and fucking. You can live out a fantasy scene jerking off with another man (or two?) that would be either impossible or difficult to create in reality. (You don't really want to give up your job at the telephone company to become a cowboy.) Some men get off on masochistic or sadistic fantasies but find the actuality of S/M distasteful; a J.O. buddy may be the perfect solution for them. Still others first got turned on by jerking off with a friend when they were younger, and this form of sex recalls for them their steamy, spermy youth. For others it may represent a temporary, sexually satisfying, trustworthy relationship until they find a permanent lover.

Possibly the only drawback to jerking off as a dominant sexual habit is that it can become a substitute for the greater intimacy of lovemaking. Still, jerking off with a friend is a way of connecting with another man but maintaining distance. Limited to jerking off, it's even safer than having a fuck buddy (see *Fuck Buddies*). Now you can be excited, get off sexually, and still enjoy completely safe sex.

J.O. Clubs

J.O. clubs existed before the AIDS crisis made safe sex absolutely necessary, but have become far more popular recently. Such clubs originated during the seventies, and were often an outgrowth of private parties organized by gay guys who were into masturbation. They invited others who shared this interest to orgies where no sucking or fucking took place, only kissing, caressing, and jerking off. The group expanded, was named the Jacks (i.e., "those who jack off"), and attracted not only exhibitionists and men with large penises (especially members of the eight-inch club), but also those attracted to them. J.O. clubs soon became so crowded they had to move their biweekly parties to large loft spaces.

What makes J.O. clubs different from back rooms (which continue to exist, though in much reduced numbers) is that penetration is forbidden (see *Tearooms and Back Rooms*). One member of Jacks says that it is for "cocksmen and cock worshipers" only. He explains that any penetration "hides" the cock.

Generally, J.O. clubs require total nudity, although some guys slip through with underwear. This isn't necessarily for modesty; some guys apparently like the look of their engorged dicks straining at the cloth barrier of Jockey shorts or a jockstrap. These joints are usually in the basement of old factories, and the amenities are a few rolls of Bounty and a couple of well-used jars of Abolene face cream. There is music, and usually free soda or beer comes with the price of admission.

While a generous-sized schlong will generally fill one's dance card faster, surprising pairings go on—old with young, fat with thin, hairy with smooth. In a microcosmic way, J.O. clubs can challenge one's sense of the hierarchies that one assumes govern gay erotic attraction. There are, to be sure, a fair contingent of well-hung gym buddies looking for same, but there's more democracy than you might imagine. We've noticed some modestly proportioned members working on their more massively hung brethren (see *Cock Size*). As for unsafe sex, the occasional finger finds its way into a (not always unwilling) bunghole. It is remarkable how well people observe the rules, perhaps because the restricted activities are almost liberating. One may also find affection and physical closeness.

The arrangements are fairly fluid with occasional threesomes and foursomes, but one-on-one action is the most common. However, there is a lot of "change partners and dance," one of the attractions of the J.O. club, as well as one of its frustrations—particularly when you've bagged a stunner, only to find that he has roaming eyes.

Lately, some J.O. clubs have evolved into sex clubs where *unsafe* sex is making a reappearance (see *Sex Clubs; Safe Sex; Barebacking; Condoms*). You should be extra careful there. Keep this in mind: The men you're having sex with probably already had sex with many other men during the night. The opportunity to have sex with multiple partners is the reason they (and you) went there in the first place. But STDs and HIV are among the uninvited guests (see *Sexually Transmitted Diseases; Sex Parties; HIV Disease*). Our consistent message throughout this book is permissiveness in sex, except for the transmission of disease.

* * *

J.O. Machines

Young boys first fall in love with their cock, a romance that—to quote Oscar Wilde—is destined to last throughout their life. Jerking off under the sheets, in the bathroom, or with friends in the school yard during adolescence soon gives way to more adult forms of pulling one's putz (see *J.O. Buddies; J.O. Clubs; Masturbation and Fantasy; Pornography*). The advent of the Internet has unleashed unlimited opportunities to sit naked in front of the computer screen, with only one hand on the keyboard (see *On-line Cruising; Teenagers*). But did you know that the computer is not the first electrical machine invented to assist one in jacking off?

It's not. The first electrical machine came on the market twenty years ago. The farseeing inventor named it the Accujac, and it consisted of a large motor out of which projected a long tube that could be connected to any of a number of hollow plastic sleeves. You attached one of these sleeves to the motor, put a bit of lubricant in the sleeve, and placed it over your dick. Turning on the switch created a vacuum in the sleeve, which rode up and down your penis, which, the manufacturer claimed, would get you off.

For purposes of scientific investigation, one of the authors offered to test-drive the $300 erotic vacuum cleaner and to write about its effectiveness for a professional journal. His lover, ignoring the demands of scientific investigation, offered instead to do it for free. The offer was rejected, and so, with all the rigors of the scientific method reinstituted, the investigator placed the sleeve around his penis, turned on the machine, and—had one of the least erotic experiences of his life! The plastic sleeve quickly popped off his cock instead of popping off the author, and the entire experience demonstrated how important mental imagery, rather than tubular construction, is to sexual arousal.

A few years ago, Bill Andriette, features editor of *The Guide*, a gay travel and entertainment magazine published in Boston, wrote a review of the Venus II, a more advanced (and $669 more expensive) version of the earlier Accujac. This was not an imitation of cheap blowup fuck dolls, or the far more common penis pumps we see advertised in every sex mag in the world (see *Sex Toys*). As Bill explained, the manufacturer "promised to free the hands from masturbatory drudgery, so that they could be free to roam forth and do their own thing: stroke one's balls, pinch one's nipples, grip one's *Honcho*."

The newer and more sophisticated machine respected individual difference in a world of wankers, offering the user a range of strokes from a leisurely 25 to a frenetic 350 per minute. But, Andriette complained, the machine didn't know when to quit. Wisely observing, "mankind can be divided into those who like their cocks vigorously attended right after orgasm, and those who would rather get punched in the stomach," he found that the gizmo turned into his personal penile torture chamber. He further complained that in high gear the newer Accujac made a racket that would wake the neighbors, while at lower speeds it sounded much like tubercular wheezing. He suggested attaching a muffler.

We believe that electrical contrivances for spanking the monkey are probably a thing of the past. Neither of these two machines is available for purchase today, and to the best of our knowledge no manufacturer has jumped to fill the gaping void with a replacement. We suspect that there's just too much (and far cheaper) competition from one's own hand, or from someone else's hand, to make the purchase a required one. We suspect, too, that a prospective purchaser might worry what questionably constructed circuits, put together by exploited workers in third world countries, will actually deliver to his cock. It may be more than he bargained for.

And yet . . . some young entrepreneur, fired up with the promise of the digital marvels possible in the world of whacking off, may still surprise us and invent an effective contrivance that can comfortably jerk us off—and maybe fuck us at the same time. What a wonderful Christmas present *that* would be for the world's growing number of bottoms.

Kinky Sex

When it comes to value judgments, everything is relative. In sex, too. Let's say you are tricking with an attractive man you met via the Internet (see *On-line Cruising*). He's really into you and he's been quite passionate in bed. But he suddenly starts chewing (hard) on your nipples; or he begins to slap your ass; or he calls you "Daddy"; or he wants you to piss on him ("In my bed!?"). Or he says, "Why don't you play the coach, and I'll be the freshman" (see *Nipples; Spanking; Daddy/Son Fantasies; Role Playing; Water Sports*).

Most gay men would probably object to some or all of these scenarios (see *Vanilla Sex*). Others might enjoy the full range of possibilities in bed (see *Versatility*). "Kinky" sex is merely sex that is not commonplace.

It has nothing to do with potentially dangerous or nonconsensual sex. We are adamantly opposed to nonconsensual sex. Kinky implies a bit of naughtiness, like kids violating adult rules and enjoying it because they're "being bad."

"Kinky" to us is sexual behavior that is

1. Consensual.

2. Not dangerous or life-threatening to you or your sexual partner.

3. Not anything that feels "bad" to you or your sexual partner.

S/M activities are definitely kinky since they follow a sexual script that defines an agreed-upon, shared power structure between men, with one or more fetishes, such as leather (see *Sadomasochism*). B&D, a form of S/M, also combines sexual scripts with fetishes (see *Bondage and Discipline*). Exhibitionism and voyeurism played out in the bedroom or at a gay bathhouse or sauna are kinky, but in a more public space they can land you in jail (see *Exhibitionism and Voyeurism*).

Fetishes, in general, are very kinky, especially so since articles of apparel appeal so much to gay men. Cross-dressing is a fetish to some gays, while men's underwear (including jocks) is arousing to a far greater group of guys (see *Transgender*; *Fetish*; *Feet*). The first emphasizes the softness of femininity, while the other highlights the roughness of masculinity.

Scat and water sports, both definitely kinky, are a mystery to the majority of gay men. They cannot fathom how behavior they were taught in childhood was disgusting could have become eroticized for other men in adulthood (see *Scat*). Neither can sex researchers, nor many of the participants themselves.

We exclude from our category of kinky sex eroticized hanging—an unusual form of masturbation in which a person jerks off while hanging himself—because it sometimes ends in strangulation and death (see *Dangerous Sex*). We also do not support barebacking, since barebackers are a public menace who transmit the HIV (see *Barebacking*). Also excluded are placing potentially dangerous (sometimes life-threatening) objects up the ass, things like Coke bottles, flashlights, and boots (see *Sex Toys*). Those who do this often end up in hospital emergency rooms to the astonishment of the attending doctors and nurses. Major surgery is sometimes required. We feel the same about inserting foreign objects such as glass or metal rods up the urethra. Frottage is kinky in bed with a consensual lover, but not with some hunky but nonconsenting straight guy in the subway during rush hour.

The line between vanilla and kinky sex isn't always so sharp. The butch guy who's fucking you on your rug might push your head down so roughly that you come out of it with a rug burn on your forehead. Or he might slap your ass hard both before and while fucking you. Bottom though you may be, you may find yourself talking dirtier and more abusively to your sex partner than ever before, exposing fantasies you never knew existed (see *Dirty Talk*). Perhaps it's about time.

Men into kinky sex are no more or less able to establish long-lasting relationships. Often, however, they don't divulge this information to their lovers, reserving the kinky stuff for jerk-off fantasies and porn videos. Occasionally they trick out with like-minded kinky men, usually meeting them via the Internet (see *On-line Cruising*). We think this is a mistake, because deception is involved. Deception never helps a relationship. We think the more constructive approach is to share these fantasies with your lover. He may not be telling you about his own kinks, and if you two had this discussion, it might lead to new sexual adventures between you. At the least, it will add a level of maturity to the relationship.

Kissing

A kiss is both a romantic symbol and an erotic act, and this dual nature makes kisses deliciously ambiguous. The lips are among the most sensitive parts of the body, rivaled only by the fingertips and palms. The mouth is the baby's first organ of pleasure, and throughout adult life a person continues to suck, taste, lick, chew, and swallow as ways of deriving enjoyment (see *Licking*).

A sexy kiss is not a chaste peck but a deep and varied exploration, not just of your partner's mouth but of his whole body. When you kiss, your mouth should be wet; a dry mouth is not very appealing. Run your tongue over the sensitive surface of his gums, between the teeth and upper lip. Reach with your tongue to the top of his mouth and dart the tip over those delicate membranes—penetration of his mouth with your tongue is the classic and highly erotic French, or soul, kiss. Suck his tongue; nibble his lower lip; lick his nostrils; smear a kiss from his neck to the hollow just above the clavicle. Kiss his ear, nibbling the lobe or scouring the whole interior with your tongue; then draw back and exhale warm breath onto the ear. Some gay men (perhaps straight ones as well) love to kiss and lick their partner's armpits; they find the odor an aphrodisiac (see *Sleazy Sex*). And foot fetishists want their feet and toes kissed and licked, especially after a hard day at the office (see *Feet*; *Fetish*). Kissing, like touching in general, is about heightened sensuality (see *Touching and Holding*).

Some men (unfortunately) resist kissing. This resistance is often a last holdout against a full commitment to homosexuality ("Real men don't kiss"). Hustlers who think of themselves as straight don't kiss; soldiers or sailors who offer themselves as "straight" trade refuse to kiss (see *Trade*). When adolescent boys first start fooling around with each other, they often draw the line at kissing. As long as their lips never meet, they are able to rationalize that what they're doing (and it can be anything from sixty-nining to what was once called corn holing) is not homosexual, but just "getting their rocks off." Why? Because kissing is at the heart of romance. It speaks louder about sentimentality than all the fucking in the world. In legions of B Hollywood movies, the final credits come up on a kiss. Likewise, in sex between men, the final pledge of intimacy is offered not by the degree of ardor or penetration or abandon during sex, but by the depth, duration, and tenderness of a kiss.

Of course, kisses don't have to be tender. They can be cool and contemplative or rough and aggressive. The mouth is not only for sucking and licking but also for biting (see *Nibbling and Biting*). Your partner may not like you to be rough, so ask him. Whether rough or gentle, kissing is an integral part of the entire experience of making love. Most men like to get fucked lying on their backs precisely so that they can kiss during sex. Before or after fucking, a kiss on the lips merges into a pilgrimage over your partner's body—the hot erogenous zones of the nipples, the toes and fingers, the

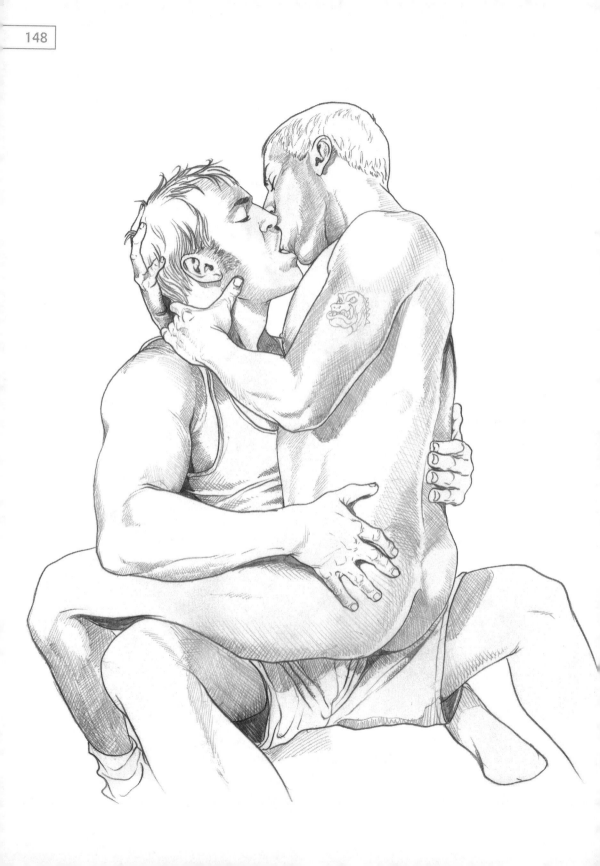

palms of the hands, or the hollows of the armpits. Your lover will tell you where he likes to be kissed; a trick probably will not, but you can usually get a good idea of what he wants done to him by noticing and imitating what he does to you.

Just how important kissing is in truly gratifying sex can be gauged by a popular slang complaint about being unsatisfied: "Fucked without a kiss!"

Letting Go

In George Orwell's novel *1984*, O'Brien asks, "What is the worst thing in the world?" For most of us it is feeling unloved and abandoned. These are all the primary feelings experienced when a love relationship ends. Sometimes the lovers have been quarreling for years. For other couples, months or years of silent distance abruptly end as one partner announces, to the astonishment of the other, that their relationship is over. No matter how long the relationship has lasted, and no matter how the end comes about, termination is painful for both parties; sometimes devastating to just one; sometimes to both.

What is worse, some men can't let go of the past. They tenaciously hold on to the conviction that "he still loves me" in the face of overwhelming evidence to the contrary. Invariably, the holder-on is obsessed with finding evidence that his former lover still loves him. These indications turn out to be flagrant distortions of the truth. The personality and character of the beloved are transformed into something approaching saintliness. Unkind acts are reinterpreted as benevolent; even abuse can be reinterpreted as love (see *Domestic Violence*). This is obsessive love, and its effects are harmful all the time.

Relationships do not always work out (see *Couples*). It may not be either's fault. Two men may have gotten together because of sexual compatibility, mistaking that for love. Over time, one or both lose interest, or one changes in important ways while the other doesn't. Even so, once a breakup occurs, both are likely to feel depressed (see *Depression*).

The obsessed man continues to pursue his lost love, while friends familiar with the situation look on with amazement. The beloved, meanwhile, may be furious and resentful over being hounded. It does no good to tell someone, "It's over," if he simply does not or cannot believe it. For him, reconciling to such rejection would be equivalent to admitting that he's no more secure than a little boy lost in the forest. At its most extreme, the obsessed (we are tempted to say possessed) man may begin stalking his former lover (see *Sexual Harassment*).

There are no cures for men who are obsessed with a former lover, or with an unrequited love. Psychologists have learned that these are the most obdurate obsessions, and the most difficult to relieve in psychotherapy. This is because the obsessed lover rejects much of the world and focuses only on his distorted belief about his beloved. The obsession is dispelled only when the man opens his life again to meeting new people. Friends can be helpful in this process, but it may take a long time.

The beloved can make things better or worse, depending upon how he ended the relationship and on his subsequent behavior. If you are ending a love relationship, tell your lover why. Don't leave it to his imagination. Make your complaints as specific as possible. If you're willing, try couples therapy, but not if you know in your heart that you want to be free of him. Otherwise you'll only breed further resentment. Be as clear as you can about what further contact you want with him. Avoid ambiguous statements, since they give birth to misperceptions. If you don't want any contact with him in the future, say so. Make it clear that you won't allow friends to be used as intermediaries, and stick to it. Tell friends that if they persist in conveying information back and forth, then you will have to terminate your friendship.

The problem of unrequited love is similar but not the same. Most of us have fallen madly in love with someone who either never knew of our passion or who, if he did, showed no romantic interest in return. Most of us get over it in time, but some men pursue the love object and become furiously jealous at the success of competitors (see *Jealousy, Envy, and Possessiveness*). A few men become so angry that they interfere in the life of the beloved. Naturally, the beloved sees only the insanity of it all. A madman is intruding upon his life.

If you are being hounded by an obsessed or unrequited lover, tell him without the slightest ambiguity that you are not interested in pursuing a relationship. Make it clear that you will not meet or talk to him, in person or over the phone. Do not accept cards or presents mailed or delivered to you. Let him know that you will immediately delete all e-mails he sends to you. *And don't read them.* Then inform all mutual friends not to transmit any information between you.

Last, cross your fingers and hope that all this works.

Grieving over the death of a lover or a close friend is a particularly painful part of letting go. HIV disease has produced a legion of young widowers who need to grieve for their losses while continuing to function effectively in the world. Some survivors have a terrible time of it; they suffer deep, long-lasting depression. A few accuse themselves of not doing enough and end up guilt-ridden (see *Guilt*). It's also common for the survivor to feel abandoned by his dead lover and resentful toward him. Others refuse to throw out or give away any of the dead man's possessions. Finally, some men launch themselves into frequent sexual encounters. All these are ways to cover up the pain.

If you have trouble letting go, join an AIDS organization. They often have support groups for survivors, which may suggest particular techniques for accepting the loss. Friends can help to an extent, but they sometimes feel inadequate to the task.

It's common for survivors to talk to the dead lover. If you do this, don't stop. Tell him how you feel, what life is like without him. Express whatever feelings well up in you, both the loving and the angry ones. And cry—or break something. Begin to throw out his things. Take some minor possession of his (nothing with emotional significance) and, while throwing it out, tell him you're doing so. Tell him (and yourself) that the physical object has nothing to do with your love for him. Another day, throw out or give away another possession. One day, when you're ready, you'll dispose of most of his belongings, but keep items that remind you of the good times, such as photographs and birthday presents. Disposing of possessions is the easy part. Recognizing that a part of you has also died is more difficult.

Memorial services are a good way of letting go. They allow you to publicly express your love toward him for the last time.

Licking

When we say that some guy we meet looks good enough to eat, we're not being cannibalistic. What we really mean is not that we want to chomp down on an arm or a leg, but that we'd like to kiss and suck on his nipples, then run our tongue along that single line of light hair running from his chest down across his tummy, around (or maybe *right in* for a second) his navel, then farther south across his lower abdomen, resting only at his pubic hair and his cock, which ought by now (if we've truly licked our way to our desire) be standing erect and ready for more tongue action.

Some guys prefer licking only around the face and the head, spending time at the nose, ears, even the closed eyelids. Others are "neck men," licking from the chin down and around the back to the sensitive nape of the neck. Others simply turn their lover on his front and, beginning at the ears, lick all the way down to the heels, then toes, of his feet, stopping for longer or shorter periods at specific localities, such as the two indentations below the spine where the buttocks blossom out, or lower down inside the buttocks themselves (see *Rimming and Felching*). Some guys prefer the somewhat astringent flavor between the anus and the balls (called the perineum in polite society), a muscular cord that some men can't get enough of. Others prefer armpits and will do a better job than any deodorant, while still others go for the delicate backs of the knees. Fingers and toes are by no means exempt from the male licker's attentions; some men are most passionate there (see *Feet*). And then, of course, there're always the balls. A good blow job is only good, never great, unless you've spent some time licking his balls. An extra reward of that activity is the increased flow of semen when he finally comes.

Heterosexual men usually have to pay a great deal extra to professional sex workers for a head-to-toe licking; but if you're a gay man, you're probably getting it for nothing. If you've never been licked all over prior to or during sex, you're missing something special. And if you want to arouse someone who seems not that interested, someone who seems nearly dead, giving him a tongue bath is sure to bring him roaringly alive and ready for whatever sex you're planning. *Bon appétit.*

Living Wills

The living will is a relatively new legal instrument that clarifies your wishes regarding medical treatment if, because of a serious accident or severe illness, you are unable to make such decisions yourself. What's at stake is the control, upkeep, and maintenance of your body when you're not in a position to make your wishes known. The living will stipulates which, if any, life-sustaining mechanisms you want used to prolong your life, and for how long. Currently only about thirty-five states permit one to make a living will. Some people feel that treatments such as breathing machines, liquid nutrition, and cardiac resuscitation are unnatural and only draw out the death agony. They also feel that extended dying increases lovers' and family members' pain, as well as needlessly depleting bank accounts.

AIDS patients and men suffering from other life-threatening illnesses or mental disorganization almost always make out living wills. All of us should do so, in addition to a traditional will (see *Wills*).

You can designate anyone you want to have medical power of attorney to make these decisions if you're incapacitated. Some states have a health-care proxy law that allows you to declare specific health-care decisions and name a surrogate to make dispositions on your behalf. Some states allow you to name a conservator, empowered to make medical, financial, or business decisions in your name. Nomination of a conservator is the most powerful protection, assuming the conservator is trustworthy and makes wise decisions. These alternatives should be discussed with an attorney who understands the social and legal problems of gay people. If you cannot afford a lawyer, many AIDS clinics and gay community centers have pro bono attorneys on staff who can help.

You should *not* keep your living will secret. Copies should go to your family, your lover, your physicians, and your hospital. But that's not enough. Speak to each in person. Make certain they clearly know your intentions. Be careful about choosing a hospital under the auspices of a religious group. Some refuse to curtail treatment no matter what legal documents you have. Others have no guidelines for abiding by living wills; they decide case by case. You or your caretaker may be forced to take the hospital to court to ensure your right to die.

Finally, don't confuse a living will with a will. You can think of both of them as documents that speak for you, but a living will speaks for you only until your death. After that, only a will speaks for you.

Loneliness

Feeling alone can be frightening and depressing. No matter how much money or status a man may have, no matter how many friends and tricks he can point to, he may still be besieged by an intolerable sense of alienation. Even a man with a devoted lover may experience profound isolation.

There are three kinds of loneliness—two that must be accepted, and a third that can be fought. First is the loneliness caused by the death of a close friend, lover, or a member of one's family. The resulting sadness is always appropriate because the loss is real, not symbolic (see *Depression; Letting Go*). A second isolation that must be accepted is "cosmic" loneliness. Often an individual in his thirties or forties who has buried the ghosts of his past, freed himself from any neurotic aspects of his relationships with his parents, his boss, and his lover, and achieved a clear-eyed view of himself—often this person will suddenly be hit hard by the full force of cosmic loneliness, what William James called "vastation" in *The Varieties of Religious Experience*: the adult recognition that we are born alone and will die alone, and that many of our private experiences will never successfully be shared with other people. There's nothing to be done about that.

But the third kind of loneliness can be combated. Though we don't think of it this way, the usual kind of aching loneliness is something we ourselves have created. This loneliness is our rejection of other people, our refusal to let them become a significant part of our life. A lonely man might say, even when he is surrounded by thousands of other gays, that he cannot relate to any of them. He will claim that all they want is sex, not intimacy, whereas it is he who demands sex and fears affection. To keep intact his conviction that no one loves him, the lonely man will seek unloving men. He may marry and live a double life, then curse his inability to find male love because he is imprisoned by his marriage, a situation of his own making (see *Married Men*).

One of the most common forms of loneliness among gay men, even in these days of HIV infection, afflicts those who consciously desire to have nothing but anonymous, quick sex. Having contrived a world of quick sex for themselves, they complain that quick sex is all that gay men ever want. Since they lack respect for themselves, they show an equal disrespect for their sex partners by not respecting safe sex guidelines and therefore endangering both lives. (Of course there are also gay men who have nothing but anonymous sex, enjoy it, and don't complain about it.)

If you are caught in a trap of loneliness of your own devising, you ought to consider changing your habits. Plan purely social times with your friends, rather than going out cruising. Love and friendship are not airtight compartments; if you can achieve intimacy with a friend, you may also be preparing yourself for eventual closeness with a lover. Meet new people in new places, or approach new people in the old places in a different way. Perhaps you shouldn't jump into bed with someone you meet at the gym; ask him out for dinner or a movie, talk to him, and court him. If trying out new approaches frightens you, no matter. Better to feel anxious about change than to remain safely in a neurotic pattern that one poet has characterized as "old, inadequate and flourishing."

Lubricants

Essential for fucking, often a real help when masturbating yourself, fun for a "slip and slide" jerk-off session with someone else, lubricants come in many varieties. Some are expensive, flavored, scented, and marketed under coy or erotic names. Others are cheaper, more practical, and as close as your grocery shelf or drugstore. Take the water-soluble lubricants, such as K-Y, a favorite among gays as it's easily washed off bodies and sheets; while some men like it for jerking off, they find it a bit sticky for fucking. The only trouble with water-soluble lubricants is that they can dry out in midecstasy. Petroleum jelly (Vaseline) and vegetable shortening are cheap and good bets, since they stay greasy for hours, but they are not water-soluble, and therefore they should never be used with latex condoms because they degrade the latex; it will tear. Note that silicon lubes can be expensive and aren't kind to your sheets.

Crisco is the favorite of fisters (see *Fisting*). Serious bottoms prefer a lubricant that's less likely to stain their sheets, especially if they're being hammered by a donkey dick. Two other lubricants, one named ID (we suppose a reference to Freud's concept of the animal-like id of the mind) and another named WET are better for them. You can also use them on your sex toys. If sexually active (we mean very sexually active), you might as well get the industrial-size pump bottle and use it to replenish the smaller pump bottle on the nightstand next to your bed.

Some lubricants claim to contain spermicides (sperm killers) that kill many of the bacterial agents that cause disease, but these claims haven't been proven in research (see *Sexually Transmitted Diseases*). Nonoxynol-9 was long touted as one of them, but it, too, should not be depended upon as a spermicide, since recent research has failed to demonstrate its effectiveness in killing the HIV. Another downside to nonoxynol-9 is that some men are sensitive to its repeated use; their cocks become chafed. Take the following scene: A man is about to fuck you. He squirts nonoxynol-9 inside a condom, puts it on, and fucks you. After he comes, you take off the condom, wipe the come off his dick, and suck him. Some men have reported numbness in their mouth. It is (forgive us) a matter of taste.

Buying lubricants won't break the budget, so you might as well try out a number of them. Just remember to carefully read the list of ingredients. It's probably best to stay away from lubes that list dyes and perfumes. For jerking off, either by yourself or with another man, use any kind of lubricant. But use only water-soluble lubricants when fucking.

Male Sexual Response

What is the primary sexual organ in your body? No, it's not your cock, even though it may seem to control much (possibly *too much*) of your life. Your brain is actually the main center of all sexual activity. Acting like an electrical control panel (and, some complain, at times like a circuit breaker), the brain and its nervous systems are the arbiters of what and who turns you on, what you want to do with him or them, and even your concept of love and the kind of men you fall in love with—or don't fall in love with.

The brain is by no means an inert organ. Three elements determine how the brain affects your sexuality. The first is genetics (see *Mythic Beginnings*). The genes determine your sexual orientation: gay, straight, bisexual, transgender. We believe genetics also influences your feelings of maleness and femaleness, what has lately been called gender identity, a term first used by sex researcher John Money. The term *gender* was popularized by the women's movement. They proposed that "sexual identity" had its origin in biology, whereas "gender identity" had its origin in socialization. Feminists prefer a social rather than a biological explanation for gender. We disagree; we believe that maleness and femaleness are biologically determined (see *Gay Politics*).

That is not to say that socialization is of no importance in human development. What is given biologically still must be molded and shaped by a social structure, otherwise a person's development would be profoundly abnormal, like those feral children occasionally found in India and elsewhere. So, secondarily, one's social role as a man, one's concept of love and attachment, and one's expectations and responsibilities in society are all learned (or mislearned) during childhood socialization, and they are coded in the brain.

The third element of the brain as the primary sex organ is our own personal and specific sexual experience in life. Our early sexual fantasies, our first experiences of sexual pleasure, our moments of sexual pain (such as being raped)—all are recorded in the brain, and all come into play and influence how we perceive and act in any new sexual situation (see *Rape; Sexual Harassment*). For example, gay men who, as children, were sissies and were teased mercilessly by their peers, will inevitably look upon other gay men and gay sexual opportunities somewhat differently from those of us who were not humiliated. Pleasant sexual experiences are also coded in the brain, such as a mutually satisfying love affair with another adolescent boy, or good feelings about being gay.

Of course the three elements of the sexual brain are not mutually exclusive—they're mixed together. We simply don't have the scientific sophistication to know

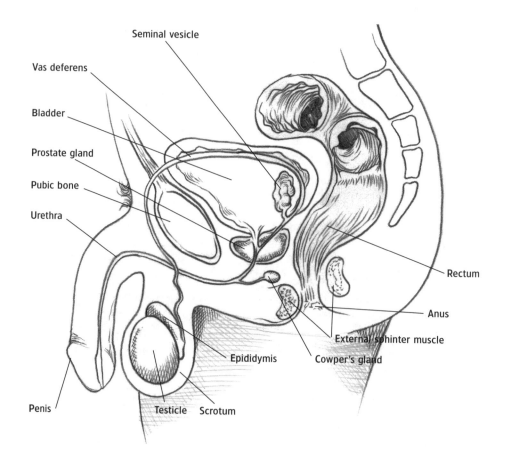

Seminal vesicle

Vas deferens

Bladder

Prostate gland

Pubic bone

Urethra

Rectum

Anus

External sphinter muscle

Epididymis

Cowper's gland

Penis

Testicle Scrotum

where one ends and another begins. What we do know is that this biosocial interpretation of sexual response is exceedingly complicated.

According to Masters and Johnson, there are four stages to the male sexual response. The first stage they call *excitement*, during which your breathing becomes heavier, your heart rate and blood pressure increase, your scrotum (the sac that contains your balls) thickens, and your testes are elevated. This is the stage during which you feel sexually excited (horny) and your cock gets hard.

The second stage is called *plateau*. It's an advanced state of arousal just before orgasm. Your cock is filled with blood to the limit of its capabilities, and your hard-on, accordingly, is at its maximum length and width. Your balls are also engorged with blood and they are about 50 percent larger than in an unexcited state. A clear lubricating liquid is secreted through the urethra and bathes the head of your cock; it is a secretion from Cowper's gland, commonly called precome. Some men secrete little precome; other men quite a bit (both are normal). Some gay men have learned to prolong this plateau state considerably through practice or via specific sex acts, while some Eastern spiritual disciplines consider this plateau state to be the highest form of human sexuality and they aim toward never going beyond it, which requires enormous mental and physical control (see *Spirituality*).

The third stage is *orgasm*, which can be broken down further into two phases. The first, called ejaculatory inevitability, is the point of no return. Contractions of your internal organs involved in orgasm have begun. The second phase is the orgasm itself, rhythmic contractions of your muscles at the base of your penis and the urethral canal (the duct in your penis); orgasm usually consists of about three to seven spurts of fluid at 0.8-second intervals. The amount of ejaculate varies, too. Shooting more or less come has nothing to do with your virility. Nor does how high you can shoot your load (although aiming for and hitting a target may be fun). Some gay men swear that the more fondling, sucking, or licking the balls receive before orgasm, the greater the amount shot out, or the farther it can shoot; while various male porn stars have gone on record attesting that letting a stimulated erection go soft once or twice before orgasm increases both the range and flow of semen shot. But be careful not to linger so long that you get blue balls.

The fourth stage is *resolution*. This is the period following orgasm when your body reverts to its normal state. Heartbeat, blood pressure, and respiration return to normal. Your balls relax to their customary position. Your erection is lost after orgasm, and your cock gets soft. Some men, mainly young men, maintain an erection after they come and go on to a second orgasm. Most of us, however, need a period of rest before we can have sex again. As a rule of thumb, the older we get, the longer the rest period needed between sexual episodes, although this, too, can vary based on how long it's been since you've had sex and how excited you are by the person you're with.

All four stages noted above are controlled by our double nervous system. Yes, we have two. The first is the *central nervous system*, serving the voluntary movements of the skeletal muscles and numerous other functions. The other is the *autonomic nervous system*, which controls the involuntary responses of the internal organs such as breathing, maintaining body temperature, and for our purpose, your genitals.

The autonomic system is further divided into two subsystems: the *sympathetic* and the *parasympathetic*. Generally speaking, the sympathetic and parasympathetic divisions are antagonistic to each other. For instance, the sympathetic division speeds up the heart rate, whereas the parasympathetic slows it down. The principle of "antagonism" functions in many parts of the body. It provides checks to prevent one function from getting out of control. Sometimes, however, the two systems work cooperatively. In the male sex act, for instance, the parasympathetic nerves control erection, while ejaculation is a function of the sympathetic nerves.

This division of labor produces significant effects. For instance, the parasympathetic system is highly vulnerable to physical trauma, substance abuse, and to certain diseases such as diabetes. It's in charge during quiescence or peacefulness. Anxiety, which triggers and is moderated by the sympathetic division, can inhibit functioning of the parasympathetic division—and so stop you from having erections. Young gays first coming out may find themselves so frightened by their early sexual experiences that they can't get hard. Being scared inhibits the parasympathetic nerves and may prevent an erection regardless of how much you are dying to get laid. However, ejaculation is controlled by the sympathetic part of the autonomic system, which means you can blow your load even if you are anxious and unable to get hard. Even so, the amount of sensory stimulation needed for ejaculation can vary according to many factors, including your emotional conditions. If you are not highly aroused, if for any reason you are inhibited, if you are sedated, if you have just come, or if you are in psychological conflict about this sex act with this partner, even if you are erect, repeated and intense thrusting and stimulation will probably be necessary to bring on ejaculation.

It would be a mistake, however, to leave you with the impression that sex is exclusively handled by the autonomic nervous system. The central nervous system also has an important role to play. In fact, few activities involve so many different parts and structures of the body as sex does. The visual and auditory stimuli that lead to arousal are affected by the central nervous system and are, in certain respects, both learned and conscious. If you see a tempting pair of buns or hear a dirty story and get turned on, you're responding with that part of the brain that entertains conscious thoughts (cognition), part of the central nervous system. Another part of the brain, the hypothalamus (a pea-sized organ on the base of your brain), seems to integrate the central nervous system, the autonomic nervous system, and the hormonal system—all called into play in human sexuality.

What about the genitals themselves? Let's take a closer look. The testes are the male reproductive glands. They produce sperm (the reproductive cells) and testosterone (a male hormone responsible for such secondary male sexual characteristics as your beard, your deep male voice, and the growth of your genitals). The testes are inside your scrotum, a sack designed to maintain sperm at the proper temperature — what most of us call your balls or nuts. To conserve heat in cold weather, your scrotum shrinks and hugs the testes close to your body for warmth; or conversely, your scrotum expands to move the testes away from your overheated body to cool off.

After they are formed in the testicles, sperm cells are stored in little tubes called *epididymides*, which are coiled tubes on the backside of your balls. You can easily feel them. The epididymides connect to long tubes called the *vas deferens*; there's one vas deferens on the left side and one on the right. These tubes, each about sixteen inches long, wind from the scrotum through the lower pelvic area of your body and empty into the prostate gland and seminal vesicles. During an ejaculation, sperm moves up the vas deferens until it reaches the prostate and seminal vesicles, where it mixes with the secretions they manufacture. The combination of these secretions with sperm cells makes up the semen that flows out of the head (*glans*) of your cock when you come. Some gay men swear they can identify what their lovers have eaten in the past twenty-four hours by the taste of their semen. We don't believe that this gustatory phenomenon has been scientifically investigated.

Moving on, the *urethra* is a tube that leads from the bladder to and through the penis. It carries your urine and, when you are having an orgasm, semen. The penis contains three tubes of spongy erectile tissue called *corpus cavernosum* (there's also erectile tissue in your nipples and nose) that fill with blood to make your dick hard. Yes, you can break your penis, and some gay men actually do, particularly during extremely rough sex. Other men bend and snap their hard cocks against their body, enjoying the sound of a hard dick banging against their belly. It makes them feel butch. Either activity, however, can form scar tissue in one or more of the *corpus cavernosum*, leading to *Peyronie's disease*. In this disease your cock looks normal when soft, but when it gets hard, it curves off to one side. A certain amount of curvature can be useful: Some guys love having their prostate pounded by a downward-curving dick, but the curvature could also be in the wrong direction and so severe it becomes difficult to have sex with another person, and reparative surgery may be called for.

Moving away from the genitals, we arrive at the asshole or anus, and its sphincters (see *Anus*). These are two ringlike muscles at the opening of the anus, called, appropriately enough, the *internal* and *external sphincters*. Gently and slowly expanded by a finger, the anus can be relaxed and opened up (see *First Time*). A bit behind and above the internal sphincter is another set of muscles—the *pubo-coccygeus*. They form a slinglike cradle from the coccyx to the hipbone holding the pelvic organs, and they act somewhat like shock absorbers. When the rectum is stretched by getting fucked, these muscles pull back and generally stimulate the pelvic organs. Beyond the sphincters, the finger or penis (or dildo) enters the rectum, a cavity six to eight inches long. Beyond the rectum is the sigmoid colon, the terminal portion of your large bowel. Usually only fist fuckers come into contact with the sigmoid colon during sex (see *Fisting*).

Is there danger in homosexual fucking? No, not if the sphincter muscles are properly relaxed, and if you aren't suffering from seriously infected hemorrhoids, an anal fissure, prostatitis, or some other STD (see *Sexually Transmitted Diseases*). If the muscles are not opened gradually, however, the sphincter *can* be ripped or the tissue inside the rectum can be damaged. Symptoms include bleeding from the anus, bloody stools, pain, and fever. Go to the doctor. Some of these medical conditions can lead to serious systemic problems.

Therefore, fucking with dildos (and other nonhuman objects) should be done with caution (see *Sex Toys*). If the dildo does not have large fake balls on one end, it could actually get lost in your lower intestine, a potentially serious problem in which major surgery may be called for. The dildo should be made of soft, flexible rubber, and *not* of hard plastic or metal. Nor should it be longer than ten inches, or else it could penetrate the sigmoid colon, which is lined with fragile, easily broken tissue. A puncture of the sigmoid colon is bad news: It can lead to internal bleeding and death. Serious, even life-threatening, physical damage can occur if you fuck yourself with sharp objects such as turkey basters and glass bottles. (Don't snicker, men have done both and have suffered the consequences.) If you are getting fucked with a dildo, tell your partner how it feels; remember he is not getting any direct feedback from the dildo, since it has no nerves in it and is not part of his body.

The Ins and Outs of Gay Sex: A Medical Handbook for Men by Dr. Stephen Goldstone is the best book published about how the sex organs work, and problematical medical conditions. We advise you to learn about the potential problems, as well as the pleasures, by reading Goldstone's book. A terrific resource on-line is www.gayhealth.com. It's the best site on the Net to keep you abreast of new developments and research in the field of gay health.

Married Men

For centuries gays have married to perpetuate their name, to please their family, or to achieve respectability in business and in the community. Homosexuality was the love that dared not speak its name for so long that marriage seemed necessary to create a family. Many men still marry for these same reasons and lead a double life. This is especially true in foreign lands where homosexuality is severely repressed. If you are abroad, especially in Asia, the Middle East, or in the macho Latino cultures of Central and South America, there's a good chance the man you are having such a hot romance with may be married with children. And he intends to remain married (see *Travel*).

In North America and parts of Europe, the pattern is changing. Some men divulge their homosexuality to their wife so as to enrich the marriage and make it more honest. Such confessions are usually painful to make and painful to hear. If resentment, recrimination, and bitterness overwhelm the couple, the marriage will end in divorce. Other men declare themselves to be bisexuals, which has its own problems (see *Bisexuality*).

Why do gay men marry? There are several reasons. Many gay men arrive at adulthood having already had intimate and erotic relationships with women. A surprising number of "childhood sweethearts" fit this pattern. Although they sleep with their wife with pleasure (or not, as the case may be), they're not sexually interested in other women. For extramarital adventures they turn to men and may have been doing so since adolescence. Some of these men have married to fulfill family and cultural obligations. Others marry because of a longing for children (see *Gay Politics*). Both children and family obligations can be elusive in gay life, although gay adoptions are becoming more common.

A second group of gay men marry out of (not entirely groundless) fear. They may have had some experience with gay life and found it limiting, unpleasant, or too unconventional. Many of these men have been frustrated in their search for love. Unable or unwilling to not conform, they please their parents and their social network. Many gay men have deluded themselves into believing that their homosexuality will vanish once they find the right woman and become a family man. Nowadays, many conservative and religious fundamentalist groups are devoted to the false and specious doctrine that being homosexual is a "lifestyle choice" that can easily be changed. Among their most insidiously destructive activities is the insistence upon hooking up gay men and straight women, or straight men and lesbians, to have sex, become engaged, marry, and have children. Surrounded by an encouraging religious community, these marriages often succeed for a short while, but in time the old gay feelings invariably resurface, often with a greater hunger than before. When the gay man realizes the fraud perpetrated upon him, he's often stuck in an unsatisfactory and sexually frustrating marriage, hostile toward those he followed, and angry with himself for going along with the marriage.

Generally speaking, married gay men knew they were gay at an early age. They often had gay sex before and after they married. They make time for their extramarital sex life by rearranging their work and leisure-activities schedules. Accordingly, they frequently lie to their wife about their time, but as in all deceptions they experience anxiety and guilt. As a result, their work, social life, and family may all suffer.

For years, gay sex for some married men meant only anonymous sex. Some cruising spots seemed designed for married men (see *Cruising*). Arrests at these spots brought in "respectable" men rather than the expected perverts. Since Stonewall and gay liberation, married men have found a wider range of choices (see *Gay Liberation*).

One possible arrangement is for a married gay to have an affair with another man whom he visits periodically and regularly (see *Fuck Buddies*). Occasional anonymous sex is another possibility since it avoids emotional entanglements that may become hazardous to the marriage. In both cases the possibility of carrying STDs into the marriage bed is an ever-present danger (see *Sexually Transmitted Diseases*). The Internet has become a major new choice for married gay men who want to meet sex partners. On-line, men seldom ask difficult questions about others' personal lives, and it's sometimes quite easy to set up meetings or, if the married man is fearful of that, to just "talk dirty" and get off at the computer. Of course, the married gay man will have to be extra-alert to ensure that his wife and children cannot access the porn sites, gay chat rooms, and any saved conversations or e-mails that would let them know he's gay.

Clearly, married gay men face daunting problems, especially those who conceal their homosexuality from their wife and family. They must constantly hide their comings and goings, address books, clothes for cruising, and responses to certain innuendos they pick up but aren't free even to quietly chuckle over. These men feel isolated, as indeed they are. They're cut off from the gay community and sometimes know little about the men they have sex with.

Many single gay men also reject married ones, refusing to participate in a sexual relationship that involves fraud and lying. They reason that the married gay man is just as likely to cheat on them as he is with his wife.

Trouble may arise if a married gay man falls in love with someone single. The gay single will probably pester his married lover for more time together—always difficult to arrange. He may even ask the married man to leave his wife. This can severely test and often end the gay relationship, with deeply hurt feelings on both sides.

For the unattached gay man, the dangers of being in love with a married man should be obvious. All the back street movies ever made suddenly seem appallingly real instead of cheaply sentimental, and nothing in the world will compensate for his being with her when you want him with you! Especially difficult are those times he may be late or not arrive at all. Often you aren't allowed to, or can't, phone to find out if he's merely being held up or indeed if he was in an auto accident. It's not difficult for your relationship to become frustrated, and you, bitter.

If any combination of gay single and gay married men is to work, probably the best is the horny, younger, married gay man with the older, career-driven, or otherwise strongly involved single gay man. They should most appreciate each other's limited time, sexual involvement, and company—without the heartaches and the messy emotional housecleaning afterward.

One solution for the married gay man is to start an affair with another married man. Each understands the problems and limitations of the relationship. If their wives (or their respective children) become friends, the men can travel on vacations and go to parties together. The downside of this, of course, is that if one of the wives discovers the truth, the emotional trauma could be spread between two families, including the children.

Today, married men can join support groups with other married men. These groups are usually organized by gay community centers throughout the country. There are also support groups for the children of gay and lesbian parents.

Massage

There are two basic kinds of massage. One is primarily intended to reduce muscle tension and might be administered by a masseur at a gym or spa. It might be recommended by a doctor to a patient who carries around enormous tension in his body, or for a more specific reason, say, a lower-back problem, or for therapy following a sports or automobile accident. This type of massage may range in intensity from a standard hour-long session to much longer and repeated deep-muscle massages such as Rolfing.

The other kind, our concern here, is an explicit attempt to bring sensual pleasure to the person being massaged. It can be done by a lover, a friend, a fuck buddy, a hired professional from newspaper or on-line listings, by a skilled hustler, or by a sexual surrogate.

The sensuous massage gives people permission to accept pleasure. In ordinary sexual situations, many people are uptight about receiving pleasure: They can give it, but they have trouble accepting it (see *Pleasure Trap*). When a person is receiving a massage, however, accepting pleasure becomes a specific and conscious *assignment*. A sex therapist will handle such patients firmly, ordering them to lie passively on a bed (or massage board or floor) and to soak up the sensations offered. The therapist, in other words, has taken charge of the situation and assumed responsibility for whatever happens. Pleasure-resistant people are finally able to relax by submitting to "the doctor's orders." This clinical arrangement can also be adapted to informal massage sessions between friends, lovers, or fuck buddies.

After someone has learned to relax, he should indicate when something feels good and when it doesn't ("More light stroking over there, please"). People need to ask for what feels good, and sensual massage opens the door for that. By learning to ask during a massage, they prepare to make their desires known to their sexual partners.

All massage reduces anxiety and tension, but sensual massage also turns the acceptance of pleasure into an assignment, oddly enough, because it explicitly excludes sexual activity. It thus averts performance anxiety—the dread that you won't function adequately during sex—a fear that can become entrenched and self-perpetuating after repeated failure. Sensual massage is a way of overcoming performance anxiety by bringing two people into physical contact under a ban against sex. If you know that no matter how aroused you become you will not be permitted to have sex, your performance anxiety will gradually ebb away.

There are several types of sensual massage, described in ascending order, up to the most sexually arousing. Often, during therapeutic sensual massage, this specific order is adhered to. You should be naked while doing sensual massage.

The first calls for the two participants to take turns rubbing each other. The man giving the massage moves with light, caressing strokes from the head and face down to the feet and toes. You might want to use a soft powder to smooth out your hands.

At every point, the person receiving the massage gives instructions for more or less pressure on this or that part of the body. The erogenous zones are scrupulously avoided: The masseur does not stroke the nipples, balls, cock, or asshole. If the man being stroked becomes sexually aroused, he should not be allowed to shift into sex play. After the first man has been massaged, they switch places.

The second type, the genital massage, permits the masseur to rub the erogenous zones, but he must stroke the genitals in exactly the same way he strokes other parts of the body. The masseur should not linger more over the cock, say, than the thighs or arms, and he should by no means masturbate his partner. The object is not to induce

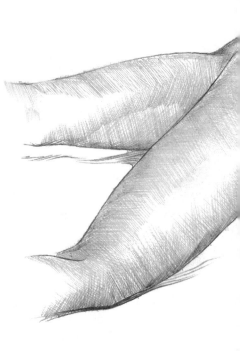

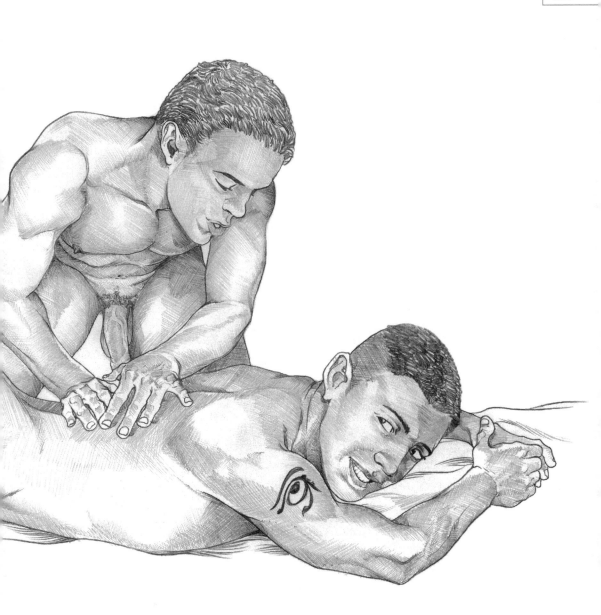

an erection or to bring about climax, but to provide pleasure, pure and simple. Both men should take note of their erotic fantasies.

Afterward both participants compare their fantasies. Some men's inhibitions about having fantasies and communicating them interfere with a rich, satisfying sex life. By becoming aware of and reporting their fantasies (even the most fleeting erotic thought) during massage, they can begin to overcome their reticence.

After the participants have tried the light, sensual massage and the somewhat more arousing genital massage, they might move on to direct sexual massage. Sexual massage may be the prelude to more intense sexual activity. The couple can use aromatherapy, "healing" oils, and powders; they can stroke each other not only with hands but also with mouth, lips, tongue, vibrators, dildos, or whatever suits their fancy. This form of massage need not be as gentle as the other two: It can get as rough as they like. The participants may take turns or rub each other simultaneously or combine massage with sucking, fucking, and other sexual acts.

Masturbation and Fantasy

The ancient Egyptians believed that the Nile River rose each year because of the continual masturbation of the god Osiris, and that his semen created all living things. It's unfortunate that this positive view of masturbation didn't survive into the Judeo-Christian era.

For centuries, masturbation has been condemned and persecuted in Western society, first by religious authorities and then by those modern watchdogs of morality, the medical profession. In the eighteenth century, the moral condemnation of masturbation was reinterpreted as a medical issue: Masturbation became an illness as well as a sin. A widely influential French physician, Tissot, said masturbation destroyed the nervous system, inevitably leading to madness.

In 1834, Dr. Sylvester Graham wrote that the loss of semen during sex was injurious to health (a popular idea at the time). Men, Graham wrote, should not have intercourse more than twelve times a year. And no jerking off in between. Masturbation was especially pernicious because it led to an enormous number of terminal diseases. To reduce sexual craving, Graham advised mild foods to decrease sexual appetites. The graham cracker was the result! In 1884, this curious connection between food and sex appeared in another guise. Dr. John Harvey Kellogg created cornflakes to curtail children's inclinations toward masturbation. Kellogg, a bit of a flake himself, wrote, "The *use* of the reproductive function is perhaps the highest physical act of which man is capable; its *abuse* is certainly one of the most grievous outrages against nature which it is possible for him to perpetrate."

From this period on, parents told children that awful things would happen if they touched their genitals: Hair would grow on the palms of their hands, or their brains would become "soft." Since even "good" children might masturbate in their sleep, some fearful parents enclosed children's arms in cardboard cuffs to prevent it.

Still, the warnings were ignored, and children went on playing with their genitals. The protests (somewhat hysterical) continued. William Acton, a prominent physician, wrote, "There is now in Pennsylvania—it seems unnecessary to name the place—a man thirty-five years old, with the infirmities of 'three score and ten.' Yet his

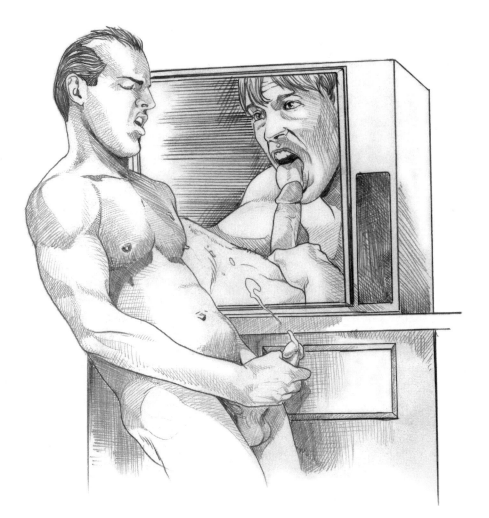

premature old age, his bending and tottering form, wrinkled face, and hoary head, might be traced to solitary and social *licentiousness*."

Between 1856 and 1919 the United States Patent Office granted patents for forty-nine antimasturbation devices. Thirty-five were for horses and fourteen for humans (horses could masturbate?). The human devices, intended for boys, were placed around his cock and consisted of either sharp points turned inward to jab the boy's penis should he get an erection, or an electrical system to deliver shocks. We don't know how many of these devices were actually used, or what effect they had on the children.

Although masturbation in men was repeatedly denounced, female masturbation was opposed with even greater ferocity. Women who masturbated were regarded by nineteenth-century medical professionals as manifesting dangerous masculine appetites. Starting in 1858, some women were subjected to a clitoridectomy, which effectively removed all possibility of clitoral pleasure. This operation continued as a treatment for female masturbation until 1937, even though it had been discredited by the medical profession a half century earlier.

In the twentieth century, masturbation was rediagnosed by psychiatrists as a sexual perversion. Though they did not go so far as to say masturbation would lead to insanity, they did suggest it led to "abnormal" sexual development, and, some feared, homosexuality—which some psychiatrists *did* believe was a form of insanity. Until 1968, masturbation remained as a mental disorder in the American Psychiatric Association's *Diagnostic and Statistical Manual*. Even today, many psychiatrists say that masturbation is not in itself a disorder—unless practiced too much. In other words, it's accepted as a substitute for heterosexual intercourse when that is unavailable, but anyone who chooses to masturbate rather than to have sex with another person is regarded as infantile or disturbed. (Read *Homosexuality and American Psychiatry: The Politics of Diagnosis* by Ronald Bayer.)

The goal of all this diagnosis was to create internalized feelings of guilt about masturbatory behavior, thereby marshaling people to police their own thoughts and actions. "No self-indulgence," says the superego (the Jiminy Cricket sitting on one's shoulder), "or I will punish you by making you feel like shit" (see *Guilt*). Men who don't start masturbating until their twenties have learned that lesson particularly well, but few can claim to have grown up in our sexually repressed society without any hang-ups about jerking off.

A view that seems to us much more rational, productive, and realistic is that masturbation is not a substitute to be tolerated, but a required behavior for proper psychosexual development. Only if boys and girls are permitted to masturbate freely and shamelessly will they be able to chart the contours of their own sexual desires. The physical reactions and imaginative ideation produced during masturbation allow the individual to define his or her sexual tastes and build confidence. The enjoyment derived from masturbation promotes greater acceptance of physical pleasure in general and of one's own body in particular.

A gay man incapable of fantasizing during sex is probably not very passionate. More than likely, he sticks to a rigid sequence of acts and is frightened and bewildered by the extent of other people's sexual inventiveness. Fantasies, therefore, are highly desirable, and masturbation is the best classroom for developing the faculty for fantasizing.

One helpful teaching aid is pornography. Some gay men are turned on by photos, others by sexy, stylized drawings, still others by stories or videotapes (see *Pornography*). Discover which media and/or styles excite you: Naked or clothed figures? Alone or engaged in sex with others? Which sexual practices do you prefer to look at? Of course, some men prefer to use their imagination to relive a stimulating episode or summon up an exciting person from their past. Perhaps they saw some really sexy guy walking on the street this morning or had a really hot sex scene with someone last week or looked at a beautiful body at the beach or the gym. It's not unusual for vigorous and horny men to vividly recall and jerk off less than an hour following a particularly exciting sexual encounter.

Pick a quiet time and take the pornography you've selected to bed with you. Create a soothing environment, with low lights and music or whatever relaxes you. Look through the pictures and choose one that turns you on. Concentrate on that picture and invent a story about it, one that also involves you. As your cock starts to get hard, continue the fantasy and begin to masturbate. If you've never used a lubricant, try one, such as K-Y, baby lotion, or Vaseline—everyone has his favorite (see *Lubricants*). Be sure to keep up the fantasy until you reach a climax. Your stories may become as elaborate and as kinky as you like (see *Kinky Sex*; *Sleazy Sex*).

If you practice fantasizing while masturbating for several days, you can attempt to transfer sexual fantasizing to encounters with other men. Some partners, you'll discover, are particularly adept at collaborating in your fantasies (see *Dirty Talk*). They talk during sex, expanding on the things you say and do, and will even act out quite elaborate scenes involving costumes, fetishes, and let's-pretend situations (army barracks, a locker room, the men's room on an airplane, and so on).

Jerking off with a partner has become the highlight of some men's sexual lives (see *J.O. Buddies*; *J.O. Clubs*; *Mutual Masturbation*). Still, men who feel guilty about jerking off ask, "Am I doing it too much?" You'll know you are when your body tells you. The skin on your cock shaft or glans will become chafed, or your dick may ache from being handled too much. Frequency of masturbation, like frequency of sex in general, is a measure of libido, boredom, anxiety, and a number of other factors, none of which is harmful. There can be one problem, however. Sometimes, a man will so finely tune his masturbatory technique that no one else can get him off. A partner often feels inadequate when that happens. One way of dealing with the situation is to cup your hand over your partner's hand and use his hand to jerk yourself off. That will show him how you like it done.

Having said all this, we should point out that the function of masturbatory fantasies is not simply to rehearse for playacting with sexual partners. Many men like to keep their masturbatory fantasies private, and the things they conjure up during masturbation they would never do with anyone else. The links between fantasy and reality are subtle and complex, so sharing your fantasy with another person might not suit you at all. Of course, if a lover understands, he will recognize that the roles you play in bed do not need to be carried into the rest of your lives. For instance, many gay men fantasize being raped. They like *pretending* to be overpowered this way in bed, but don't want to be raped in real life. But if you want to keep your fantasies private, fine; their only function is to redirect your focus from the mechanics of sexuality to its creative spirit and to shift your attention from meeting someone else's expectation to fulfilling your own.

Finally, we end this essay with a quote from another physician, Dr. Thomas Cogan, who, in 1589, wisely wrote:

> *The commodities which come by moderate evacuation thereof [that is, of semen] are great. For it procureth appetite to meat and helpeth concoction; it maketh the body more light and nimble, it openeth the pores and conduits, and purgeth phlegm; it quickeneth the mind, storreth up the wit, renewth the sense, driveth away sadness, madness, anger, melancholy, fury.*

What modern writer could have said it better?

Mirrors

Not the mirrors you look into while shaving or to check the crease in your trousers. Mirrors used in sex can be any size and shape and can be placed anywhere. One mirror or several, placed around the bed or staring down from the ceiling, can double your pleasure. To the joy of direct sexual involvement with your partner, they add another pleasure, that of watching yourselves. You can pretend you're a porn star. Mirrors can show you intriguing new angles on yourself and your partner during what may have become boring positions and activities. They can turn a duo into an illusory foursome. The more mirrors you have, the more fully you can see details and the whole scene; no matter what position you choose, you'll otherwise miss an angle or two. Some men like to look at themselves in the mirror while jerking off. They particularly like the image of their tensing muscles at the moment of orgasm.

Men have become such looking-glass addicts they've mirrored their bedroom, dressing room, and bathroom. But others are afraid of being branded narcissists and therefore avoid mirrors as though they cast evil spells. A bit more narcissism would make most men more secure about their body, especially when they check out exactly what each part looks like, from different perspectives, in various positions, aroused or not.

Mixed HIV Couples

With the advent and widespread use of various kinds of chemical "cocktails" to control the HIV from progressing as quickly as it did in the beginning of the AIDS epidemic, several unprecedented social, psychological, and medical situations have arisen. In addition, several conditions already in place have now become much more common among gay men and in gay life. One of these is relationships between people of mixed HIV status, where one of you has tested positive for the HIV and the other has tested negative.

Coming inside your lover, or having him come inside you, has always been one of the joys of gay sex. For the last two decades, these pleasures have largely been replaced by safe sex practices (see *Safe Sex*). If you or your lover is HIV-positive, it doesn't make any difference whether you are a long-term couple, fuck buddies for a few months, or just meeting. Simple yet practical measures such as wearing a condom and using spermicide lubricants while fucking ensure that the virus isn't transmitted from one to the other. If you're living together, it's probably best also to keep toothbrushes and razors separate (perhaps by color-coding?), and it's still recommended that you not kiss after flossing your teeth. Such practical measures are easily undertaken. However, it's the emotional upheaval of HIV that most threatens relationships.

For many gay men, an HIV-positive diagnosis can be shocking. While some men are capable of ignoring the implications of such a diagnosis and carry on with their life and their lover much as they did before, most men are thrown into turmoil and need time to come to terms with the consequences of this new knowledge. A preexisting couple, whether committed lifelong lovers or occasional fuck buddies, can be threatened by the sudden and often overwhelming fear of illness and death. There is also the terrible fear that the HIV-positive lover may transmit the virus to his HIV-negative lover. Historically, many new infections have indeed been transmitted in this manner, especially if the infected lover is barebacking (see *Barebacking*). Perhaps one member of the couple didn't know about his seropositive status and inadvertently passed on the infection. Others, concealing their secret out of various real and imagined fears, go ahead and risk exposing the other partner. Or perhaps the seropositive person is terrified that he will be abandoned by his lover at the very time he feels he needs him most. The HIV-positive person isn't likely to mention this fear to his lover because he realizes its irrationality or its uselessness. These may all sound like good excuses for unsafe sex. They're not.

Guilt is another ingredient in this emotional stew. The seropositive man may feel guilty about his former sexual behavior. The seronegative partner, on the other hand, may feel guilty not for what he's done, but rather for what he feels. His first reaction may be panic (though he's not likely to show it). "I want out of here," he may say to himself, "but I'm trapped." He's frightened that he may become infected, yet he feels that he can never leave the relationship. The healthy lover, who is frightened for himself, often compensates by taking charge of his infected lover's life, treating him as if he's physically and mentally crippled. This is likely to drive both men crazy.

Love in a relationship means many things. One is the freedom to ventilate feelings and reveal vulnerabilities that surface when danger threatens. The combination of guilt, depression, abandonment, and resentment can only be handled when lovers talk about these feelings truthfully. It's a scary but necessary process. It's also a good idea for both men to have support networks to help them with their feelings and to get advice from those in a similar situation. This is a time when friendship can be most valuable. Occasionally, a therapist may be called in to aid communication.

Lovers need to agree about who should be told about the diagnosis. Some seropositive men want to keep the information close to home and divulge it to very few, while others tell everyone. There is no right or wrong here. Occasionally, however, a seropositive man will ask his lover not to talk about it to anyone. This is unfair. The healthy lover needs to be able to express his fears to someone other than his lover.

What about sex? There is no reason to curtail it, so long as you are safe. In fact, some imaginative lovers use a new HIV-positive status to branch out, and to begin experimenting more with sex toys, kinky sex, uniforms, bondage, S/M. Problems will occur, however, if the uninfected lover starts to treat his partner like fragile porcelain, while the other lover still wants to have the same sort of sex they shared before the diagnosis. If he liked a rough fuck before, it's highly unlikely he wants to be touched like a sacred virgin now.

An HIV-positive man doesn't want to be treated like fine crystal *outside* the bedroom either. If you've always complained to him about some aspect of his behavior (say, not helping around the house), don't stop complaining now because of his diagnosis. Hard though it may be, don't show an exaggerated concern over every cough, groan, or pimple.

If you are a committed couple, at some point you'll feel comfortable enough to talk about the future. You'll want to get your financial and health plans in order (see *Insurance; Living Wills; Wills*).

It's a little different socially and emotionally—although not sexually—if you are an unattached HIV-positive gay man, especially if you are recently diagnosed. At first you'll probably think you'll never have sex again and wonder who out there would ever find an HIV-positive person desirable.

Luckily, many health clinics and gay community centers have substantial spaces and programs for meeting and associating with other seropositive men. If you are HIV-positive and in a sensual relationship with another HIV-positive man, safe sex is still critical. One of you may be using a series of cocktails that have side effects that affect him differently. Or your HIV may be "undetectable" by testing, while your partner's is still quite high.

Sometimes when you're HIV-positive, you meet someone who is seronegative or whose HIV status you do not know. Ideal though it would be, most people don't swap HIV status on first dates. Some encounters happen so quickly you may not have time to get the information or to let yours be known. Many men are afraid to let others know they are seropositive for fear the other man will lose interest, even if your status is positive but undetectable. Unfortunately that's a chance you have to take. If you lie and he finds out, not only will it probably end whatever relationship you've had, but he may feel justified in going around and telling friends about it, and in causing you other kinds of trouble—lawsuits, for example, aren't unheard of. Besides, he may have a perfectly good reason for being skittish around HIV-positive men. What if he's lived with, nursed through many bouts of ill health, and then *lost* a lover or best friend to AIDS or another disease? Few men not actively seeking sainthood are willing to take on that kind of task a second time. When you are together (but *not* while having sex), discuss the subject. Find out his ideas, his fears, how much information or misinformation he has. Once you've gotten to know each other better and you think he can handle it, tell him your status. If your relationship is genuine, it ought to survive the news. On the other hand, going around blurting out your HIV status indiscriminately—as some ham-fisted gay men tend to do—seldom attracts lovers.

Some gay men find that the easiest way to talk about HIV status is to ease slowly into the sexual part of the relationship. They'll only kiss, neck, and maybe, at most, mutually masturbate on a first encounter. At the second encounter, they may add some oral sex into the date. If pressured to have anal sex, they have a golden opportunity to say something like "Sure. Got a condom?" This is bound to bring up the subject of HIV and health. If your partner says he won't use condoms and refuses to discuss the situation or his HIV status, it's a good time to cool off the date and maybe even your new relationship.

Whatever you do, don't allow yourself to be pressured into having unprotected anal sex by someone who is either HIV-positive or who won't reveal his status. No matter how famous, good-looking, "out of your league," or "A-list" he may be, or you think he is, the truth is that *your* health and *your* life is on the line. No matter what he says or what you may think, you deserve better.

Mutual Masturbation

Back in the "medieval times" of the mid-1970s, psychiatrist David Ruben actually wrote and got away with a best-selling sex guide that said homosexual males only masturbated each other. Gays of his day used to read his section on homosexuality aloud at parties, trying to finish this short section while deflecting howls of laughter and lewd comments (amidst a hilarious good time for all) from fellow cocksuckers and sodomites.

Naturally, then and now, some gay men did (and do) prefer to jerk each other off. Especially in circumstances where privacy is difficult if not outright impossible, jerking each other off really is the easiest, fastest, and most effective way of having sex. Interviewed U.S. sailors and marines reported having this kind of sex, sometimes with other gays, sometimes with straight men, while awaiting action, or even while being shipped en masse into battle during World War II and the Korean and Vietnam wars. Partly they did it, they said, to pass long waiting times, and partly to release pent-up tension.

Today, mutual masturbation is unquestionably the preferred sex act of the health conscious, or if you are unsure of your partner's HIV status. It's also common if you are having sex with someone you just met and don't know much about. And if you're on a first date or still in that transitional period in which you are dating someone you're not totally comfortable with, it's a great way to have a good time without fear. Needless to say, mutual masturbation is a popular method of sex in public places.

For many gay or bisexual teenage boys, this is the only generally accepted kind of mutual sex, so if you are not certain you're gay and want to try sex with another guy, mutual masturbation is probably your first step. You can do it sitting, standing, lying down in bed, with one of you sitting and one standing, with one kneeling and the other standing. You can rub against each other while jerking each other off. You can look at each other's face, and body, and of course at each other's cock and balls. You can kiss, lick, nibble, or bite each other. You can do it naked, seminaked, clad only in underwear or jockstraps, or with only your cocks sticking out of your flies. And if you become very excited, you can instantly move from jerking off to other sex, say giving a blow job (see *Blow Job*).

Those who are expert in masturbation—and yes, some do call themselves jerk-off artists—are very expert indeed, and putting yourself in their hands leads to some of the best sex in your life (see *Masturbation and Fantasy*; *J.O. Buddies*; *J.O. Clubs*). Some men prefer to use no liquids while jerking you off. Some will utilize a little (or a lot of) saliva. Others have their specialty "lubes," which range from what you can find at your grocer's to what you can find at your local sex shop (see *Lubricants*). Olive oil, butter, K-Y, and all kinds of other oleaginous substances are used; it all

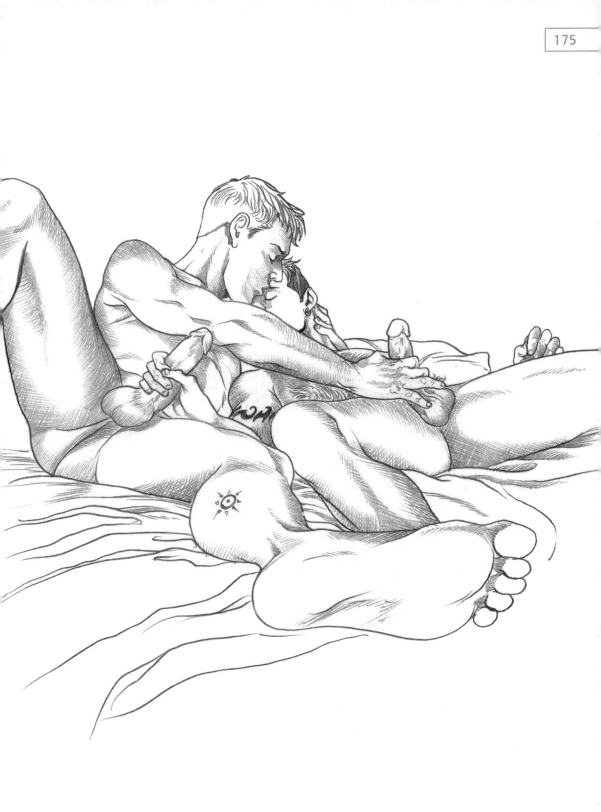

depends upon your "taste" during sex. One particular expert acquaintance of the authors, a corn-fed Midwest-farmboy type with particularly soft hands, swore by Corn Huskers lotion, and he made an excellent case for its repeated use.

Your only real consideration will be to give as good a time as you get, and if you are clothed, try to remember to point his cock head away from your Armani trousers when he comes.

Mythic Beginnings

One tribe in New Guinea believes that homosexuality results from eating the meat of uncircumcised pigs. Before you laugh, keep in mind that the Western world has invented other theories no less imaginative, and none have been substantiated. For that matter, no scientist has ever explained how people end up heterosexual, a matter every bit as mysterious.

Theories about the origin of homosexuality can be divided into three categories: folk, physiological, and psychological. The most common folk theory holds that boys become gay if they are molested by experienced older homosexuals. This is called the recruitment theory. But childhood seduction has no demonstrable influence upon the later sexual preference of the child. The trauma of childhood sexual abuse may make the individual fearful of *all* sex later in life, but it will not influence his sexual orientation (see *Early Abuse; Sex Phobia*). The recruitment theory is in reality nothing more than a smoke screen, designed to hide that most child molestation is heterosexual and occurs within the family.

A second folk theory holds that boys grow up to be gay if their fathers are weak and ineffectual. Such a theory equates homosexuality with inadequacy, a dubious identification. Moreover, it ignores that more than half of marriages end in divorce and a substantial number of children grow up without a father in the house. There is not a shred of evidence that sexual orientation is influenced either by divorce (no matter how bitter) or by the absence of the father.

Still another folk theory holds that gay men are afraid of women. This idea is sometimes called the *vagina dentata* theory; it is based upon the notion that a gay man hates his mother and transfers that hate to all women. Needless to say, there is no better support for this folk theory than for the others, and it ignores that many gay men have had and will continue to have satisfying sexual experiences with women.

The first person to propose a biological theory for the origin of homosexuality was the philosopher Aristotle. He wondered why some men (they were called catamites) liked to get fucked. In explanation, he suggested that such people have an extra nerve that ran to the rectum, which, he hypothesized, was stimulated during intercourse. No biological genius, Aristotle's extra-nerve theory doesn't hold up anatomically.

A nineteenth-century French doctor, Tardieu, claimed that active pederasts had a slender, underdeveloped penis tapered like a dog's, and that those assuming the "passive" role in anal intercourse had smooth rectums. One wonders how anyone could come up with anything so preposterous.

A number of other biological theories were proposed throughout the twentieth century to explain homosexuality. The simplest was genetic: Homosexuality is inherited.

The next biological theory was based upon hormone levels: Gay men were supposed to have excessive female hormones (estrogens) circulating in their bodies, but were deficient in male hormones (androgens). After decades of research that theory was found to be completely in error.

There have been just as many psychological theories. The first (and the quaintest) we know of was suggested by a Persian physician a few hundred years ago. He wondered why so many Persian men preferred to have anal intercourse with young boys rather than vaginal intercourse with their wife. He believed that the preference for vaginal or anal intercourse was determined by how a man learned to masturbate. He said that men were either "pounders" or "flippers." Pounders held their dicks tightly and in adulthood preferred the tightness of a boy's asshole, while flippers held their dicks loosely and therefore enjoyed the wideness of a woman's vagina. While obviously incorrect about the origin of sexual orientation, the theory allows us a small window through which to view a past society that was more positive than our own about both masturbation and anal intercourse.

Of the twentieth-century psychological theories, the most discussed are those of Freud and his successors. Describing what he called the Oedipus complex, Freud wrote that a boy of four or five wants to have sex with his mother. The boy is afraid, according to Freud, that the father will discover this incestuous wish and castrate him. To defend himself, the boy either identifies with his father, becomes heterosexual, and thereby enjoys a vicarious sexual relationship with his mother, or he identifies with his mother and becomes homosexual.

Later psychoanalysts rejected Freud's theory, which was based on the belief that everyone is born bisexual and is potentially either heterosexual or homosexual. These sexist psychoanalysts were uncomfortable with the notion of bisexuality and proposed, instead, that boys are turned into homosexuals by "castrating" or "engulfing mothers," women who are seductive toward their sons. Neither Freud's theory nor the later revisionist theory has the least bit of scientific evidence to support it, although this hasn't stopped the vast majority of psychoanalysts from trying to "cure" their homosexual patients.

It should be clear that there is no generally accepted theory to explain the origin of homosexuality. Researchers are still split between those who hold a psychological and those who hold a biological explanation. Research in endocrinology may one day reveal the secret of sexual orientation. For the moment, biological explanations of homosexuality remain hotly contested. Recent anatomical studies have suggested differences between male and female brains, and between the brains of gay and straight men. How data from anatomical studies will fit in with that from prenatal hormonal research remains to be seen.

But is there any reason to "explain" the origin of homosexuality? Whenever society, through its medical experts, has tried to "explain" homosexuality, such explanations have merely been pretexts for attempts to "cure" it. The cures have included castration, electric and chemical shock, imprisonment, and ostracism. Who can blame gays for being skeptical of the motives of straight authorities investigating the "etiology" of homosexuality? Don't let anyone try to change your sexual orientation. It's as natural as your need for food and drink.

Nibbling and Biting

Sensuality requires unpredictability. Just as a good conversationalist varies his tone, alternating humor with seriousness, small talk with big ideas, the full exposition with the abrupt transition, so a good lover keeps his partner slightly, wonderfully off balance. During a long, tender encounter, slow and dreamlike, a bite or a nibble can be the sudden flash of light amid the misty gray.

Your partner, say, is kissing you deeply, meditatively—but then he bites your lower

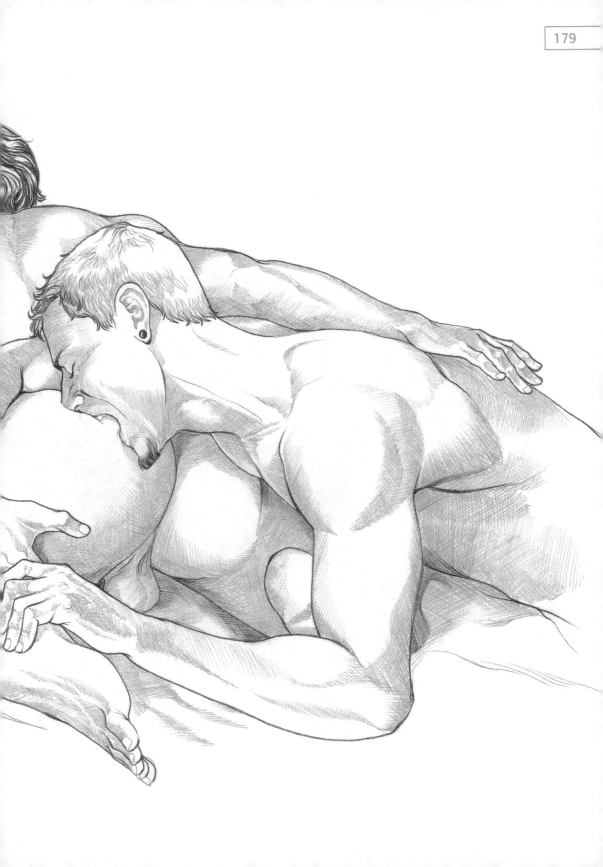

lip in a short, sharp nip. Or he is licking every square inch of your body, from your forehead to your toes, but when he reaches the tender flesh on the inner side of your thighs just below your crotch, he nibbles you playfully. Or you are alternately bathing his ear in saliva and blowing a cool stream of breath over the hot, wet skin—then you dive in to nibble his lobe.

Some people believe the ultimate is to nibble and worry one spot with a prolonged kiss and leave a hickey there, something he must hide the next day with a high collar or makeup toner. Others think hickeys too adolescent and prefer instead to nibble a partner's balls, nipples, or the cheeks of his ass. Each tastes different, and using lots of saliva while nibbling will cause your partner to writhe in delight.

Obviously you need to be careful about any behavior involving nibbling and biting that goes on too long. But as a rule, love bites can add the proper spice to a sexual meal.

Nipples

The Canadian poet Ian Young calls nipples "Corks bobbing / On a hot sweet sea." We agree. One of the hottest sights around is a pair of ripe nipples on proud pecs straining against—or even bursting through—the material of a tight T-shirt. To get your pectorals just right for that, you'll probably have to go to the gym and sweat through a lot of exercise. But to achieve outstanding nipples, you can exercise right in your own home. If you do it regularly, little by little, tit play will increase their size.

Doctors tell us that men and women have the same nerve endings in their nipples. There has been an increasing interest in tit play by gay men as they catch up on what women have always known: Your nipples are tight little bundles of sensation just waiting to be awakened. Erotic nipple play has become so popular that there are now Web sites and clubs on the Internet devoted exclusively to nipple action.

Gay men like nipple action every way, from feathery, soft kissing to biting and chewing to heavy S/M using "alligator clips," clamps, and weights—tit torture. Tit play is fun with a partner or by yourself while you're jerking off. If you are with someone, work on his nipples during foreplay, while you're sucking him off, or while you're fucking him. And consider this: You can play with someone's nipples before, after, or even instead of genital sex. Some guys love to play with each other's nipples after they've come: It's intimate and sexy.

When working on a trick's tits, start gently. Some men have extremely sensitive nipples, and a gentle touch to one guy is the equivalent of a bite to another. Don't assault nipples: Stroke them gently with fingers, lips, and teeth; and work up to more intense sensations. Listen to what your partner says: If he likes what you're doing and wants it harder, he'll definitely let you know, either by his physical reactions or by his words.

It may take you a while to discover the pleasure your own tits can provide when you're by yourself, but it's worth the effort to find out. Try brushing them lightly with your fingers or hand; then alternate that with kneading and massaging, while you masturbate. Start with a gentle touch and slowly increase the intensity. Fondle them, pinch them gently, then pinch a little harder. Tug the hairs around the nipple one at a time. Gradually work up to rougher stuff.

You may come to like some fairly rough chewing on your tits. Don't be surprised. Your response is perfectly natural. Babies have been chewing on their mother's nipples for millennia. Or you might want a more permanent kind of nipple action. If so, pierce one or both of them and put rings or bars through them (see *Body Decoration*). Should you come to prefer heavy workouts on your tits, you'll be rewarded the day after a session: As you walk around town, the sensation of your shirt against your sore tits will remind you of the man who worked on them.

Noisemaking

Making love without noise is like playing a muted piano—fine for practice, but you cheat yourself out of hearing the glorious results. There are, it seems, no studies on the effects of shouting, moaning, gasping, and whispering on the quality of sex, but many people report that noisy sex is richer and wilder then silent sex (see *Dirty Talk*). The sound of passion, apparently, releases greater passion, in much the same way that flamenco dancers or gospel singers spur one another on to new heights of frenzy by shouting their excited approval.

If you're inhibited about vocalizing your pleasure, you might try this exercise with your partner: Let him masturbate you. You should not reciprocate for the moment, but rather concentrate on your bodily sensations. Become conscious of your breathing. Inhale deeply, and then when you exhale, make a sound (as soft or as loud as you like). As your partner masturbates you, tell him what feels good. If you want him to go faster or slower along the shaft, tell him so. As you become more and more excited, allow your vocalizations to become louder. The point is to express your feelings. And when you come, don't hold your breath. Make as much noise as you can on a single deep exhalation. You'll also notice, as you arise from your swoon, that your partner is in a fever of excitement and ready for his turn.

After you've had noisy sex a few times, you'll probably make a few observations. First, vocalizing is a way of relaxing your diaphragm and throat and releasing your entire upper body. All too many people who are accustomed to furtive, silent sex freeze their upper body and confine their erotic sensations to below the belt. Second, you'll learn that your vocalizations excite your partner and let him know, moment by moment, what you are feeling; this enhances communication and establishes greater intimacy.

Zoologists who study animal behavior in the wild have pinpointed many *innate releasing mechanisms*, reciprocal signals that mating animals send one another to trigger the next behavioral sequence in sex. No one knows for sure if the sounds of passion function this way in humans, but at the very least, making noise seems to work in some analogous fashion. As your excitement rises, you make excited sounds, which in turn raise the level of your partner's passion until you are both caught in a reverberating cycle of pleasure.

On-line Cruising

The Internet has become the single most common place for gay men to cruise, but the most important thing to understand about on-line cruising is that most gay men who do it never took a course from Miss Manners. Don't expect politeness and empathy (see *Etiquette*). However, there are advantages to on-line cruising. It can be an alternative to going out to bars and clubs. Some men don't like drinking (or smoking) and prefer to be away from that kind of environment. It's also cheaper; you don't have to buy drinks. Somehow rejection via the Internet seems to be less hurtful than being rejected in person. And if you're not hooked up to a Webcam, you also don't have to look or dress your best (see *Webcams*).

You'll need to choose a screen name for the purpose of sending and receiving e-mail. We suggest three screen names. The first is for your family and straight friends—probably a variation of your name, squeaky-clean, dull, and unerotic, such as Roger235, indicating that there are 234 other Rogers who registered before you (and God knows how many after). The second screen name will be for your gay friends, used for when you gossip, joke, and talk about whatever interests you. BangBang-Roger is an example of one with some humor, and its ambiguity doesn't tell who's doing the "banging."

The third screen name is your on-line sex name. That's where marketing skills come in handy. In just a few letters you need to convey your sexual preferences and perhaps your geographical location. Top55SF, and Fuckmyfacenow are examples.

(Sites like Yahoo! and AOL are unlikely to allow you to use Fuckmyfacenow, but the gay sex sites will.) The first one indicates that you're a top in bed (and that there are fifty-four other tops also registered, or that you were born in 1955) and you live in San Francisco. Other tops are unlikely to apply. The second example indicates the urgency of your demand for sex. Humor in a sex screen name is to be avoided, as humor and lust seldom travel well together. Where humor does appear in the screen name (and in the profile), it usually indicates a sparkle to the gay man's personality—a turn-on to those gay men who want to get to know their sex partners, and a turn-off to those who don't. Some gay men have two sex screen names: They may use one for vanilla sex and the other to act out their raunchier sex fantasies (see *Vanilla Sex; Kinky Sex; Sleazy Sex*). We remind you to keep your e-mail names separate. It's seldom cool when, say, your mother or younger sister has to reply to Fuckmyfacenow's mail.

We repeat a caution you'll see in other entries in this book. Do not look for your lover's screen and e-mail names on his computer. To paraphrase Oscar Wilde, the second-worst thing in the world is not finding his screen names. Allow him his jerk-off fantasies, just as you'd like him to allow you your own (see *Couples*).

Depending upon the site, you may be allowed to do a search, specifying exactly whom and what you're looking for, for instance, a top if you're a bottom, or versatile guys if that's your thing (see *Bottom; Top; Versatility*). The search will generate a list of matching profiles. You'll then be able to e-mail the guy whose profile you've chosen, stating what piqued your interest. It may have been his picture, or his profile. "I like your profile" is a perfectly inane opener; tell him what you *liked* about it. You may be ignored if he already looked over your profile and wasn't interested. Obviously on-line cruising is not for the faint of heart.

Chat rooms are another great place for on-line cruising (see *Chat Rooms*). You'll see a list of the screen names of the people in the room at the time. According to the server, you may also be able to check their profiles. If you see one you like, introduce yourself to the guy. Perhaps respond to his screen name or to something he just said in the chat room. "I love come," you might say to Gymslut, and follow that up by talking about the come in your balls waiting to get out. Gymslut will either like it or he won't. But if he doesn't, someone else in the room might. At some point you (or he) will ask, "Are you looking to hook up?" Getting this far can take anywhere from ten minutes to many hours.

While many gay men say they use the Internet to meet other men for potential relationships, the truth is that dating results from on-line cruising a lot less frequently than do sexual connections. This has a lot to do with the nature of the Internet and the anonymity it supplies. "Let's get it on now or forget it altogether" tends to be the operating theory. Most of the time, questions asked and answered are about sex, not about your personal life. In the Brave New World of on-line cruising, a potential trick telling you he wants you to shove a twelve-inch dildo up his ass while squeezing his tits hard, then pulling on his balls with ten-pound weights, and pissing on him afterward is not considered personal—asking where he went to school is! On the other hand, there are tales of lovers who first met on-line. Anything's possible.

Many men who may be shy in public or feel at a disadvantage in one-on-one verbal exchanges often blossom on-line. It's true that you need to be something of a wordsmith on the Internet. Paint a picture in words of yourself and of what you want in someone else. Practice beforehand, or afterward, too, if you realize you've screwed up a potential connection because you fumbled over the words. The Internet is a great place to practice dirty (or sentimental) talk, if you and your partner are into it (see *Dirty Talk*).

A lot of married men are on the Internet. For obvious reasons, married men lack freedom and spontaneity of action, i.e., they can't generally leave home to have sex with you immediately. Gay men usually have strong feelings about this: Some like the idea of having sex with married men, others detest it.

The Net also has some annoyances. Particularly bothersome is the character who gets his jollies from "conquering" you. His object is to get you to desire him, after which he'll reject you and sign off. Should that happen to you, don't get even by doing the same thing to someone else. Just don't be caught a second time, and if you're in a chat room, let others know about this joker's game.

Let's say that you and Gymslut have met on-line and maybe spoken on the phone and decided to hook up for actual sex, and that you've reached agreement of what you're going to do. The final decision about having sex usually occurs when you show up at his door (or he at yours). What happens if there's no chemistry between you? Some gay men will simply say, "No thanks," and leave. But other, perhaps more socially conscious, guys argue that as long as you've gone this far, and as long as he doesn't look as if he lives under a rock, and he hasn't lied too wildly about his statistics, and he doesn't want to pour hot wax on your cock and balls—well, why not try him out? Given this situation, it's your call whether to have sex with him or flee and go home, where you'll jerk off to fantasies of your favorite stud. We offer no advice on this question; it's really up to you.

If we haven't already mentioned it, it's a pretty good idea to agree before you reach his place that the two of you will practice safe sex, and that you will not drink or use drugs. They interfere with good judgment, something you need when meeting anonymous men.

· · ·

Open Relationships

We're told that geese and other waterfowl have lifelong monogamous relationships. It's good to learn that there's at least one animal that does. We humans have a harder time being faithful to our lovers throughout life. It's not that long-term monogamy doesn't exist in gay relationships. It does, but not often.

Many unproven theories explain why men (gay or straight) have problems remaining with one sexual partner. Evolutionary psychologists maintain that the cause is genetic, the effects of evolution over tens of thousands of years, starting with the cavemen. Their impregnating as many women as possible in the shortest time was the most efficient way of ensuring the propagation of the species. Most mammals seem to behave the same way. Feminists adamantly reject genetics (and biological theories about anything), suggesting instead that our cavemen behavior is the result of social learning in a patriarchal society and our inability to form intimate relationships. A few of them call us sexual pigs.

Most men who are just entering into a love relationship assume or explicitly insist on sexual exclusivity. They only have sex with each other (see *Fidelity and Monogamy*). An open relationship often occurs after years of being together. It takes many forms. Some couples will seek a third man for a threesome so that they're together when having sex with another man (see *Three-Ways*). The Internet has made finding this person much easier nowadays (see *On-line Cruising*). Other men prefer the relative anonymity of getting together at either a jerk-off club or a sex club (see *J.O. Clubs; Sex Clubs*).

If one partner goes away on business, both might have the freedom to trick, but there are generally rules about whether the one staying at home can bring a trick home ("I don't want your trick in *my* bed!").

Many conflicts about tricking occur, including whether to adopt a "Don't Ask, Don't Tell" policy. There are minefields everywhere. Some lovers allow each other the freedom to occasionally trick in the belief that horniness is nothing more than "an itch that has to be scratched" and does not imply failure in the relationship. This policy works best if sex between the lovers remains exciting. It's also less threatening to the relationship if the outside sex is anonymous, such as in steamrooms and bathhouses (see *Baths*). "I don't want to know" is the most common response by that lover who doesn't trick out often, and generally that's a good choice. It's hard for any of us to keep our own feelings about competition and abandonment under control while hearing the details of a lover's outside sexual encounters (see *Jealousy, Envy, and Possessiveness*). One sometimes finds the lover who stayed home becoming intrusive by wanting to hear the graphic details of his beloved's sexual adventures; a voyeur to his lover's sex, becoming sexually excited listening to the account. The lover could feel intruded upon unless it leads to sex between them. More often, however, it leads to resentment in both: The voyeur may be angry because his lover has a different kind of sex with a stranger than at home, and the lover may resent the intrusion on his privacy and may also sense hostility.

In fact, most (but not all) couples go through alternating periods of monogamy and tricking. For many years, the AIDS epidemic was a good enough reason for couples to maintain monogamy. The possibility of bringing home one or more STDs is still a good reason to avoid tricking (see *Sexually Transmitted Diseases*).

We have said this before, but it bears repeating: Do not steam open your boyfriend's snail mail; do not figure out his password to anything; do not decide whether or not a profile on a sex board is his; do not to read his e-mail; do not listen to phone messages on his answering machine. If you suspect that he's tricking out, ask him (see *Couples*). But be prepared to have a real discussion about your feelings as well as his; about your feelings of envy as well as jealousy, about your fears as well as his. In other words, don't be a parent or schoolmarm; be a loving friend.

Out on the Job

You've just finished school—high school, GED, or college—and you've decided, or your and your family's circumstances have decided for you, that you have to join the workforce. Some of the first questions that are going to arise, among the many in dealing with this ordinarily difficult new situation, are whom you do come out to, how do you come out, and when do you come out?

Notice we didn't write *whether* you come out or not. In an earlier edition we might have put it that way. But not now. The reason, of course, is that we believe in gay liberation, and we believe that one of the best ways to achieve full civil rights for gay people is to come out to family, friends, colleagues, *and* coworkers (see *Civil Rights; Gay Liberation*). There are several reasons behind this imperative. First, many people who have been brought up to fear and loathe gays and lesbians for religious reasons still have not had *any* kind of relationship with homosexuals. These unfortunate people simply have to face living in a world with open, uncloseted gays. Whether you asked for the job of educating them or not, it is your job. They then will have the choice of how to respond to you. They can change jobs, ignore you, make trouble for you (and given today's sexual politics, much more trouble for themselves), or become your friend.

Second, you have every right to be recognized by your coworkers for who you are, without having to hide your sexuality. And if anyone tells you that telling someone at work that you are gay is being overly "political" or too "in their face," tell them you were brought up to believe that lying is even worse, and that's the only other alternative.

Third, if everyone in our life came out to friends, family, and colleagues, the straight world would be able to see how many GBLT people there actually are. This gives us a distinct psychological advantage; after all, there is strength in numbers.

In the United States today, there's probably only one good reason why you should *not ever* come out at work—if you have joined the U.S. armed forces. With their horrendously bigoted and intolerant Don't Ask Don't Tell policy, the military is a fag-baiting and homo-hunting group. If you think you'll get through your service unharassed, you'd better be very butch, extremely discreet, an expert liar, and really love the military.

In virtually any other federal job, including the State Department, the CIA, and the FBI, you can be openly gay. You can be a gay electrician, gay plumber, gay explorer, gay dogsled driver in the Arctic Circle, gay construction worker, gay oil-rig worker, gay dangerous-animal handler—you name it, there's a place for you, and don't let anyone tell you otherwise. It's about time the straight world accepted that while some of us are hairdressers or ballet dancers, others prefer traditionally male vocations.

Probably the best way to come out on the job is carefully. Check first to see if your city, state, or county has any rules on their books that make it a crime for you to be discriminated against for sexual preference. If such laws have been enacted, you're on totally safe ground. If they have *not* been enacted, ask other gay men about how *they* have handled such situations in the past. Don't go on what one person says; take a consensus. Many Western and Southern U.S. cities and states are hurling themselves headlong into the twenty-first century, and while they may not have legislated the required protections, they do understand the need to draw gays and lesbians to revive or enliven their workforce, inner cities, and tax base. Lawmakers in these cities will probably bend over backward to accommodate you. On the other hand, if you find yourself in a small town in a Bible Belt area, believing that your coming-out news will be greeted with a casual shrug of the shoulders is wishful thinking. Use your knowledge and your common sense. And in the latter case, unless you are bound to the place by unbreakable ties and believe your life and health would be in danger if you come out, you might consider getting protective legislation enacted, or at least begun, if only for your own future happiness and defense. We're sympathetic to gays who live in right-wing religious communities who choose not to come out because of harassment by employers, police, homophobic teenagers, and their families. But we would ask this: Why are you staying there?

Let's say you learn that your employment rights as a gay man are protected or that there is a casual attitude toward gays. How do you know the right time to come out? In an ideal world, the best time is probably during the initial job interview. But unless you are being hired by a gay firm, or a firm known to be friendly to gays, you will probably not find the time or opportunity to mention it, as the process will probably be tightly focused on work and experience. Let's say it is a gay-friendly firm; how would you come out in an interview? An easy and offhand way is best. Look for an opening. Say the person hiring tells you the company has a great softball team. You might answer, "Well, my boyfriend and I (or my partner and I) love softball," or some such phrase, keying him in that you're both a team player *and* gay.

If you are unsure that the initial interview is the time to come out, then try the first few days on the job. Orientation procedures, general training, and direct training are probably the easiest places to do it. Your supervisor during this time will likely *not* be your permanent chief, so it usually puts less pressure on you to tell her or him that you're gay. Again a low-key, casual approach is best. "My partner—or boyfriend—and I love Chinese food. Is there a good Chinese restaurant around work?" Or some such phrase will convey the information with as little threat as possible. And if you don't have a partner, you can say, "A guy I used to date for a while," or even, "this couple of guys I know who live together and I . . ." What is most important is that you say it boldly (not aggressively) without hesitation. To do otherwise will suggest that you're still upset about being gay.

Another good way to come out is if you are in a relationship and have exchanged rings. Someone will probably ask about your wife. Reply "My husband . . ." or "My partner . . ." and answer the question. If they're still dim-witted about what you're saying, be a bit more specific, using the pronoun *he* until they get it.

The last possible time you can come out *naturally* at work is when you are assigned to your permanent desk, unit, group, or office. Within a few days you will meet and get to know your colleagues. Some of them will end up feeling betrayed if you're gay and they *don't* know it. You don't have to call a general meeting for this; you could tell one person, the one you feel closest to or that you may trust the most. Follow your intuition. Within days, if not hours, everyone else will know.

Okay, you've come out at work. What happens next? Coming out at work entails, besides the initial process, several other potential hazards and pitfalls you may or may not be prepared for, many of them seemingly harmless at first. Say several coworkers invite you out for dinner after work. If you have a lover, tell them so. Allow both them and your partner to decide if he will be included. Or your coworkers may invite you to dinner at their home or out on a special occasion. Again, if they don't include him, you have to say something like "I have to check with Tom." If they don't ask who Tom is and/or don't make an immediate effort to include Tom, but plan to include other spouses, then it's best to decline the invitation. Don't make a fuss. Just say no. In time, they'll learn to ask Tom along or to stop asking you alone.

Another potential pitfall of coming out at work is that you will doubtless encounter what we call "professional homosexual lovers." Much like the Holy Roman Empire, which Voltaire quipped was neither holy, Roman, nor an empire, these people are neither professional, homosexual, nor do they love you. Well-meaning or ill-meaning—it makes little difference which—you can spot this type easily. They generally come up to you and say something apparently sympathetic if ham-fisted like "I never met a homosexual before, will you tell me all about being gay?" A good response is "I don't really have all that time, but I'd be happy to recommend *The Joy of Gay Sex: Third Edition*, where you'll find out all you want to know." Or recommend some other, less overtly sexual text, say George Chauncey's *Gay New York*.

Other professional homosexual lovers will appear to be more accepting, intelligent, and subtle at first, but will then do something that makes you feel totally stereotyped, such as asking you for decorating tips, fashion ideas, recipes, or your endorsements of the best plays and ballets in the area. To avoid being locked into an uncomfortably clichéd relationship with them, you might want to suggest a periodical you read containing the info. Better yet, tell them "I'm a lousy cook" or "I'm color-blind" or "I haven't seen a play since high school. But how about them Packers [insert your local professional football team here] last week?"

Another possible pitfall to coming out at work is that if you are single (and sometimes even if you are *not* single), straight coworkers will try to fix you up with the one other homosexual they know. Now it may not matter to them that he's nineteen years old, a weekend deer hunter who avidly collects submachine guns, and his idea of a good time is putting down a six-pack in record time, then bungee-jumping off your local Suicide Rock; while you're thirty-six, into bargello embroidery, African-violet gardening, and Russian films of the 1930s. They'll still assure you both that you're made for each other. If you agree to a date, this will cost you a single embarrassing night, along with a word or two afterward or the next day at the office laughingly pointing out how this combo couldn't possibly work, but you appreciate it anyway, thanks. You might want to add that your tastes in men are very, *very* fussy. The best prevention is to be appreciative but totally skeptical of being set up on a date by someone straight.

And of course there's one more possible pitfall to coming out at work. Someone, probably a guy, and probably an attractive guy—one you may have had your eye on from the first time you noticed him—may take you aside one day and quietly reveal that he's "interested" or "intrigued with this gay sex stuff," but has never done anything about it. Should that not get you equally intrigued, he may then or later move on to more suggestive topics, such as how he's always heard that gays are better cocksuckers than women, but hasn't been able to prove it; or some such not too subtle come-on. Many straight men are in fact attracted to other men, especially to gay men; and many straight men really love having gay men attracted to them, and they will flirt outrageously with gays on a level they'd never consider doing with a woman. But few of them will actually do anything physical about it, despite your giving them all the opportunities in the world. He'd rather be safe: have the fantasy of being with a gay guy while having sex with his wife or girlfriend. The chance that you can have sex with this man is probably about 20 percent. And that one in five who *does* end up having sex with you? Well, chances are, it'll be a onetime thing. He's done the experiment and now he's satisfied. So be prepared for that. It'll probably be more trouble than it's worth, as virtually all coworker sexual relationships turn out to be, heterosexual or homosexual. When will it *not* be more trouble than it's worth? If (1) he's unmarried and unattached, (2) you're unattached, (3) you are having really good sex, (4) you can stand being with him outside the bedroom, and (5) one of you is willing to find another job.

Parents

Coming out to parents can be difficult, especially if you are still living at home. The desire to come out to our parents is a measure of the growing self-esteem of gays. This wish is not only based upon a decision to be honest but also arises out of a need to communicate the good things that are happening in our lives.

A few tips about coming out to your folks: First, practice by coming out to some of your straight friends; study their reactions and examine how you feel as an out gay man. You should definitely consult your gay friends about their own experiences coming out to their parents.

If you feel you want to come out to your parents, it's best to choose a moment when you're alone with them, away from brothers and sisters or other relatives, and unlikely to be interrupted. However, if you're already out to your siblings, let them know what you're about to do. They can be helpful afterward. Also, make sure that you choose a time when they are relaxed. During this disclosure, do not confuse the issue of homosexuality with other matters ("No wonder I'm gay, Dad, you never paid attention to me"). No blame attaches to anyone for your being gay, so you should not allow your parents to accuse themselves, each other, or you.

Your parents may accept your homosexuality easily, or they may need a lot of time to accept it. Be sure to give them all the information they require; you may be surprised how little they know. Your disclosure, however, is likely to stimulate new worries about you. Two of the most common questions are (1) Won't you be lonely? and (2) What are you doing to prevent getting AIDS? Be prepared to answer them. You'd also be wise to bone up on research about biological and learning theories about the origin of homosexuality (see *Mythic Beginnings*). It's smart to get your folks a couple of books about homosexuality, especially those written specifically for parents. If there isn't a gay bookstore near you, check out the Internet (see Appendix). There are also gay book clubs on the Internet—insightoutbooks.com is a good one. Don't expect your parents to read books immediately; they'll need time to work up the courage. You might also tell them about the nearest branch of Parents, Families and Friends of Lesbians and Gays, a support group for parents. You can get a list of branches by writing to PFLAG, P.O. Box 27605, Washington, D.C. 20038. Since your parents are likely to feel shy about joining the group, you might offer to go with them. On the other hand, they might be uncomfortable if you accompany them, so don't feel resentful if they choose to go alone.

Your parents are going to need support and reassurance since your news may come as a big surprise. Tell them you're disclosing your homosexuality to them because you love them and want to share this important area of your life. Tell them you're the same son you've always been. Tell them you love them; they need to hear you reaffirm your affection for them, since they may have heard that homosexuals usually reject their family (a myth, but a common one). If they ask embarrassing details about your sex life (they usually don't want to know), just quietly tell them that your sex life is as private as theirs. You should accept the responsibility for telling your brothers and sisters and other close relatives that you're gay; don't leave it to your parents.

Another dimension of coming out to parents is introducing your lover. More and more parents are accepting their son's lover, but one still finds some attacking the relationship, usually with the panicked rationalization that "he" made you gay, or if it weren't for "him," you'd marry that nice girl around the corner.

A visit to one's parents during a holiday is often full of skirmishes. "You're coming home *alone*, aren't you?" from a parent is not so much a question as it is a command, which usually means "Don't bring that bastard into my house!" Some gay men need their parents' approval so badly that they leave their lover home. A different kind of gay man will say, "We're a couple, and we go places together. If that's not satisfactory, we won't visit you. Think it over and call me when you've decided what you want." Some gays find it helpful to invite recalcitrant parents to visit them and meet a lover before visiting the parents' home.

Often the difficulty comes from only one parent. Try to avoid playing one against the other, although naturally you want to enlist as much support as possible in helping you win acceptance from the recalcitrant parent. In some cases it's a sibling who reveals unsuspected depths of prejudice. This must be confronted. Don't worry that one or both parents will be so shocked that they will have a heart attack. That's an absurd notion. Your homosexuality cannot kill anyone. Even though it's anxiety-provoking, coming out to parents has its rewards. Not coming out to them cheats you out of that.

For many years, AIDS or one's HIV status has increased the pressure on gay men to divulge their homosexuality to their parents. A seropositive gay man may no longer want to hide his lifestyle, even if the cocktail has contained the virus (see *HIV Disease*). Some gay men have come out to their parents only after being diagnosed with HIV disease. The most conflict-laden scene occurs when a gay man lying mortally ill in a hospital tells his parents that he is gay and simultaneously that he has contracted AIDS. This is a classic double whammy. As a son, recognize how difficult this will be for your parents to absorb, and help them by directing them to friends, social workers, or medical staff who can answer many of the questions they're sure to have.

The HIV crisis has confirmed what we know about parents and their capacity for love. The majority of parents respond with compassion for their son. They support their son emotionally, financially, and physically. So do other relatives. These parents have also recognized the value of their son's lover and friends, who share the burden of caring for the ill son by cooking for, washing, and crying with him. In these cases, parents, lovers, and friends also provide important support for each other.

Unfortunately, not all parents are loving people. In fact, a shocking number of them have turned out to be selfish and narcissistic in their reaction to the AIDS crisis. "How could he have done this to *me?*" is a typical comment from such a parent. These parents totally abandon their son. They refuse to visit a son who is ill; they refuse to phone or to write. Frantic calls from the son's lover or from other family members are ignored. If a sick son wants to visit them, they refuse to see him.

After the son's death, these selfish parents swoop down and steal his body without informing the son's lover or friends, the very people who cared for him throughout his illness. They dispose of it in a private ceremony so that they won't be embarrassed by a funeral. They certainly don't attend the memorial services held by the lover or the friends of the son. Often, their final revenge on their son for his homosexuality is to violate the terms of his will.

The HIV crisis has not created these monsters; they were there all the time. But AIDS has forced us to rethink our relationship to our parents. We are reminded that some parents do not love their children and possibly never loved them—or anyone else, for that matter.

Some gay sons should *not* come out to their parents ever; they should refuse to have anything to do with them. This is not said lightly. Gay men who come from spiteful families must (and doubtless will) seek support and love elsewhere, because in their cases, love never has and never will come from their parents (see *Gay Families*). It's hard enough to give up parents when they die; oddly, it appears to be even more painful emotionally to give up unloving parents. Perhaps it's terrifying to realize that you were right about them all the time.

· · ·

Phone Sex

Ma Bell was heavily into the sex business until the Internet arrived on the scene. Every gay newspaper and magazine carried advertisements featuring hunky models with big dicks encouraging you to call them. For just a dollar or two a minute, you'd find a dreamboat of a man who's impatiently waiting for you. Thousands of men called for two reasons: to jerk off or to meet men. While the Internet has made connecting a lot easier to meet men for sex, phone lines still have their appeal.

On the phone, you don't have to look your best, and the guy talking knows how to help you get off, as you do him. It's a cooperative venture. Some gay men have so fine-tuned their voice and manner of speaking they still prefer phones to computers even if it costs more.

Jerking off on the phone has many advantages: For one, there's no need to worry about unsafe sex. Another reassuring aspect is the safety you get with anonymity. Phone sex is not threatening, and while other callers can reject you, it seems to hurt less than it does face-to-face. And there's always someone else to call and talk to. With the fear of rejection diminished, gay men are free to stretch their imagination to the limit.

Phone sex might even teach you about some aspects of the mysteries of Eros that you never thought about before. Do you love light, boyish voices and turn off to deep, masculine tones that smack of your father's cold authoritarianism — or do you tremble and grow weak in the knees when a guy's deep voice has the comforting authority of your favorite radio or TV announcer? A Midwestern accent may fill you with thoughts of rolling around in a meadow with a corn-silk-blond farm boy, even though you're aware that the body attached to the voice is that of someone who works in a three-piece suit. To one man, a sleepy, slow Southern voice may summon up visions of long, lazy nights of tender lovemaking, while to another it's a reminder of homophobic rednecks.

There's absolutely no truth in advertising on the phone. Any cock that measures from four to seven inches is described as eight inches long, cut or uncut, depending upon what the owner thinks you want to hear. If it's actually eight inches, the proud possessor will boldly proclaim it's a nine- or ten-incher. He may even have given his cock a name in honor of its imposing size, although to our knowledge no one has fully cataloged the nicknames of people's peckers. Inversely, as additions are made to cock size, subtractions are made from age. The general rule seems to be a five-year discount, so a thirty-year-old claims to be twenty-five, a forty-year-old claims to be thirty-five, and so on. Contrarily, younger guys, in their teens or early twenties, sometimes increase their age a few years so as not to frighten away older gentlemen (in their thirties).

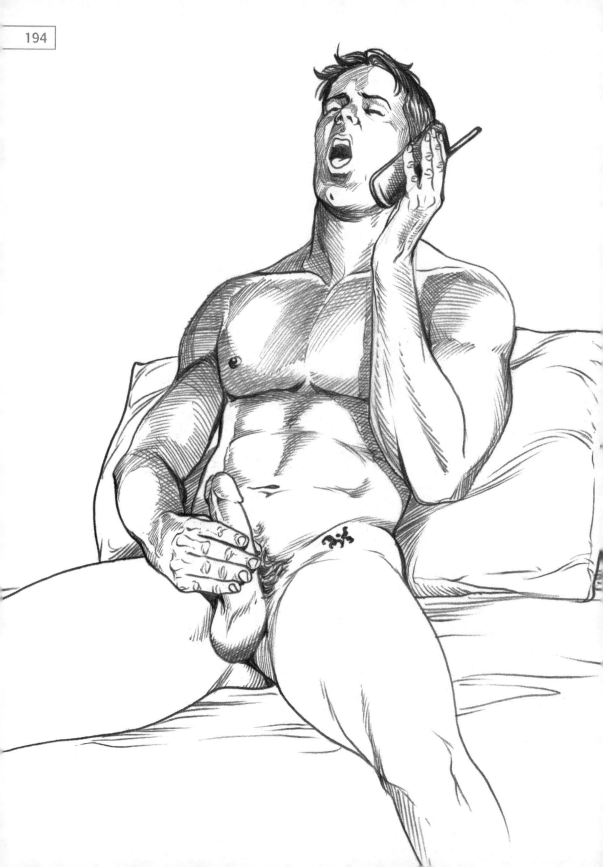

Other physical descriptions are usually equally imprecise. A man who describes himself as a football player is probably overweight. The caller who claims to have a swimmer's body may be thin, perhaps very thin—unlike professional swimmers.

All this exaggeration (and blatant lying) is perfectly all right, even preferable, if your intention is simply to use phone contacts to jerk off. Under those circumstances, why let any inhibitions keep you from describing yourself as perfect, whatever that may mean. Embellish your fantasy with whatever sexual desires you've been suppressing. Many gay men, for instance, have rape fantasies, but fear telling lovers (or gay friends) about them. The phone is the perfect setting to indulge this scenario. Your temporary sex partner will be delighted to "rip off your clothes, throw you on the bed, hold your hands down, and fuck the shit out of you." Don't bother to wonder whether his description is accurate. It's all make-believe, just for fun, to get a load off.

On the other hand, you may actually want to meet people through the phone sex lines or phone calls made from ads. In this case, we advise you to describe yourself accurately. If you're standing in the rain at 3 A.M. ringing someone's doorbell, and you have described yourself over the phone as looking like Tom Cruise, don't expect to get in if, instead, you resemble Henry Kissinger. It makes no sense to lie if you want to meet men over the phone. Lying indicates you're insecure about your body, which turns people off. And you may find someone who's aroused by the very thing you feel insecure about in your body. Find him, and you'll not only have a good time, but you'll end up feeling better about yourself.

It does make a difference when you call. For example, on weekdays, from 7 to 9 A.M. is when you're likely to hear someone say, "Can I take care of your morning load?"—i.e., it's jerk-off time. Then you're off to work like everyone else. The afternoon can also be jerk-off time, but with a different group; that's when horny artists, freelancers, and waiters frustrated with work take to the phones. Early evening is slump time for phone sex. People are going about their business, meeting friends, having dinner, going to the movies. Prime time for phone callers is 11 P.M. to 2 A.M. These are "the relentless hours." From 2 to 6 A.M., weekdays, you may hear from people who've been partying all night on drugs and alcohol and have artificially heightened desire. Often, because of the drugs, they can't get hard-ons and would be dreary sex in person, but not necessarily over the phone (see *Booze and Highs; Drug Abuse; Drugs and Sex*). The post-club-going crowd, high on ecstasy, may also call at this time.

Weekend nights on the phone are often not about jerking off, but about setting up a meeting. Phone lines are at a premium on weekend nights, and busy signals are common. Couples looking for a third party to spice things up at home most often use phone lines then.

If you invite to your home someone you've never met, check through your peephole to be sure only one person shows up. Unless you planned it that way, if there's more than one, don't let them in. Some men believe it's less dangerous to go to the other man's house. Others prefer a neutral place like a street corner or coffee shop, where they can look over and talk with the guy before bringing him home.

Having phone sex is simple. Dial the number. If you reach your party, start talking.

If, instead, you get a *recorded message* asking whether you prefer a one-to-one or group line, it means that no matter what the sex-ad said, you have reached a pay phone service. The recorded message should tell you the cost of using it. If it doesn't, hang up immediately.

If you continue, you'll hear a beep, which means you're connected. Start talking, perhaps saying "What's up?" or "What are you looking for?" Don't expect men using these phone lines to chat or get to know you. If someone responds, find out whether he's interested in jerking off or meeting. If you want to meet, find out where he lives; you may or may not want to go to his neighborhood, or travel may take too long. Find out what he's into, what type of sexual scene turns him on, and make sure you are compatible. You may also ask what he's wearing. Attire (or lack of it) is extremely important for men into jockstraps, specific kinds of uniforms, underwear, rubber, latex, or leather (see *Uniforms*). If something turns you on, say so, describing exactly what you like about it—and how your hard cock feels. Don't be shy.

To reduce phone bills (which can reach astronomical heights if you're not careful), some men give their phone numbers and hang up. If you do this, be prepared for sex calls anytime, day or night. Caller ID and cell phones are useful in screening callers—if that's what you want to do. Some gay men have two phone lines under different names: one for friends and family, the other for sex.

On the phone, your attitude is important. Being nasty or overly aggressive is usually rewarded with a dial tone. On the other hand, sounding like a top or being authoritative may be just what someone is looking for. There is a fine line between them. On the phone, being verbal is crucial. Use adjectives describing yourself and your favorite sexual scenes. If you don't know which words to use, watch a porn video and note those words that turn you on. You're trying to conjure up an image for the other guy. Having a sexy voice helps. If yours is high-pitched or odd in some way, practice talking with a hushed, lowered voice, or with a slight accent of some kind to change its sound.

Finally, in phone sex, as one phone habitué puts it, "the come-audio is very important." Since you won't actually see each other ejaculate, only the sounds you make while coming provide the image of your coming to your phone partner. If you usually come quietly in real life, turn the sound up until it's a missile exploding. If your come dribbles in real life, on the phone pretend it hits the walls—or better yet, all over your face—"And I want you here to lick it off." Coming over the phone should take much longer than in actuality. The exaggerations make it more sexual, and more fun.

Along the way, some guys may hang up. Don't take it personally. Some will say good-bye, others won't, and after all, time really does mean money if you're paying. You may not fit his fantasy, or he may want to meet someone in his own neighborhood.

Is using the phone for sex psychologically harmful? If you use it to get your rocks off from time to time, it's a minor diversion, no problem. But if phone sex is a persistent, expensive habit, and if you use it instead of meeting other gay men and forming relationships, then it could be a real problem. Jerking off on the phone can become so specialized it interferes with your ability to have a face-to-face physical relationship. If that happens, or if you go to it when you're having personal problems with a lover, then you're becoming dependent and you should probably stop having sex on the phone for a while. After all, you can't settle a conflict with someone you care for by hanging up on him. No, that requires exposing your emotional vulnerability, a type of behavior scrupulously avoided in phone sex.

So avoid the trap of using your phone to avoid intimacy or evade real human companionship. The trials and tribulations in actually meeting guys face-to-face and crotch-to-crotch can be avoided by using phone lines, but don't forget the phone is just an inanimate object and in the long run no substitute for coupling, kissing, sucking, fucking, and a real-live beating human heart.

Pleasure Trap

A man caught in the pleasure trap is willing to give pleasure to others but does not seek his own sexual gratification. He says he doesn't mind if he doesn't have an orgasm; all he wants to do is make you feel good. In tricking, such a person seems an ideal partner, completely unselfish and giving. But in a long-term relationship his refusal to express his own needs becomes (or at least is perceived as) a form of hostility. A relationship always implies reciprocity, and the man caught in the pleasure trap refuses to allow reciprocity.

What causes some men to give but not take gratification? They may be attempting to blackmail their partners into loving them by acting so unselfishly; the unconscious bargain they are proposing is "I will satisfy your sexual needs if you will take care of my emotional ones." Or they may be afraid to feel the full force of their sexual impulses, fearing that if these needs were ever unleashed, they would become all-devouring. Or they may suffer from poor self-esteem or body image, believing that they don't deserve sexual pleasure and surely don't have the right to ask for it (see Body Image; Guilt). Or they may be martyrs, hoping to demonstrate their long-suffering patience (and thereby manipulate their partner). Some men suffer from the pleasure trap because of their own homophobic hatred.

Whatever the origin of the problem, it *is* a problem and should be treated. Not only does it cheat both lovers out of the thrill of mutual sex, but it also causes the afflicted individual to feel alienated from his own body. Working with a lover on the problem can help, though most people will need to enter psychotherapy.

Pornography

But I warn you, with yet more solemn emphasis, against EVIL BOOKS *and* EVIL PICTURES. *There is in every town an undercurrent which glides beneath our feet, unsuspected by the pure; out of which, notwithstanding, our sons scoop many a goblet. Books are hidden in trunks, concealed in dark holes; pictures are stored in sly portfolios, or trafficked from hand to hand; and the handiwork of depraved art is seen in other forms which ought to make a harlot blush.*

So wrote Henry Ward Beecher, a hundred and fifty years ago, about the dangers of pornography. Even earlier, in 1675, a group of young dons at All Souls College were caught using the Oxford University presses to print copies of Giulio Romano's engravings of Aretino's *Postures*, the most famous, possibly the only, illustrated sex manual of the day. We don't know what punishment they were given for their pornographic (or commercial) interest. And in 1889, the novelist Henry James wrote in a letter of some sadness that young men in front of him at Westminster Abbey were passing around photographs of naked Italian men (probably by Von Gloeden) at a memorial service for the poet Robert Browning.

Gay porn is divided into soft-core and hard-core. Soft-core consists of photos of men dressed, partly dressed, or naked, but usually alone and without erections. Hard-core pornography, on the other hand, consists of photographs, stories, films, or videotapes of guys masturbating, sucking, fucking, and actively engaging in sex. Besides rental videos, porn can be found in porn theaters, on TVs at some bars, sex clubs, baths, and private parties, and more recently, on the Internet.

The object of pornography is to sexually turn you on. Most people use pornography to excite themselves to a point where they will either jerk off or have sex with a partner. In fact, lovers often use pornography as a prelude to having sex together. Some feminists claim that pornography has another purpose, to demean women, while right-wingers say that porn is designed to destroy the nuclear family. These groups have their own political agendas. It is, however, true that men are more easily aroused sexually by visual means than most females are; whether this is biological or the result of socialization is still hotly debated.

Almost anything can become pornography. An underwear or swimsuit ad in a magazine, an International Male catalog, even an ad for beer or a soft drink can be arousing. Some are turned on by drawings in which specific physical details (rounded buns, big cocks, massive chests) have been emphasized. Many young boys get their first glimpse of nudity by thumbing through old *National Geographics*, conveniently found in most school libraries. The Internet provides easy access to thousands upon thousands of porn sites, ranging from personal photo collections to subscription sites with interactive features, downloadable video clips, live sex shows.

Videos, however, are where gay pornography remains the most sophisticated. Gone are the days of amateurishly shot, grainy, black-and-white, 16mm flicks. DVDs and videotapes have replaced films, and a whole new array of porn stars has been acclaimed.

Few videos or photographs leave much to the imagination, and as a result, some men turn to written pornography. That the protagonist's looks are only suggested can be a real stimulant to the imagination. A whole genre of quickie gay novels is available in most pornography shops, along with true-story anthologies of gay sexual experiences from military scenes to boarding schools, prisons, and travel. Some of these books, with their memorably suggestive covers, are offshoots of the "homo" paperbacks of the fifties, the golden age of gay pulp, before gay literature, magazines, and videos became generally available. What few photos there are in these newer versions are mostly either of young, blue-collar semihustlers or bodybuilders. At their best, these books are not only sexy, they're informative, intriguing, politically and socially savvy.

The only psychological disadvantage to pornography is that it could easily give rise to unrealistic expectations and dissatisfaction with the looks and performance of a sex partner. In the constant interplay between the need for intimacy and the need for fantasy, neither should crowd out the other.

Problems of Ejaculation

There are two kinds of ejaculatory problems—*premature ejaculation* (coming too fast) and *retarded ejaculation* (coming with great difficulty or not at all). While people with retarded ejaculation exercise *too much* control over their sexual responses, those afflicted by premature ejaculation lack control—or rather, have too little awareness of their bodily cues. A man who ejaculates prematurely is not aware of what's happening inside his cock and particularly in the muscles surrounding it.

One self-help technique for coming too fast is this: Choose an understanding partner to jerk you off to the point of coming. Concentrate on your sensations and be on the alert for signals of imminent ejaculation. When you think you're about to come, tell your partner to stop masturbating you. Once the urge to come has abated, ask him to start jerking you off again. Once more stop him when you're close to climax. Repeat this exercise twice more; then go ahead and come. Sex therapists call this the stop/start technique.

During the next class (school was never like this!) your partner sucks you off to a point just short of climax. When you feel you're about to come, stop him. Repeat three times, then come. The final step is fucking.

When fucking, the best way to start out is with your partner on top (see *Sitting on It*). He should make slow movements up and down on your cock while you concentrate on your own physical sensations. When you feel that orgasm is near, stop him. Repeat three times. On the fourth time, go ahead and come. After you have overcome premature ejaculation in this position, you can switch to the side-by-side position (see *Side by Side*). Always go slowly. And remember, safe sex guidelines should always be followed during these exercises.

Men who suffer from retarded ejaculation—i.e., they come very, very slowly or not at all—perform adequately until it's time to come, and then they can't. As a rule, they usually have no problem coming while jerking off in the privacy of their bedroom. Other men have no problem coming when someone else jerks them off or sucks them off, only when fucking.

The immediate physical cause of retarded ejaculation, it is believed, is involuntary muscular overcontrol. The muscles around the genitalia appear to lock shut and there is nothing you can do about it, since they are under the control of the autonomic (involuntary) nervous system (see *Male Sexual Response*). That means that the problem originates, like almost all sex problems, in the brain. It's a common response in men who are extremely tired (this is also true of impotence). But it may also occur in a man who's been fucking for a long time but trying not to come. He may succeed all too well. In these cases the problem is situational, and not chronic.

The deeper, psychological cause, however, is probably anxiety. Fear of sex, guilt about homosexuality, anxiety about pleasing one's lover or about giving in to the loss of psychological and physical control during an orgasm—all are possible factors. A number of psychologists also suggest that a strong unconscious hostile element may be involved. Whether anxiety is channeled into impotence, retarded ejaculation, or the inability to get fucked may depend upon one's psychological makeup. An impotent man will become flooded with anxiety; a latecomer, by contrast, probably doesn't feel anxious at all (see *Impotence*).

If retarded ejaculation is persistent and long-standing, this exercise should help. If you have no problem masturbating alone, be sure to continue your jerk-off sessions.

One evening, ask someone you completely trust to sit in the next room while you jerk off to orgasm (see *Fuck Buddies*). The next night invite him to sit in the next room while you masturbate for a few minutes. As you approach climax, he should enter the room, *but not look at you*. The next day he should come into the room while you jerk off, at first with his back to you, the next time facing you.

Stagy and contrived as this procedure might sound, it follows a sound principle — psychologists call it *desensitization*. In any set of desensitization exercises you start with a situation that provokes no anxiety, then slowly move, step-by-step, toward the situation that alarms you. In overcoming retarded ejaculation, you are moving from jerking off alone, a relaxed situation, to jerking off in front of a partner. Once jerking off with him in the room and facing you is comfortable, he ought to come closer, and just as you're about to climax, he should take over (the crucial moment) and jerk you off.

Latecomers habitually study themselves and watch their partners for reactions. This scrutiny only makes the problem worse. Turn out the light and surrender to your fantasies (see *Masturbation and Fantasy*). Forget about your cock, forget about what your partner is thinking, and picture a mouthwatering scene. If no fantasy springs to mind, use dirty pictures or a porn tape (see *Pornography*). As you get caught up in this distracting whirl, your partner should jerk you off to climax. Concentrate on the video or the story, not on what he's doing (see *Dirty Talk*). On the next evening he should go through the same procedure. Finally, try fucking him after you're midway through jerking yourself off.

Psychotherapy is not especially recommended for ejaculation problems, though sex therapy may be quite useful. Find out the name of a professional sex therapist and consult him or her. If you or your lover have become anxious in your attempts to cope with the problem, you may both welcome the assistance of an objective third person.

Temporary problems of ejaculation are notorious side effects in men taking certain kinds of antidepressant medications (see *Depression*). One of the new classes of these medications is the selective serotonin reuptake inhibitor, more commonly called SSRI. It includes such drugs as Prozac, Paxil, and Effexor. They have been lifesavers for some men, reducing feelings of depression, and making life livable again. But the downside is that they lower your libido and your ability to get erect and to come. The higher your dosage, generally the lower your libido. Some men experience all these effects at once; others still feel aroused, but no matter what they do, or how much a partner helps, they can't come.

It's a shame some depressed men feel they have to choose between being depressed and having a sex life. Many simply stop taking the drugs. That's a mistake.

There are two ways of handling the problem. If an SSRI is effective in treating your depression, ask your doctor for another medication that will alleviate the sexual side effects. If that doesn't work, switch to a non-SSRI antidepressant. Wellbutrin is one of the most popularly prescribed substitutes. But don't become worried about your problem of not coming; it's only temporary. Stopping the antidepressant will bring back your usual genital responses.

Party drugs present other problems for those wishing to have a normal sex life (see *Drugs and Sex; Drug Abuse; Booze and Highs*). Some of the most popular drugs may make you feel good, but your sexual functioning will be reduced to zilch.

Profiles

Your profile on a gay site or chat room is your marketing tool, the hook written by you in such a way as to entice other gay men to meet and have sex with you. For some profiles, you may be asked to answer a list of questions, while others are more open-ended, allowing you to be more creative.

When putting together your profile, first are your screen name, your age, height, weight, hair and eye color, type of build, and your location, which might be the name of your town if you live in a rural area, or your neighborhood if you live in a city. There's no point in lying about your physical characteristics unless you never plan to meet anyone in person. Many gay men interpret lying as a sign that you feel uncomfortable about yourself and your body, and they'll reject you because of that. Remember this is not an exercise in trying to look like Adonis; it's about marketing yourself. If your ears make you look like Dumbo, don't hide the fact, celebrate it. Make them a part of the sex scene.

Next in your profile are your hobbies, sexual and otherwise. Some gay men want to be appreciated as a total being, not only for the size of their cock. They'll talk about hobbies, travel, life experiences, and that may be appealing to other gay men, particularly those looking for personal relationships. On the other hand, for some men lust is 100 percent of the game. They'll only talk about sex, making every attempt to turn you on by their sexual fantasies. They may neither know nor be interested in your "real" name. You're just a trick (see *Cruising; Tricking*).

You would be well advised to practice writing out your profile before you actually post it. See how it looks and sounds, but always remember, you're not filling out a résumé for a new job—you're trying to attract guys! Don't use too many words; someone browsing profiles is usually incredibly impatient. At the slightest sign of boredom he's on to the next profile.

Men are turned on by images; the sight of a cute body actually releases testosterone, and other men want to see what you look like. Should you picture yourself dressed or undressed? Depends upon what you're hoping to get out of posting your profile. If you have a perfect body and are looking for identical, godlike guys, show as much of yourself as possible. Ditto if you are hairy and looking for bear admirers, or if you are heavy-set and trying to attract chubby chasers, or older but in great shape and want primo young guys interested in a daddy, or if you're well-hung and looking for "cock worship" (see *Bears; Daddy/Son Fantasies*). Also use a naked picture to demonstrate what kind of sex you're interested in—lying on your stomach with your naked butt in the air should spell out *bottom* to all but the brain-damaged, while showing yourself trussed up from the ceiling with a hard-on unequivocally spells out *bondage* (see *Bottom; Bondage and Discipline*). But also keep in mind that a single piece of clothing worn well—Jockey, jockstrap, or whatever—can be more provocative than nudity.

There's also the question of context; whether only you (and your bed) can be seen in the picture, or whether you want to show a background such as your sailboat (and your chic or funky marina), or a mountain trail you're hiking, wearing butch, ankle-high boots, or a beach you're relaxing on, in nothing but a revealing Speedo. The context of the photo can provide a great deal of information about you and the values you hold dear. A picture of you sitting on the front porch reading a hardcover book makes a different statement than one showing you jerking off on your bed while drooling over a porn magazine. Neither one is right or wrong. But the Internet being what it is, the jerk-off picture will doubtless get more responses, while those who respond to the book will choose you more for your character than for your cock.

Some guys browsing on-line will not respond to a profile that doesn't have a picture. Rightly or wrongly, a percentage of them will interpret its absence as a sign that the person is ugly and ashamed of his body; while others can't be bothered to stick around and read a profile unless they see exactly what they're getting themselves into.

We believe your profile should include the words *safe sex only*. That cuts out barebackers, men who are seemingly dedicated to perpetuating the HIV disease epidemic (see *Barebacking; HIV Disease*). If you don't specify safe sex, you're likely to have to answer the question of your HIV status; you'll be surprised how many gay men are smart enough to ask.

You'll also have to state whether you're "chemically friendly." That means how open you are to drug use. You might as well be up-front about this because men who respond to your profile will want to know. Drug use can be as mild as a few tokes of pot or a glass of wine, or as heavy as using crystal meth, coke, even heroin (see *Drugs and Sex; Drug Abuse*). We believe you should avoid heavy drug use, not the least because of their association with HIV disease and STDs (see *Sexually Transmitted Diseases*). Getting zonked out on drugs isn't a good way of protecting yourself from being robbed or worse while tricking. We think your profile should state: "Not chemically friendly."

* * *

Promiscuity

The word *promiscuity* is usually used pejoratively, as in loaded statements such as "The AIDS crisis is a direct result of promiscuity in the gay community." It's not a neutral description but a moral condemnation, and it's used against gays by anyone or any group that condemns homosexuality. What constitutes promiscuity depends upon the speaker and his value system. One person will call a man who has two sexual partners promiscuous; another will reserve this condemnation for a regular frequenter of brothels. As a rule, gay men call someone promiscuous if he has sex with a lot of different guys.

Such a man is often called a slut or whore (sometimes by himself) because he has a greater sexual appetite than most of us. People say he is promiscuous because he won't "grow up" and "settle down" with a lover. Interestingly enough, the word *promiscuous* is seldom applied to men who have a chain of relationships over a period of years—what is usually called serial monogamy—because these relationships occur only one at a time.

The word *promiscuous* should be retired from the vernacular. As a rule of thumb, if a gay man is unattached, there is no harm in his having as much (safe) sexual experience as he wants. If he has a lover, they should decide how much sex, if any, they will allow outside the relationship, and under what circumstances (see *Couples; Fidelity and Monogamy; Jealousy, Envy, and Possessiveness, Open Relationships*). One lover having sex without the other's knowledge is not promiscuity but dishonesty; this situation is best viewed as a failure of communication rather than a moral flaw.

On the other hand, some men's obsession with sex is so severe that it threatens to take over their life (see *Compulsive Sex*). Sexual desire becomes the tail that wags the dog, and these men's lives are disrupted by the incessant search for sex, regardless of time or place, the partner or the pleasure. This runaway sex can significantly interfere with their work and social life. Such men often go into debt to pay for phone sex lines, subscriptions to multiple gay Internet sex sites, or to buy hustlers and sex paraphernalia. They may even put their life in danger by seeking out potentially dangerous men or harmful types of sex (see *Dangerous Sex; Sex Toys; Hustlers; Phone Sex*).

For those who spend the better part of the day in sexual exploits and who don't enjoy it, the question is, why? The problem, we believe, is not sexual at all. Their sexual extravagance is really a smoke screen. Some psychologists believe that fear of abandonment lies behind the excessive pursuit of sex and that such activity serves as a substitute for love and intimacy. The multiplicity of sex partners prevents the development of a strong attachment to another man. Such gay men eventually feel sexually unfulfilled and emotionally desperate and should look into counseling.

Racism

Racism is insidious and pervasive in American life. Unfortunately, ignoring and excluding people of other races are aspects of gay life, too. In the gay community, racism operates in a subtle, covert manner. Certain people are not welcomed into organizations or included in activities. Questions about this are deflected with the insulting rationalization "I didn't think you would be interested." Such exclusion is particularly pernicious because people can get away with it. One comes across what are in effect whites only, Latinos only, and African-Americans only bars, clubs, and community groups. There is little mixing.

A less covert, but equally pernicious, form of racism is carding. This can occur wherever identification is required for admission to a bar, club, beach, pool, or concert. Originally intended to keep underage persons out of places where liquor is served, carding is now used by management and staff to keep out Latinos, Asian-Americans, or African-Americans. Usually everyone will be required to show one piece of ID, say a driver's license, as proof of age. But a person of color might be asked to show two, three, or even more pieces. Often the same African-American or Latino who is cordially received when accompanied by a white person is carded when he's alone. In this way, people are, at the very least, hassled. Even if permitted to enter, they have been made to feel unwanted and unwelcome. At the worst, they're discriminated against and kept out.

Racism also varies by geographic location. Moving from North to South in the United States for example, one discovers that many Southeast Asian immigrants are treated as badly as blacks used to be. While in the Southwest of the country, people of Mexican descent are scorned, joked about, and put down, even by Asian- and African-Americans. Various white "Aryan purity" groups, also antigay, have been revealed to have homosexual members who target other races with beatings and death. For years it was believed that at home Europeans were not racists. That might have been true when other races formed such tiny presences. When that region's boom economy in the eighties and nineties began attracting greater numbers of non-white immigrants looking for work and better living conditions, things changed. Now Germany has its "Turkish problem," Eastern Europe its "West African problem," France its "Algerian and Congolese problem," while English skinheads are nick-named Paki-bashers and dot-busters because of the frequency with which they attack peoples from the Indian subcontinent (see *Traveling*).

We call racism the exclusion of any race or ethnic group by any other race or ethnic group. We believe African-Americans who exclude Asian-Americans, and Latinos who exclude African-Americans, are as racist as whites who exclude blacks, though the latter is by far the most common form of racism in our society.

Some gay men worry that their sexual interest (or lack of interest) in blacks and Latinos is racist. Unless the person is overtly racist, we think this is not the case (see *Types*). On the other hand, white men who sleep with blacks and Latinos but exclude them socially are expressing racist attitudes.

Rape

In recent years, the incidence of rape of men by men has significantly increased. In fact, many cases of rape are forms of gay bashing, perpetrated by straight men (often in groups) against gay men. Feminists and sociologists have called our society a culture of rape. Its characteristics are sexual inequality, exploitation of sex in commerce and entertainment, and rigid concepts of sin and retribution. The attacker invariably blames the victim by saying that she or he dressed, acted, or spoke "provocatively" or in some other way "asked for it."

"Rape is about power, not about sex" has become a commonly heard statement. Yet sex and power are intimately related. What changes sexual intercourse (in its widest sense) into rape is not the force used, but rather the lack of consent.

Which leads to one of the dirty secrets of recent gay life—date rape. This used to be rare among men, often the result of crossed signals. An experienced man, for instance, might pick up someone who is just coming out and, misled by the inexperienced one's flirtatiousness, thinks he wants to have sex. In fact, however, the inexperienced man is just looking for a conversation and cuddling. The experienced man may fail to respect his partner's limits. Overcome by the combination of resentment and lust, he may force sex on his partner.

The increased frequency of date rape in recent years seems to be directly correlated to the fear many gays feel about contracting AIDS. Less willing to be sexually active, yet attracted to their partner, they appear indecisive; another may interpret the indecision as flirting. Should misunderstanding continue, the partner may feel frustrated. If he has a violent streak in his personality, sexual assault may be the result. As a response to this threat, some men leaving bars or clubs with a stranger have taken up the practice of introducing him by name to a friend or even to the bartender—for safety's sake.

Rape has always occurred in prisons. In recent years, potential victims have been placed in special cell blocks to decrease the incidence of rape. Unless segregated, the younger, slighter, more attractive male in prison better be ready to defend his asshole. Recently a slew of lawsuits against prisons and prison employees by men who were raped and as a result contracted AIDS has received much publicity. The victims contend they were subjected to "cruel and unusual punishment," forbidden by the U.S. Constitution, and they are demanding civil and criminal recompense.

Rape is assault and can produce physical trauma as well as psychological harm. If you have been raped, you should report it to the police and seek medical care, even if you suspect that cops in your area may be unsympathetic to a raped man. Many larger cities have rape crisis lines that can advise you on how to handle the police, to get medical treatment, and to seek counseling. If such crisis lines or clinics do not exist in your area, check your local gay center or gay-info hot line. Or you can always call the New York City Gay and Lesbian Anti-Violence Project twenty-four hours a day at 212-714-1184.

Seek medical treatment whether you report the rape or not. This may include a rectal exam to check for internal tears or bleeding. If tests for STDs and AIDS as a result of the rape are *not* part of the exam, be certain that you get tested for them (see *Sexually Transmitted Diseases*).

Again, whether or not you report the rape as a crime, you ought to look into counseling. Male rape victim clinics using group sessions are psychologically useful. Many rape victims end up feeling powerless and out of control in completely unrelated areas of their life (work, sports) as a result of the attack. Some victims feel partly responsible for the assault, an idea often fostered by their attacker—"I know you want it. Why else would you wear those tight jeans!" Group sessions, one-on-one counseling, and talking it through with friends are needed to free you from the emotional pain.

An even more painful kind of gay rape occurs when a father (or a stepfather) sexually assaults his son. There may be anal or oral penetration. These assaults often begin before puberty and may continue for years. Sons who have been sexually assaulted by a parent or baby-sitter are sometimes terrified of divulging the secret. They are often rightly afraid of paternal violence against themselves or other members of the family. Particularly reprehensible parents will make threats such as killing the child's pet if they tell.

If your father has raped you, don't keep it a secret. You owe it to yourself to confront the problem. You also owe it to siblings who may still be at home. Find someone you can talk to, perhaps a teacher or a friend's parents; definitely see a psychotherapist. If a friend confides information like this to you, be compassionate and guide him to people or organizations that can help.

Gay men also have fantasies about being raped, but these are quite different from the foregoing acts of exploitation. Gay men sometimes masturbate to the fantasy that another man (or the entire college football team) is forcing sex upon him (see *Masturbation and Fantasy*). Some find the scenario arousing and even act it out with tricks or lovers. There's also an extensive genre of pornography founded upon these ideas. Don't feel guilty if you enjoy the fantasy. It doesn't mean that you want to really be raped. Part of the fun in gay life is the ability to let go during sexual fantasies, and to become passive in the arms of another man. The "rape," we suspect, is but a transformation of the desire to be taken care of by another man, and that leads to feelings of intimacy.

Rear Entry

This is the classic gay fucking position, the reality behind those old jokes about turning your back and facetiously saying, "I kept dropping my soap in the shower—hoping something would happen." This position entails standing, or leaning forward slightly, and spreading your ass cheeks to provide entry. Or you can do it doggy style, dropping to your hands and knees while he kneels and enters you from behind. For some men it's the preferred position: After all, it's the one doctors have you assume for a rectal examination, because it affords the easiest entry. For the top, doggy style enables him to make pelvic thrusts at the fastest possible rate; for pure speed it can't be beat. And due to the angle, for many men it is the best position for fucking deeply and over the longest period.

It's also a sexy position. The man on top has a full view of the buns he's penetrating, and he can watch his cock slide in and out of his partner's asshole. He can let his gaze wander slowly up his partner's back and stop at the tensed shoulders and straining triceps, or he can lean over and wrap his arms around his partner's waist or chest and nibble at his exposed nape or ear. The guy getting fucked is possibly more conscious of his own body in the doggy position than when he is lying on his back or on his stomach (see *Face-to-Face*; *Bottoms Up*). The fuckee is also more active in this position. He can push back onto his partner's cock; he can rest his weight on one forearm, freeing his other hand for masturbating himself. Or he can easily drop down from all fours to stretch out on his belly and from there roll his partner and himself onto their sides (see *Side by Side*). Or while still up on all fours, he can raise his

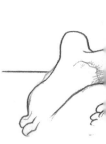

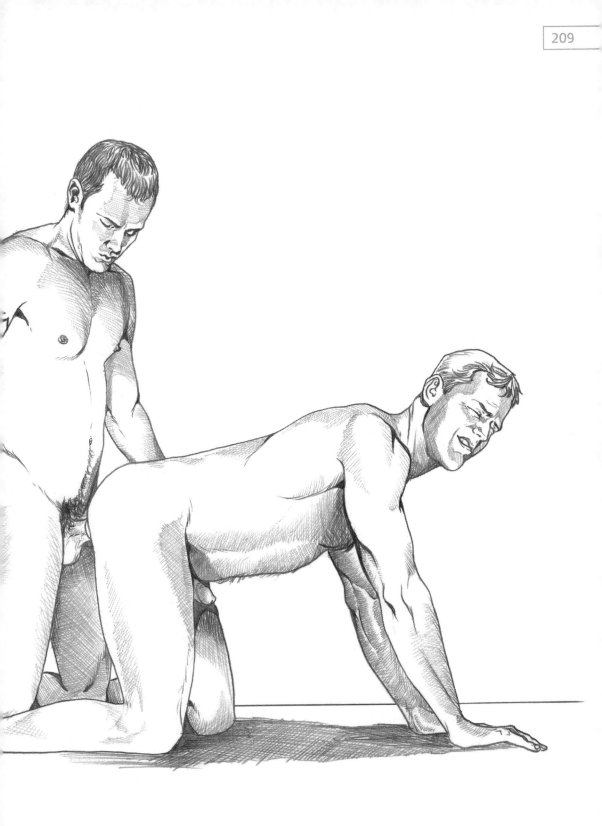

upper body until both he and his partner are kneeling, hips, torsos, and heads vertical.

Kissing, however, is a casualty of fucking doggy style. Unless the bottom has a rubber neck or the top is extraordinarily tall, a full mouth-to-mouth kiss is usually impossible (see *Kissing*).

Rejection

Being rejected by a stranger in a bar on a Tuesday night at 11:30 P.M. is not a final judgment on whether you are attractive. Ask yourself what his reasons might have been. He might be tired, have a cold, or have a lover waiting for him at home. Perhaps he's just finished having sex, or you're not his type because you have a beard (or because you don't). There's no way you can ascertain his motives, but bear in mind that they may have nothing to do with you (see *Types*). Try to remember all those who have said yes to you over the years, as well as your achievements, both personal and professional.

How should you handle hurt feelings when someone turns you down? Since no one gets used to rejection, there's likely to be momentary shock. Three responses should be avoided:

1. Immediately finding fault with the man who rejected you ("He's not so great" or "I'm sure that tan is out of a bottle"). Revenge or spite only serves to keep you obsessed with a rejection best forgotten.

2. Going around rejecting others. Having been shot down, you decide to put a few notches on your own gun. After letting someone squirm until he works up the courage to ask you home, you have the (perfectly hollow) pleasure of rejecting him. But the worst response is:

3. Depression. You indulge in self-pity. You decide that your personality is dull, your looks repellent, and your life meaningless. You have five more drinks and then stagger home, feeling old, ugly, and hopeless (see *Depression*).

If rejection is so wounding, you should ask yourself what past experiences you may be unconsciously reliving—rejection by a parent, a childhood friend, or first lover. One occasionally finds men who are accomplished at setting up rejection by picking out the coldest man in the bar, the one most likely to turn someone down. Such self-defeating behavior needs to be faced squarely and dealt with in therapy or self-analysis.

Perhaps it's time for a change, time to move on to a new spot, a new meeting place, and a new group of people. You'll be surprised how being a "new face" can pick up your social life and cut down rejection. On the other hand, maybe you do need to make some changes in yourself. Make an honest evaluation of your behavior in social situations. Perhaps your anxiety is being expressed in a hostile or rigid attitude. If so, change this. We all have to make adjustments in ourselves from time to time.

Relaxation

Sometimes people become overwhelmed with anxiety just before or during sex. If you have this problem, take time to relax. Although you may fear your partner will be insulted if you don't jump right into sex with him, he himself may welcome a breather.

One relaxation technique is, paradoxically, to tighten sets of muscles deliberately. Start with your hands. Make them into fists, then open them and say to yourself, "Relax." Next, tighten your arms and then relax them. Pay special attention to the tension in your neck and stomach. Throughout your exercises breathe deeply. Psychologists call this *progressive relaxation.*

Another technique is to call to mind a scene that is totally calm, maybe one out of your past or, alternatively, one you have made up. It might be a beach or a forest or a picture-book castle, but whatever it is, if you tune in to it, it will relax you.

You might ask your partner to help you. Lie still, trying to relax your body as much as possible. Imagine it is so heavy it will sink through the bed, or so limp that you are like a rag doll. Then your partner should pick up your hand or foot and drop it back to the bed. Alternatively, you can lie back, concentrate on breathing deeply, and have your partner masturbate you as you exhale. Each time you breathe in, you should be able to inhale more easily and more deeply.

Once you are fully relaxed, you can ease into sex. If, however, during the sex you become anxious again, don't be afraid to stop for another breather. *Taking the time to relax is much sexier than being tense during lovemaking.*

• • •

Rimming and Felching

Though often used as a preliminary to fucking, rimming is fun in itself and an effective way to relax the two muscles of the asshole, called the anal sphincters (see *Male Sexual Response*). Unfortunately, rimming is also an easy way to contract several serious diseases, including hepatitis A, amebiasis (and other parasitic diseases), and venereal diseases, such as syphilis and gonorrhea (see *Sexually Transmitted Diseases*). Therefore, rimming is clearly considered an unsafe sex practice. It should not be practiced with tricks, since their sexual history is unknown to you. Do it only when you are absolutely certain of the health of your sex partner.

There is no evidence that rimming, or being rimmed, has transmitted HIV. However, using dental dams (thin plastic or rubber squares used by dentists to protect the mouth during orthodontic surgery) is sometimes recommended. Don't use Saran Wrap or the like. It's porous, allows bacteria to pass through, and won't prevent disease.

Here's how to rim: Gently run your fingers along the curve of your partner's back until you reach his buns. Knead and cup them; just barely touch the crack. Knead your partner's cheeks and give him a few light nips with your teeth. Some men like to slap their partner's buns at this point to heighten the excitement, assuming he likes his ass whacked (see *Spanking*). Run your fingers down the crack, and draw a line with your tongue all the way to his balls.

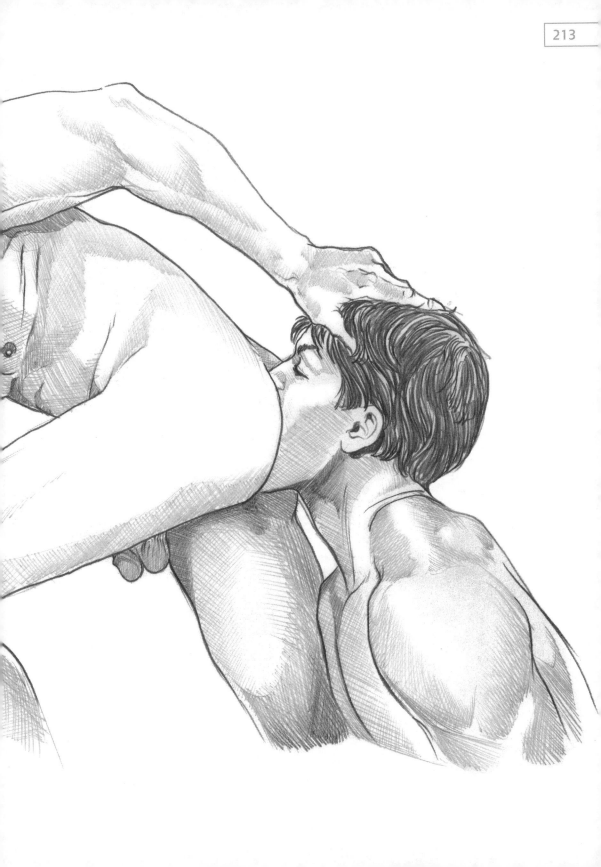

Reach between his legs and play with his cock. Simultaneously work your tongue into the crack of his ass. Lick a circle, making smaller and smaller arcs until the tongue can feel the difference between the skin around the hole and the muscle. Dart and flicker in and out.

Rimming can be done in many different positions. Your partner can be on his back, with his legs in the air. You can be in a sixty-nine position (see *Sixty-Nining*), you sucking on your partner's cock while he rims you. Or he can be flat on his stomach while you lift his legs and feast on his buttocks (see *Sit on My Face*). Rimming can be passionate; the man rimming feels his partner's ass contract and relax, which spurs him on. The man being rimmed can push back toward the tongue or rotate his hips. He'll sigh; his breathing will come faster and sharper—responses that usually delight his partner and encourage him to new efforts.

Felching happens after you've fucked your partner and then rim him, either inadvertently or purposely sucking out the semen you just ejaculated into him. We do not recommend it in these days of AIDS, because it would mean that you fucked without a condom. This is not a new sexual practice, although a new generation has apparently rediscovered it. The practice is obviously limited only by your attitude and sense of danger. Keep in mind, however, that not everything that comes out of an anus is necessarily something that you personally put into it.

Role Playing

In the past there were psychological advantages to social role playing. It reduced anxiety by defining social behaviors: "You do the dishes, I take out the garbage. You invite the guests, I support the family." Role playing, therefore, established ground rules governing the relationship between two people.

Today, such role playing scarcely works even for heterosexuals, although they have been carefully coached from childhood on what constitutes proper male and female behavior. The gay couple has no stake in preserving the male-female social dichotomy.

Sexual role playing is something quite different. A gay man may decide to assume a specific but temporary sexual role. On occasion, he'll want to dominate a cute "kid," and the next night he may want to be the kid himself. There is little or no carry-over from the bedroom to the rest of life. Lovers may take turns assuming sexual roles with each other (see *Versatility*).

Many gay men dispense with roles altogether and do not connect fucking, say, with dominance, or sucking with passivity. To them, sexual pleasure is the main goal, and they do not attach much significance to who was doing what to whom. Still others enjoy deliberately playing a particular part. Often these games are called scenes—captor/captive; delivery boy/householder; sergeant/recruit; ticketing policeman/offending driver; or examination giver/test taker. But the men remain ready, willing, and able to swap roles midstream, thereby developing maximum flexibility in their role-playing repertoire (see *Bottom; Top; Sadomasochism*).

Pornography is also a good outlet for various sorts of role playing, or at least for experiencing role-playing fantasies (see *Pornography*).

Sadomasochism

Sadomasochism is a sexual variation that celebrates virility, ritual, and pain. Its proponents adhere to sharply defined roles based upon power: master and slave, or "top man" and "bottom man." The word *sadomasochism* itself is derived from the names of two men: the Marquis de Sade and Leopold von Sacher-Masoch. De Sade (1740–1814) believed that pain, not pleasure, was the highest goal of sexual activity. His *120 Days of Sodom* is a compendium of examples. Sacher-Masoch (1836–1895) was a historian and a novelist. All his novels contain whipping scenes, and he himself preferred to be whipped by women wearing furs, especially older women.

Many examples of sadomasochism can be drawn, curiously enough, from the history of the Catholic Church. The flagellants, for example, were a twelfth-century mass movement that encouraged people to flog themselves until blood flowed. The lives of the saints are also replete with instances of masochism. In 1920, Saint Margaret Mary Alacoque was canonized. A seventeenth-century nun, she carved the name of Jesus on her chest with a knife, but because it didn't last long enough, she burned it in with a candle. At least as bizarre was Saint Mary-Magdalen dei Pazzi, who used to roll in thornbushes in the convent garden, then go into the convent and whip herself. She also forced novices to tie her to a post, insult her, whip her, and drop hot wax on her.

Although many gay men have dismissed S/M at one time or another, a large segment of the gay population continues to walk the streets of cities garbed in black leather and chains or in uniforms such as those of motorcycle cops or marine MPs (see *Uniforms*). Some men pull this off superbly. A guy with a three-day growth of beard, a torn T-shirt, muscled biceps, and wearing leather chaps and motorcycle boots can attract a lot of attention.

There is no simple explanation for the increased popularity of S/M, nor of its attractions. We offer as possibilities the following: First, this phenomenon is not con-

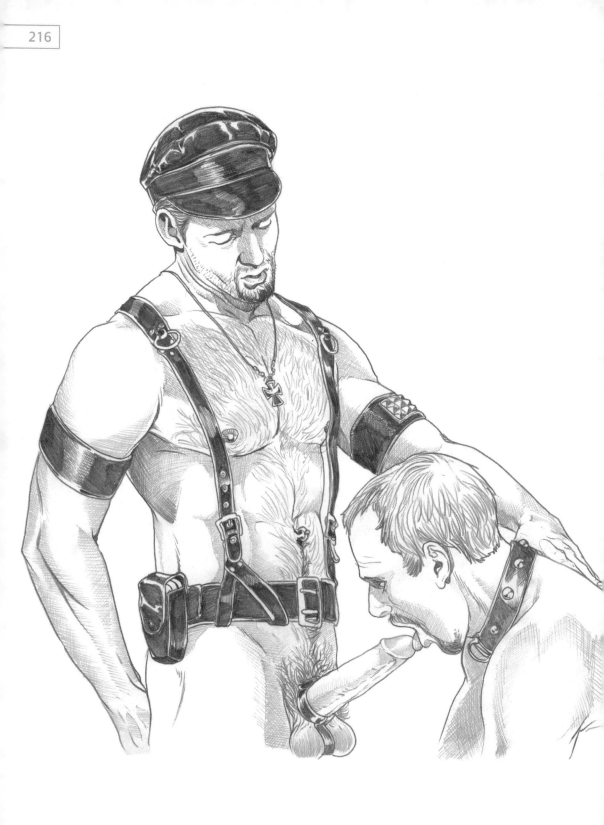

fined to gay circles. We live in an era that glamorizes tough guys; many top box-office stars are he-men. This is the popular image of male sex appeal. Second, not all men in leather are sadomasochists; for some, denim and leather are just fashion. Many men who have adopted the S/M look are not really interested in inflicting pain or suffering.

Sadomasochism has been around a long time; permissiveness has really allowed it to appear more openly; desires that were always there, if hidden, are now boldly displayed. Then, too, men in their forties and fifties have found more acceptance in leather bars. The leather look can add a strong allure to a man who has lost the charms of youth.

Our culture is a hierarchy of power, but in everyday life, power is clothed, not naked; hypocritical, not honest. Parents dominate children, men dominate women, whites dominate blacks, the rich dominate the poor, the boss dominates his employees, and straights dominate gays. S/M dramatizes these situations and even temporarily reverses them, so the oppressed accountant by day can become the oppressing sadist by night.

Tricking within the context of sadomasochism has certain advantages. So many of the attitudes, verbal exchanges, and sexual moves are ritualized and safely predictable that a one-night stand often lacks the fumbling and uncertainty that can characterize tricking in other contexts.

Finally, S/M can touch deep emotional chords. It may seem rigid, but it allows people to explore fantasies of domination and surrender, of cruelty and tenderness, of contempt and adoration.

Before getting involved in this scene, be aware that for some men real violence is not only exciting, but essential. Occasionally, genuinely harmful things do happen. If you decide to try this scene, start out with someone you know. You may be too naive to spot a potentially dangerous person (see *Cruising*; *Dangerous Sex*).

The novice often starts as a masochist. There's no way you can learn to be a good S except from someone experienced. Don't be too worried; the experienced S will let the novice establish his own limits. It's probably a good idea to agree on a *safe word*, a signal that lets the S know that those limits have been reached. If you're with someone who refuses to use a safe word, don't get involved.

Another word about signals. Keys hung on the left and handkerchiefs in the left back pocket indicate the sadist or "top man;" keys or handkerchiefs on the right indicates a masochist or "bottom man." Many men wear the insignia of motorcycle clubs, especially on the backs of denim jackets. They have no sexual significance except for the icon showing two semicircles, one above another, each penetrated by a sharp line; this is the badge of the Fistfuckers of America (see *Fisting*). Some men into S/M are also into fisting. The Hell Fire Club is a group of men into serious S/M. It operates by invitation only and holds a yearly meeting, called Inferno, in the Midwest. The club's name is probably borrowed from the

Hell-Fire Club organized by Sir Francis Dashwood in late-eighteenth-century England.

Some S/M lovers who have been together for a long time maintain a strict role division. Usually, they do not carry this role playing into ordinary life. The slave does not serve the master except during sex; otherwise he's equal. Other lovers who are into S/M reverse roles. Still others drift into ordinary gay sex with each other but play out S/M fantasies with strangers.

The dividing line between S/M and other styles of sex play isn't always clear. Most men enjoy some roughness in their sex play from time to time. A well-placed slap on the ass at the right time, or lots of dirty talk, can add excitement to an ordinary encounter. Tit clamps, dildos, ropes, and other sex toys can also be used to increase excitement (see *Bondage and Discipline; Nibbling and Biting; Nipples; Body Decoration; Sex Toys; Spanking; Kinky Sex*).

Psychologists have tried to identify the boundaries of S/M by research. It isn't easy, because S/M covers a wide range of sexual activities. Recent research has suggested that it consists of four broad sexual themes: hypermasculinity, administration and receipt of pain, physical restriction, and humiliation. But many S/M activities don't fit neatly into this classification.

Safe Sex

It's late at night, and you are partying with a friend at the most popular club in town. Perhaps you're at a gay summer resort like Fire Island in New York, or Fort Lauderdale in Florida, and men are dancing all around you. Many are in bathing suits or shorts, and the shared energy is intoxicating. As you whirl about the dance floor, you notice someone you spied on the beach earlier, a man you think is cute. You observe how he snaps his head back as he dances, trying to keep the hair out of his face, and how it just bounces back again. You wish you were assertive enough to walk over and, while looking into his eyes, brush his hair back. You imagine yourself cupping his face in your hands, delicately kissing and caressing him. But you're too shy, and you tell yourself that someone as attractive as he wouldn't be interested in you.

Only minutes later the unbelievable happens: Standing outside for a bit of fresh air with your dance partner, you hear someone say, "Hello." The voice comes from behind. You turn around. "My name is Paul," he says as he brushes his hair back. This gesture is enough to turn you on, and you blush. You're already getting hard. Your friend, diplomatically, makes himself scarce. You hardly know what you're saying as you and Paul chat together, and his words seem to float in the air but never get to your ears. If you could only hear what he's saying.

An hour later, you're holding hands, back at a nearby cottage he's rented. Only the briefest moments are spent on the couch, and soon you two are lying together on the bed, kissing, caressing—and tasting each other. Then he turns on his back, spreads his legs, and says, "Fuck me." He hands you a lubricant. You ask for a condom and he says, "I trust you."

You've gone to bed with a fool. A cute fool, maybe, but a deadly one.

The scenario might be slightly different. Paul might want to fuck you. Again, no condom. He might say, "You're the only person I've ever fucked without a rubber."

In this case he's not a fool; he's a liar. You're the fool if you believe him.

Why do men endanger their life by having unsafe sex? First, our impression is that it is younger rather than older men who are violating safe sex guidelines, believing "it can't happen to me." Other young men feel deprived, contrary, and rebellious. One youth said, "You guys [meaning the older generation of gay men] had all the fun! You got to do everything. And what are we stuck with? Rubbers and hand jobs?"

A second reason is that men are turned on by visual stimuli, by seeing an attractive face and body. It stimulates all the sexual hormones in the body. Imagine, then, how difficult restraint is when so many available men in a club or at the beach are stimulating visual and tactile senses. We also know that using alcohol and drugs interferes with good judgment (see *Booze and Highs*; *Drugs and Sex*; *Drug Abuse*). As one psychologist noted, "The superego is soluble in alcohol." Some men fear offending a potential sex partner by insisting on safe sex, especially if that partner is physically desirable and someone they've been after for a while. Other men are unable to fight peer pressure: If "everyone else is doing it," so will they, even if it hurts them (see *Dangerous Sex*; *Saying No*).

All these factors may explain why some men appear to go into something like a fugue state (psychologists call it denial), a state of amnesia, forgetting friends and lovers who are ill or dead.

Making choices about sex is important now that AIDS has caused the death of so many men in the last twenty years (see *HIV Disease*). Older gays have watched close friends, lovers, and other family members die. But most younger gay men have not; and until they do, they think it's all exaggeration. It's not; it is crucial that all of us understand the parameters of safe sex, not only to protect our own health, but also to maintain the health of our community.

Being in love can lead to life-threatening mistakes, especially for men who have come out during the AIDS epidemic. Newcomers to the gay world bring a reservoir of love with them. For the first time in their lives they can express their romantic feelings as they search for lovers. Some gay men act as though they're more terrified of being abandoned by a potential lover than by the possible transmission of the HIV. They have unsafe sex with someone they love, rationalizing, "I'm afraid he'll think I don't love him," or, "He'll leave me if I tell him I don't want to take his come," jeopardizing both their own and their lover's life. A friend might reply, "Schmuck, how much can he love you if he's willing to put your life in danger?"

Many gay men behave as though safe sex guidelines didn't exist. It's not because these men are stupid or lack information. The guidelines are fairly easy to understand. You'll find them listed at the end of this section. Most gay magazines and every AIDS organization publishes the latest information about safe sex.

Your sexual behavior is an expression of how you feel about yourself. If you respect yourself, safe sex won't be a problem. Sexual behavior is also an expression of your feelings about other men. When you cajole, exploit, or manipulate someone in bed, you're not expressing sexual needs. Your lust is a cover-up. Perhaps you're angry with all men, or you're resentful over an unresolved childhood incident or a disappointment in a previous love affair. All can be motivations for exploiting another gay man.

Gay men have three responsibilities with respect to safe sex. The first is to oneself. If you have self-respect, you won't do anything to put your own life in danger. Your second responsibility is to others. You should do whatever you can to influence the sexual behavior of your friends, tricks, and potential lovers. Tell them you want them to have a good sex life; you just don't want them to become ill. Teach them about safe sex, and show them where to get more information.

Your third responsibility is to the gay community. We hope you'll join the strug-

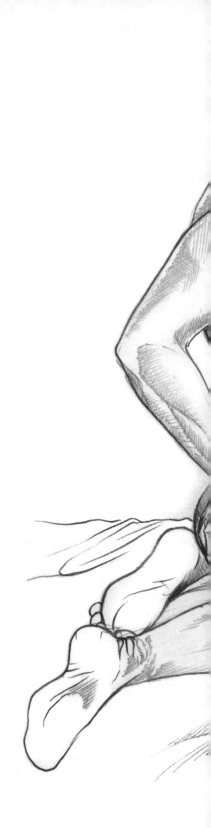

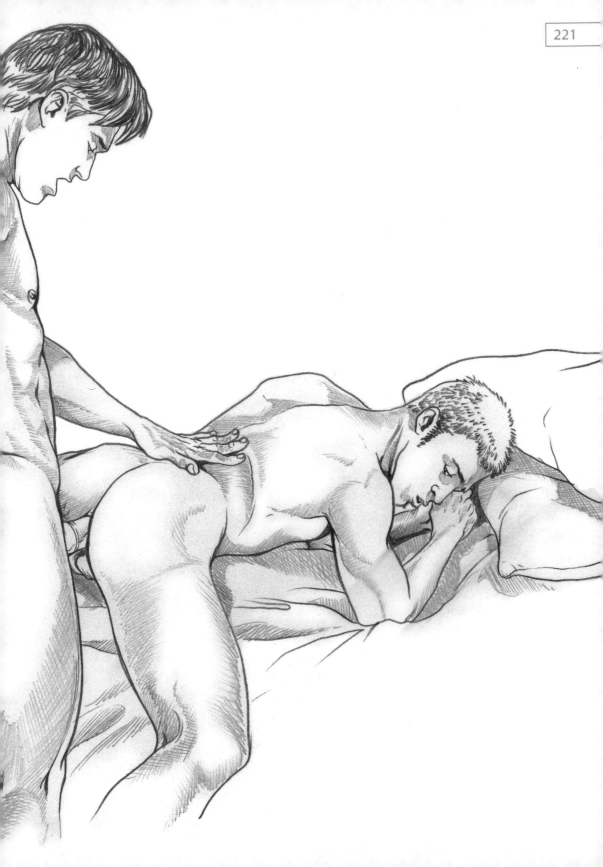

gle with other gay men and lesbians to pressure our government to find a cure for AIDS. If you can, serve as a volunteer in an AIDS organization. Keep in mind that the only way gay people have secured our rights is by demanding them. As a gay man in the gay community, your example is an important part of that struggle (see *Civil Rights; Gay Liberation; Gay Politics*).

Considered Completely Safe

Mutual masturbation

Hugging

Body rubbing

Massage

Dry kissing

S/M if without bleeding or bruising

Sex toys used only on self

Considered Possibly Safe

Anal intercourse with a condom

Wet kissing

Sucking, but stopping before climax

External water sports (no swallowing)

Fisting (with latex gloves)

Considered Unsafe

Swallowing semen

Anal intercourse without a condom

Water sports in mouth or on skin with sores

Sharing IV needles

Sharing enema equipment or sex toys

Rimming

• • •

Saying No

Many men are so afraid of offending other people that it is only with great difficulty that they can say no to a sexual invitation. This liability can lead to touchy situations.

Directness is always best when you're saying no. Lengthy and complicated excuses rarely work; they tend to get taken at face value, and often all you achieve is putting off having to deal with the same guy later. Softening a negative response with smiles, shrugs, and equivocations—"That's a really nice invitation, but I don't think I really should, at least not this time, I guess"—is horribly ineffective. Equivocation betrays uncertainty on your part and invites renewed appeals from the other person. He pressures you, and more often than not, you give in.

There's only one solution: Take a deep breath and, politely but with no trace of hesitation, say no. A firm "No, thank you" to a sexual advance is much kinder than an unnecessarily rude response, or no response at all. He may not be your cup of tea, but he's still a person with feelings, and he dislikes being rejected as much as you do.

The AIDS epidemic has added a new dimension to saying no. We're now forced to say no to men who excite us sexually, but who won't respect safe sex guidelines. These men should be avoided even though they may stir the greatest passion in us. One needn't say no to another man who's seropositive or who has AIDS, because with safe sex you can protect each other from transmitting the virus (see *Body Fluids and Disease; Safe Sex; HIV Disease*). But someone who acts as if there *isn't an epidemic* and proposes what you know to be idiotic activities, such as barebacking, is himself ensuring its continuation. If you still feel such a man is hot, go home and jerk off while fantasizing about having sex with him. Whatever you do, don't take him with you.

Scat

A small minority of gay men like to make feces part of the sex scene. The word for this—*scat*—is derived from the Greek word for dung. It has also come to mean references to something filthy or obscene, as in toilet jokes. Scat is probably more talked about than performed.

Some guys who are into scat shit on each other or eat each other's shit or smear it over their bodies. For others, it's not the physical aspect of shit so much as its symbolic value that counts. Rather than using shit to degrade themselves and each other, they use it in a variety of metaphoric, even ritualistic, ways, often without touching it—experiencing it being produced by another; sometimes adoring it in almost the same way that infants play with it as a marvelous product of their own body.

Scat may be associated with S/M, although not necessarily so. A few leather guys indulge in this scene; in an S/M context the master shits on his slave as yet another way to humiliate and degrade him. Among masochists in search of extremes, scat must represent the ultimate indignity—and therefore the ultimate turn-on. There is no reason to believe that someone who eats shit during sex also invites or even tolerates humiliation in his everyday life. *Scat* really describes a sexual act, not a social role. But since scat is frowned upon so widely by sex researchers and by gays themselves, we know little about the subculture.

Scat, like rimming, does expose you to hepatitis, a variety of parasites, and bacillary dysentery (see *Rimming; Sexually Transmitted Diseases*). Fortunately, HIV has not been implicated.

The scat scene is a curious one for psychologists. They have no idea how it originates, although they assume that some psychological trauma in childhood causes feces to become eroticized. For the average person, scat is usually just downright kinky (see *Dangerous Sex; Kinky Sex*).

Seduction

The term has come to have such a negative connotation—enticing a novice so as to have your wicked way with him—that we sometimes forget that seduction can be an exciting game for both the seducer and the seduced. Seduction in consenting adults can be quite charming.

Right from the beginning, you have to choose whether to go for immediate sex or to attempt an affair (see *Cruising*). Each requires slight modifications in seduction technique. Affairs usually start with courtship. Even if you meet in a bar in an obvious pickup situation, you might ask for his phone number rather than going home with him that very night and having sex; instant sex may cut the tension between you and allow you to fall into a wham-bam-thank-you-Sam cycle. Far better, if you have serious intentions, is to phone him the next day and invite him to dinner or to a movie, perhaps on a prime-time weekend evening. Your wanting to put off sex may puzzle him, but he may also be intrigued and complimented.

On your date, ask all about him and speak freely about yourself in return. Don't stress your weaknesses and shortcomings. Later on, if you become close, you can share misgivings about yourself and talk about your problems.

Don't discuss the casual sex you've had, though you might feel free to mention love affairs. The note to sound is intimate, not chummy; romantic, not social. Engage his interests and address yourself to his hopes and anxieties. Many men in their twenties, for instance, are as much concerned with their career as with finding a lover. Make yourself doubly attractive by giving him a chance to discuss these aspirations.

If a one-nighter is your aim, the approach will be different. As soon as you meet someone at a party or a club, make your intention clear by moving the conversation toward sex. Many men are offended if you ask exactly what they like to do in bed; they prefer to let things take their course without prior discussion. Keep the conversation flirty, filled with innuendo, and pay him several discreet sexual compliments. (Don't ask him if he has a big cock.) The aim is to create an erotic tension in which you two are the only people who count, a tension that can only be resolved through sex. Before sex, you should do nothing to destroy the fantasy you're carefully weaving about the two of you.

Some men have gone a step further in their seduction technique. All they have to do is get the man home, where they've exercised their erotic imagination in designing an atmosphere so seductive few can resist. The lights are on rheostats; a stereo bathes the room in sound. The bed is low, immense, and covered with bolsters; the rug is soft and inviting should sex spill over onto the floor. The windows are curtained for privacy; the room switch dims the lights and starts a porn video (see *Pornography*). Other men think such a bedroom too contrived for their taste. Perhaps the best advice is to develop a good sense of humor, a bit of style, and lots of charm. With these traits, in the right proportions, men will be drawn to you like iron to a magnet.

Sex Ads

Sexual advertisements can be found in gay newspapers and magazines where they begin "GWM," meaning "gay white male," or "GBM," meaning "gay black male." Because personal ads are costly and outline specific requirements, an entire shorthand has developed that can provide fairly detailed information. Here is an ad taken from a newspaper:

Masculine

23 W Bott BB 6'3" br/bl vgdlkg HIV-185 7½ cut Fr A/P Gr P. Seeks prof. big Lat/Medit top hung uncut dom kinky 30s–40s HIV-. All photo/phones get reply. Box XYZ, Anywhere, CA.

Let's decode this. The man placing the ad begins by describing himself. He is "masculine," which means butch or straight-looking.

Next, he's twenty-three years old, white, a bottom, and a bodybuilder (see *Bottom*). He then lists his height (6'3"), hair color (brown), the color of his eyes (blue), and (immodestly) brags that he is *very* good-looking. He further notes his HIV antibody status (negative), his weight (185 pounds), and the length of his cock (7½ inches), adding that he is circumcised (cut). (Some ads also list the circumference of the cock.) Finally, he lists the sexual activities he prefers: "Fr A/P"—"French active or passive"—means he will suck cock and get sucked. "Gr P" means "Greek passive," that he wants to get fucked but doesn't wish to fuck anyone else. The next sentence in the ad begins with "Seeks" and details the kind of man the advertiser's looking for: a big professional man, preferably of Latino or Mediterranean background. A top man, hung (a big dick), uncircumcised (see *Foreskin*). He adds that he'd like the man he's seeking to be dominant and kinky, but doesn't specify what kind of kinky acts he prefers (see *Kinky Sex; Sleazy Sex*). Furthermore, he specifies the age of his preferred partner—somewhat older than himself—and his preferred HIV antibody status. The final sentence tells the reader that if he sends a photograph of himself and includes his phone number, the advertiser will reply without fail. He finishes with his post-office box number, city, and zip code.

Here is another ad from the same issue of the same newspaper:

Country Man

Seeks same for friendship or more. Interested in farm or outdoor worker. I am 38 5'11" 155#, gr/br. Will travel, NY, PA. Reply to Box #123, Syracuse, NY area.

This ad needs little in the way of explanation. The man is saying he has a simple life, simple needs, and simple requirements. He's less concerned with anything specifically sexual in a partner than in sharing a particular kind of lifestyle and interests. Travel is emphasized because gay men are usually so widely spaced apart in rural areas.

Obviously, ads can be as detailed or as vague, as friendly or as aloof, as professional or as giddily romantic, as you want them to be. You write them; you answer them: You're the boss!

When should you advertise for sex or romance? When you prefer it over the use of the Internet (see *On-line Cruising; Chat Rooms*). Ads allow you to meet new people and have new experiences. If you have very specific sexual needs and requirements, you may *have* to advertise to find someone in your area who shares these tastes. Or advertise if you are targeting a specific group of guys—say intellectuals via *The New York Review of Books* or those interested in agriculture through the pages of *Organic Gardening Today*.

When should you answer a sex ad? When you're a little bored with the same old people and things in your life. Some guys have had amazing luck placing and answering ads; others have had no luck at all. It's a question of marketing. Your first ad is not likely to attract many people. With experience, you'll find out what kind of description is most appealing to readers of the newspaper or magazine.

But don't ever write false advertising. For instance, the gay community has its share of size queens (see *Cock Size*). If you don't have an eight-inch (or larger) cock, don't claim that you do. While few of us meet a trick who has a tape measure in hand, most of us can see the difference between a normal-sized cock and a particularly large one. Instead, write something about another positive feature of your body and/or personality or interests. People who are lied to in ads (and on the Internet) feel betrayed and resentful. It doesn't make them feel sexy, and they're likely to walk out on you.

It's generally a good idea to talk on the phone with your potential sex partner who answered your ad or whose ad you've answered until you feel comfortable with him, which may be from a few minutes to an hour. Discuss whatever issues are on your mind, such as safety, health, HIV status. Some gay men like to have a couple of phone conversations before they meet with a stranger. Be cautious about meeting someone who refuses to discuss these matters because it suggests that your potential sex partner is hiding something, and that's a bad sign. If you feel comfortable after talking on the phone, arrange to meet with him. While some men will invite the trick to their house, others prefer to meet first in a public place such as a café. If you don't like his looks or manner after meeting him, tell him outright (see *Types*; *Saying No*). Don't beat around the bush. It only confuses him. He has a right to know that it won't work. And keep in mind that he may reject you as well (see *Rejection*). While talking, steer your discussion away from sexual topics and concentrate on general ones. There's no reason why you can't have a friendly chat (see *Etiquette*).

Sex Clubs

As the gay community became aware that the HIV was being transmitted among men in bathhouses, most of the baths were closed (see *Baths*). But gay men have always looked for private, enclosed sanctuaries of relative safety where they can meet other men for sex, and a variety of replacements soon came along. Jerk-off clubs are one substitute for baths and back rooms—they are private, popular, and being membership clubs, generally safe from police intrusion (see *J.O. Clubs*).

Another institution also arose after AIDS, at first mostly in a few large cities, later spreading throughout the country—the sex club. Whereas the jerk-off club was designed to actively discourage sucking and fucking, the sex club—based on back-room bars and various "glory hole" clubs of the 1970s—actively encourages fucking and sucking by providing an anything-goes atmosphere reminiscent of the wildest days of the baths.

In these clubs, a number of men, particularly younger men, allow themselves to be fucked without a condom—a foolish, self-destructive act—while men fucking them seem not to care that by gratifying their own needs they are perpetuating the AIDS epidemic (see *Barebacking; HIV Disease*). These clubs are extraordinarily *unsafe* environments in which to have sex. They may even be a major factor in the new upsurge in HIV infection, which is especially devastating to the Latino and African-American gay communities, which seem to account for a disproportionate number of new cases. In European countries where backroom bars and sex clubs are allowed to proliferate—France, Italy, and Spain—HIV infection has once again mounted. Two other factors contribute to the unsafe environment of sex clubs: STDs are uninvited guests, and recreational drugs interfere with good judgment (see *Sexually Transmitted Diseases; Drugs and Sex; Drug Abuse*).

People go to sex clubs for several reasons: for the excitement, for the danger, for the extremely graphic sensual ambience. Other reasons include the belief that "nothing bad can happen to me." Some younger gays feel left out, deprived of the sexual liberation of their elders. No matter that few of their elders actually survived that liberation. There are no possible rejoinders to this perspective except to say that if you must go to a sex club, by all means go and see what's going on. But we unconditionally discourage *participation* in sex clubs because they are unsafe environments (see *Safe Sex*).

Sex Parties

Most of our ideas about orgies derive from film. Biblical epics of the twenties, and especially the Technicolor fifties, set the standard with their masses of writhing unclad and semiclad bodies, their "exotic" music, and their general sense of ambivalent anything-goes. Cecil B. DeMille was a filmmaker particularly skilled at displaying masses of seminude bodies within a religious scene.

Like the best movies, the best orgies, now called sex parties, are carefully orchestrated in advance and controlled throughout with occasional adjustments. Naturally, some sex parties continue to be completely spontaneous, but these, alas, are few, far between, and all the more memorable for their rarity.

In the "good old days," most sex parties took place at a gay bathhouses. By the mid-

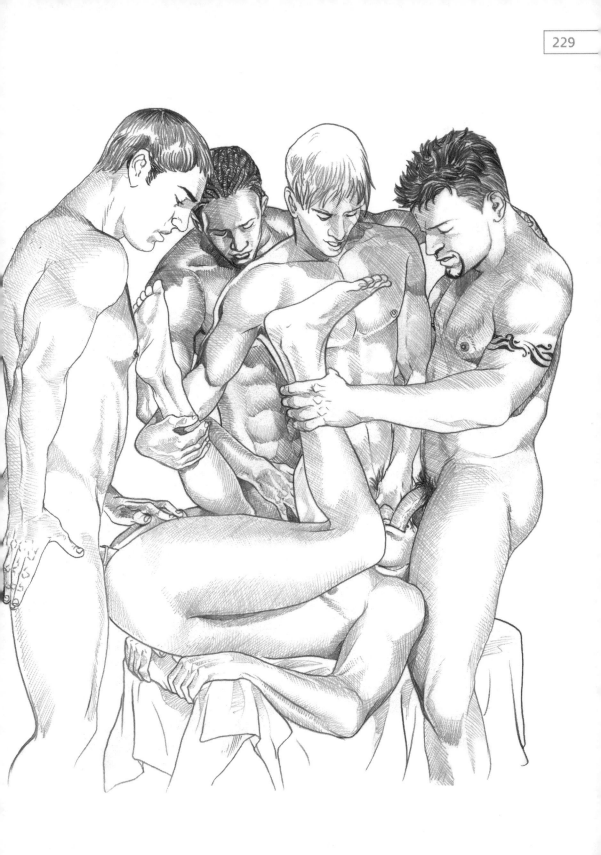

1980s, gay bathhouses and backroom bars were coming under increasing pressure to close because of the AIDS epidemic. Both gay critics and civil health authorities viewed them as one of the primary sources of contagion. Research at the time (and still today) identified multiple sexual partners as the best correlation with transmitting the HIV. The more sex partners you had, the greater the probability that you'd become infected. Virtually all the bathhouses and backroom bars closed. Not that gay men stopped having sex, but they could no longer walk from one sex partner to another as freely as they did at the baths. Jerk-off clubs arose in their place, often with "monitors" making sure that no one actually penetrated anyone else.

Perhaps the closing of the baths and the back rooms was the impetus for the rise of private sex parties. These parties are usually organized by a gay man and held at his house. They are, therefore, more controllable and, while highly sexual, are usually more friendly than the anonymity of the great masses of people who go to the few baths still in existence (see *Baths; Tearooms and Back Rooms*).

One doesn't need a large space to contain a group of naked, horny men. While a country house with a swimming pool (just like in porn videos) is aesthetically preferable since men can have sex in and around the pool, we know of successful sex parties in studio apartments. The only physical requirement is privacy.

There are a few other requirements. Men who come to these parties must be uninhibited and experienced in the gay sexual scene. Timidity is not welcome. Nor is this the appropriate setting in which to come out in the gay world. One is expected to participate sexually with the whole group; you can't pick out a boyfriend for the evening. You may be a top or a bottom and not want to switch, but be prepared to square off with a number of people before the last man leaves.

There are a number of ways of getting a sex party group together. The easiest, given that you have sex with a lot of men, is to call a bunch of your tricks (you'll need a minimum of four, preferably more) and ask if they'd like to meet one another at your house for sex. They may be intrigued. On the other hand, they may all look alike or be all bottoms or all tops, in which case they may be upset with you, since you're probably the only one who will enjoy it. Calling your tricks only works if you (and they) are sexually versatile (see *Versatility*).

Placing an ad in a local gay publication is another way of getting a sex party started. But remember, you'll be the organizer and you'll have to do most of the work. Your ad should say something like "Established sex group looking for more members. Versatility and safe sex required. Not chemically friendly. Call John at XXXX." Ask potential callers to leave information about their stats. Which stats? Whichever ones interest you. The phone number you use is generally an anonymous mailbox where interested guys can leave their phone numbers. Call them, or at least those who sound like good prospects. You should ask basic information including age, height, weight, and hair color. Some people want to know about other physical characteristics, including dick size and whether they are cut or uncut.

It's your party, so ask whatever you want, but do it in a sexy way, not like you're an agent from the IRS.

Each caller must be interviewed on the phone for a variety of reasons. First, you want to weed out potential weirdos and/or dangerous people. You also have to be certain that there aren't too many bottoms at your party. It's simply a fact that bottoms outnumber tops (some bottoms wail that the ratio is four to one), and you don't want the evening to end up with everybody "pussy bumping" (it also gives you a bad reputation). A few minutes of phone talk will give you an idea of whether the guy sounds gregarious and sexy. If he lacks confidence or sounds ambivalent, pass him by. Take at least fifteen minutes for the phone interview. You should also know the age range of the people you'll invite. There are no rules of thumb, except that all the participants should be turned on to men in that age range. People of different races usually tell you so up front as they don't want to get rejected when they arrive. Experienced organizers of sex parties prefer to invite a mixture of both experienced and novice participants. Ask for their stats during the phone interview and check to see that they agree with the message they left in the mailbox. (You'll have to be good at keeping records.) Question any discrepancies; they may be warning flags that the guy is hiding something. If you don't get a satisfactory explanation, pass him by and go on to the next phone call.

The phone interview is a perfect time to discuss safe sex and drugs. We're all for a wide sexual repertoire, but passing on the HIV and STDs isn't our idea of good hospitality. Tell the man you're interviewing that barebacking isn't allowed and have him agree to fuck or get fucked only with condoms (see *Barebacking*). That means, incidentally, that *you'll* supply a bowl of condoms next to the bowl of nuts. *Don't* depend on your guests to bring them. Accept that you have no way of ascertaining whether any of your guests are HIV-positive. Of course you can ask, but some guys lie, and others are so terrified of being tested, they might not know. For a couple of reasons, we also think you should prohibit alcohol and party drugs. Men who are alcoholic or use party drugs are more likely to try to have unsafe sex with you or one of your guests. Secondly, many party drugs, while making one feel sensual, also make dicks soft or prevent coming (see *Drug Abuse*). Guys who want drugs are generally more into the drugs than the sex. Passing around a few beers or a bottle of wine is enough to take the edge off nervousness.

Some gay men interview each potential sex party participant in person, but this can be a laborious procedure if you receive dozens of phone messages. There's no perfect number of men to invite to a sex party, except that experienced organizers suggest inviting twice as many as you actually want. For whatever reason, many won't show up.

A third way to get a sex party organized is through the Internet. Go to a gay cruising site and post a message. You'll have to leave your e-mail address. Have no fear since you should have two or three e-mail addresses (one for your mother, one for your friends, and the last for cruising the Net—and sex parties). Ask men to e-mail a photograph of themselves. You could insist on a nude photo, but be prepared to e-mail him a picture of your naked body in return. Under no circumstances should you send a man pictures of other guests unless they give you permission to do so. If you're hampered by a huge number of responses, just whittle them down to a reasonable number.

After a few sex parties you'll generate a regular guest list. Future sex parties should combine them with a few new faces.

Set arrival time at, say, 8 P.M. on a Friday night. Call each guest a couple of days before the party for confirmation that he's still committed. Give them all time to arrive; don't rush into the sex. This gives them a chance to meet, chat, and size each other up. Have a cutoff time for arrival, say, 9 P.M., and don't answer the doorbell after that; it breaks the mood (unless you're good at hopping, it's also inconvenient to ask someone to take his dick out of your ass so you can answer the doorbell). Have condoms, lubricants, and towels in plain sight. Some hosts like to provide refreshments, while others ask their guests to bring them. Some hosts ask for $10 or $20 for soda, beer, and light snacks.

Cover your furniture with "party sheets." Roll up valuable rugs, or anything else that might get come-stained. If you don't, you'll end up with too much DNA on your furniture. Come towels should be spread out. Put away anything that's breakable. A man with a cock in his mouth shouldn't have to worry about your Limoges bowl, and you don't want to hear it crashing to the floor.

Pay attention to the environment. Provide music, but not too loud and not too pounding. The lights should be dimmed, not turned off, as it destroys the voyeuristic element of the scene, and more practically, so guests won't trip and break lamps, furniture, or their own bones. Provide plastic bags for their clothes and label bags with their names. If there are only a few guests, they'll probably prefer to pile their clothes in a corner.

Some experienced hosts ask guests to wear their underwear for a while—if they are wearing underwear. Start the party with a porn tape on the VCR. This usually produces hard-ons and touching of same. Taking off underwear—uncovering a fat dick or a bubble-butt ass—will certainly heighten the level of excitement. Someone has to break the ice; if none of your guests does, then you must. Start kissing someone while caressing his cock. The others will join in.

Sex parties can last from two to four hours. Many men will chat afterward; they may go out for dinner or to a bar or dancing together. It all depends upon how friendly they want to be. The friendlier ones will exchange e-mail and phone numbers—perhaps to get together at a later time as a twosome.

There are problems to contend with. How you handle them depends on how prohibitive you want to be. It's difficult to interfere with barebacking or someone who arrives drunk, although as the host you can ask them to leave. (And don't ask them back.) Also don't invite back someone who doesn't prepare himself for getting fucked.

It's not just that you don't want little brown stains on the sheets, but a failure to douche indicates a man who doesn't take care of himself—or care about others. There's also the possibility of a rude guest who rejects everyone. While he may say that you and your guests are not his type, he's probably just scared. Quietly tell him that he doesn't have to stay; he'll be glad to hear it.

Recently some sex parties have taken place at the house/apartment of someone with a Webcam. The camera was turned on and the scene sent over the Internet for others to watch (see *Webcams; Exhibitionism and Voyeurism*). That's really pushing the envelope. Never do this without everyone's permission.

Should a gay couple join a sex party together? (See *Couples.*) Some couples can without jealousy (see *Jealousy, Envy and Possessiveness*). Others can't and are asking for serious trouble in their relationship. Remember, sex parties aren't for everyone. Many gay men prefer a more sentimental environment—sex parties are definitely not sentimental. Follow your own fantasy.

Sex Phobia (or Puritanism)

Puritanism is named after the European émigrés who arrived in America in the early seventeenth century and set up the Plymouth and Massachusetts Bay Colonies. They were the conservative Christians of their time who fled England, Holland, and other countries because they felt those places were too morally easygoing. Mocked and oppressed at home, they established a new home where they were free to oppress one another and anyone else who came under their sway, including Native Americans. Because they eventually became cofounding fathers of the United States (along with the English settlers in New York, Pennsylvania, Maryland, Virginia, and the Carolinas), their ideas about life, including sex and morality, have deeply permeated American society for better and for worse.

Essentially, puritans believe that humans are sinful at birth, and despite various mitigating rites such as baptism, people can never fully escape being sinful all their life. Human sexuality has only one function: to produce a child. Any sex act not motivated by reproduction is sinful. As a result, 99 percent of the daily sexual acts of people, no matter their sexual preference, are totally unacceptable to puritans.

What we call sex phobia is that same puritanism that assures most of us that we are eternally damned no matter what we do, but somewhat updated and clothed in twenty-first-century garb. It's best-known adherents are Baptists and Evangelicals, seen through television shows on "Christian cable networks," where the main goal appears to be to raise money and broadcast their divisive message in a sweet-as-molasses delivery. Virtually anyone who disagrees with their views is deemed a "damned sinner," condemned to burn in hell. Their major enemies are people who support freedom of choice on abortion, homosexuals, and anyone who participates in nonreproductive sexual acts. Other religions, notably Orthodox Judaism and conservative Islam, even though they differ greatly from fundamentalist Christianity in other ways, share their belief in sexual repression.

In America, large swaths of the South and the Midwest fall into what is known as the Bible Belt. Anyone born and raised there is immediately and continually subjected to this oppressive and repressive thinking; as well as subjected to the corollary belief that anyone who thinks differently is evil and in league with the devil. Breaking out of this repressed closed-loop form of thinking means learning to think independently, and it is usually accompanied by the loss of many friends, family members, and past associates. Even questioning that belief system makes you ipso facto the enemy you've been taught for years to abhor; one ends up hating oneself. For gays, lesbians, bisexuals, transgendered people, the teaching of puritanism is clear: You are a sinner and unworthy of love. Repress who you are; convert to heterosexuality.

The AIDS epidemic exhibited instances of the result: dying sons facing rejecting puritanical families expressing vituperation in the name of religion. This behavior contrasted sharply with the true loving care some dying men received from their gay families and friends, and occasionally by truly loving families (see *Gay Families*; *Parents*).

Many gay men have not escaped the clutches of their puritan ancestors. Signs of its effects show up in their attitudes about sex and in their sexual behavior. The primary sex-phobic attitude is the condemnation of sexual behavior in others, gay or straight, along with the belief that society is justified in punishing (jailing) people who participate in particular kinds of adult consensual sex. Another puritanical belief is that one kind of sexual behavior is more "normal" than another among consenting adults, even though that other behavior may cause no physical or psychological harm. While one sexual behavior, oral sex, say, may be more statistically common than another, such as fetishistic sex, puritans lump them all together, saying one is as unhealthy as the second (see *Blow Job*; *Fetish*).

Even when gay men raised under sex phobia find the inner strength to question, think for themselves, or physically escape central sites of puritanism, too often the teachings of a lifetime have become too deeply embedded in the mind. Attitudes influence behavior. Gay men who define their sexuality in extremely narrow terms, who either avoid sex completely or some of its variations, are adhering to puritanism and are probably suffering from guilt, depression, and sexual problems. For gay men it's not so much the actual sexual behavior that is affected. In other areas of their life, conflict, doubt, shame, and a constant sense of worthlessness often lead gay men of these backgrounds to internalized homophobia, drug abuse, and alcoholism (see *Homophobia*; *Drug Abuse*; *Booze and Highs*).

If any of the above seems familiar to you, remember, you are not to blame. Also remember, there are professional and nonprofessional people who are willing to help you get past the worst effects of sex phobia.

Sex Toys

Sex boutiques sell a wide range of merchandise. Among the items most commonly offered for sale are an enormous range of aids for curing sexual dysfunctions: creams to delay ejaculation; machines and salves to cure impotence; and aphrodisiacs to enhance sexual desire. They are all expensive, useless junk. However, regarded as amusements and not cures, sex toys can add variety and excitement to your erotic life. You can insert your cock into a rubber or plastic sheath, and a partial vacuum that builds and releases on the principle of a cow milker will suck you off (see *J.O. Machines*). A more expensive model will suck and fuck you at the same time, or suck you and your partner simultaneously. Electric vibrators slipped onto the back of the hand can introduce novelty into masturbation. There are battery-operated vibrators in the shape of cocks, which you can use to fuck yourself.

There are *dildos* in all sizes, some eight inches in circumference, others nearly a yard long. Don't use one longer than ten inches, or you may damage yourself. Perhaps you should start with a small one and get used to it. The dildo should be made of soft, flexible material, either rubber or pliant plastic. Hard plastic or metal dildos are dangerous, as are those that can be cranked and twisted about in your ass (a metal wire runs down the center of the tube and might poke out and puncture the wall of the rectum). Be sure the dildo has balls or a wide base so it can't slip up your ass beyond the point of retrieval, which might require surgery. A double dildo (called a double dong) is a long rubber tube with a glans at each end. Some couples coordinate their movements while using it so that each partner gets fucked simultaneously. *Remember, don't put candles, turkey basters, flashlights, Coke bottles, lightbulbs, or any other objects up your ass—and don't let anyone else do it to you* (see *Dangerous Sex*; *Saying No*). While this list sounds absurd, foolish gay men have tried them all.

An entire class of sex toys consists of gadgets associated with S/M, such as chains, belts, handcuffs, whips, nightsticks, and other instruments of authority and punishment. Others were first associated with S/M but have now become ubiquitous in the gay scene. *Cock rings* are devices placed around the bottom of the penis and sometimes around the balls while the cock is soft or semi-hard. After the cock becomes fully hard, the ring cuts off the outflow of blood and prolongs the erection. There are several kinds of cock rings: metal loops of varying size, leather straps that snap shut, and leather thongs that are tied around the cock and balls. The leather strap is the most comfortable and the easiest to get on and off, but many men prefer the hardness (and coldness) of thick metal rings. Mind you, many metal rings are thick enough to set off metal detectors. This can lead to embarrassing (or hysterically funny) situations in airports, schools, and some government office buildings as you try to explain to the authorities why you keep setting off the security alarm.

Another device often sold as a sex aid but much more useful as a sex toy is the *cock-enlargement pump*. Most of these consist of a plastic tube (into which you insert your cock) and a pump attachment. Some J.O. clubs sponsor "pump nights" for those into vacuum pumps (see *J.O. Clubs*). Essentially the pump is a device for masturbation. It will certainly not enlarge your cock, no matter what the ads promise. *Always be careful when using this device!* The cock has a rich and sensitive vascular system; abusing it can damage blood vessels. Men who use such pumps often tend to have puffed-up-looking cocks, with puffy, loose skin, as a result of the vascular damage. It's seldom attractive or good for your health. Manual machines are preferable to automatic pumps.

Tit clamps are popular. These metal clips, called alligators for their shape, and sometimes lined with rubber, boost sensation when placed on the nipples. They can also cause excruciating pain. *Snakebite kits* have rubber sucking cups that serve the same purpose. *Tit rings* are inserted through pierced nipples, just as earrings are placed through the earlobe. They are less painful to wear than tit clamps (see *Body Decoration*). Sometimes a leather thong or metal chain is strung through the tit rings and given to the sadist to play with. Many masochists enjoy "tit torture" during sex, especially when they are sucking off their master.

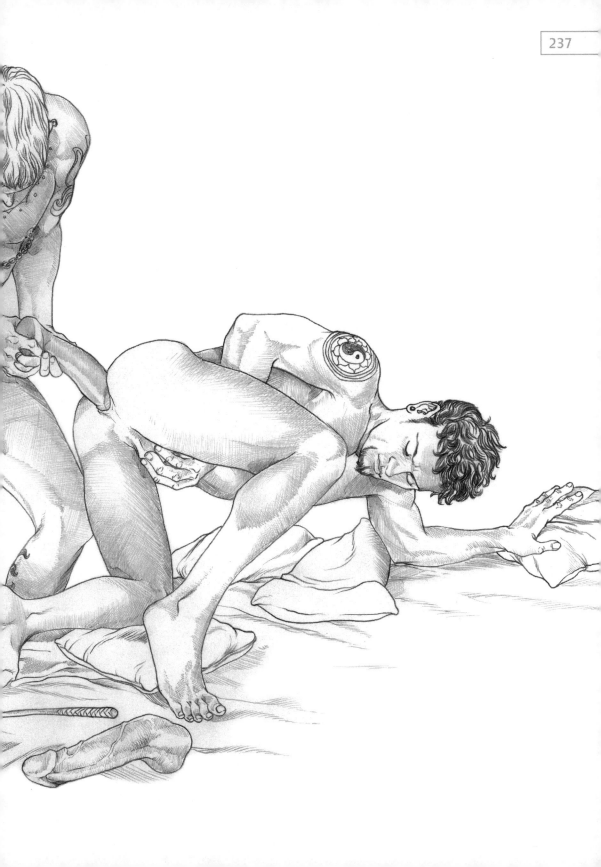

Sometimes weights are attached to a slave's balls. As he becomes more aroused, heavier weights are added. Other, more exotic gear includes leather or latex masks, gags (see *Bondage and Discipline*), dog collars, and leashes. Male "chastity belts" are also available. They consist of a leather belt around the waist, a strong snap that goes between the legs, and a dildo inserted up the ass and held in place by the strap. Some of those trim executives you see dashing about town or presiding over committee meetings are sitting on a six-inch dildo only their master can remove. Less extreme, but also popular, is the *butt plug*, a rubber object shorter than a dildo that when inserted keeps the asshole from tightening up. Use one if you have a big-cocked lover who likes to fuck you often.

Ambitious sex boutiques may offer a great many more devices and toys, including such large S/M contraptions as racks, stockades, and slings. These are all for gays with large bank accounts.

Remember, sex toys must be cleaned after use. In most cases washing them well with hot water and antibacterial soap is recommended. However, if there's any doubt, or if the skin of anyone in the scene has been broken, do the following: Wash the toy with soap and water, then thoroughly rub it with alcohol, to kill any lingering germs. Finally, give it a second wash to get the alcohol off. This procedure ensures not only your own health, but also the health of future sex partners.

Most large cities have sex shops where these toys are available. Many are advertised in gay periodicals. The Internet is an excellent resource.

Sexual Harassment

Often misused and misunderstood, the phrase *sexual harassment* has gotten such a bad rap that it's almost impossible to look at it in an unclouded way. All of us have heard horror stories about some guy who made what he thought was some innocent remark and not much later found himself on the unemployment line. The truth is different, and usually more complex. Sexual harassment is something that can affect any gay man on the job, at leisure, while traveling, and in his dealings with family and strangers, the community, or the government. The rules that were originally established to protect women from sexual harassment from men are now being used to protect straight men from sexual harassment from women and other men, and gay men from sexual harassment from anyone, gay or straight, male or female. While it is true that males still have more difficulty demonstrating that they have been victimized, enough legal cases have been won by men, along with sizable damages awards, to show that, too, is changing.

What is sexual harassment for gays? Like old-time ice cream, it generally comes in two flavors, one seemingly vanilla white and the other darker in color. The seemingly vanilla variety occurs whenever you as a gay male are being sexually bothered by a straight man or woman who is more powerful than you are or in a position to do you harm if you don't go along with his or her wishes. We call it vanilla because it presents itself pretty obviously as harassment.

How do you know you're being sexually harassed? Generally, harassment is when someone makes you feel extremely uncomfortable because of your sexuality, and this person is acting in a *sexually suggestive* or *aggressive manner.* If someone marches around your office or your school with a sign reading ALL GAYS GO TO HELL: REPENT NOW with quotations from the Old Testament, he or she is unquestionably a bigot and a homophobe, but unless (s)he's also grabbing your ass and/or crotch or offering him/herself for sexual favors, he or she is *not* sexually harassing you (see *Homophobia*). On the other hand, an avowedly heterosexual man or woman in your class, at sports, or especially at work who continually talks to you about being gay, having gay sex, or sex with you, even when you have asked him or her to stop doing so, *is* sexually harassing you. As is anyone, especially a superior, who takes you aside to tell you that you are either dressing too provocatively (when you know that you aren't) and that you're getting him or her hot; or the opposite, that you're dressing insufficiently sexy. If someone tells you that he or she has been looking forward to experimenting with gay sex or with a gay man, and you have been chosen to fulfill that particular desire, it's sexual harassment. It stands to reason also that any superior who demands sex outright in return for a promotion, for a transfer to a better department, or for not firing or transferring you is sexually harassing you.

Remember, not everyone who discusses gay sex with you is necessarily committing a crime. If you allow such discussion, encourage it, or do not stop it, then something else is in operation (see *Out on the Job*). And if your straight coworkers, male or female, go out of their way to discuss their heterosexual acts in great detail ("I ate pussy for three hours last night"), this is considered sexual harassment.

Of course, some gay men sexually harass straight men. If you're the one doing that, you have no sympathy from the authors. If you've asked the object of your attentions to go out with you and have been refused or been told he's not gay, keep your trousers and lips zipped. Remember these clichés: Life is unfair; and you can't always have what you want. And if the guy overreacts to your advances, keep in mind that you may not be the first man to have wanted a piece of him. If he's cute, he may have been sexually harassed or even sexually molested already and is afraid of having it happen again. If you discover that's the case, back off totally.

The second, darker kind of sexual harassment comes from within the gay community itself and is one of its dirty little secrets (see *Racism; Domestic Violence; Rape*). This brand of harassment happens when another gay man makes repeated, unwelcome advances toward you at work or at school. Unfortunately it's not all that different from sexual harassment by straights, except perhaps that as gay men we expect better from other gay men and it can be crushing indeed to realize a fellow homosexual is being such a louse.

Also keep in mind that if you are working in a mixed (gay and straight) office or school and you are discussing in detail your sexual activities within others' hearing, and you don't stop doing so after they've asked you to stop, you are also guilty of sexual harassment. No matter how much you think your straight boss or his elderly secretary should know about your rimming and felching habits, keep it to yourself.

What do you do if you believe you are being sexually harassed? If it's at work, go to whoever handles personnel and ask for the guidelines on sexual harassment. Don't be bullied by the personnel director either into initiating action or not initiating action. He or she may have his or her own agenda. Follow the guidelines prepared for you. If such guidelines do not exist, request that they be prepared. In either case, unless your direct supervisor is the culprit, the matter will be brought to that supervisor's attention and you'll meet and discuss the matter. Spell out exactly what's going on and what makes you uncomfortable. Your supervisor will probably speak directly to the offender. Keep in mind that *unless that person is warned* by someone in charge, he can always pretend he didn't know that what he was doing was offensive, even if you and others said so a hundred times. Let the perpetrator make the next step, hopefully to mend his or her ways.

If the person harassing you *is* your superior or your professor or someone possessing some direct economic or social power over you, then you must take action either above his or her head or go around him or her and work through the personnel office. But whoever he or she may be, let the guidelines and people in charge do what they are supposed to. Allow time for it to pass; allow an apology to be rendered to you; allow all of it to stop and blow over. It's a good idea to keep a written record of everything that transpires.

If it continues or worsens, it's up to you to report it again and this time to demand specific action. At this point, the company, school, or organization will ask if you wish their harassment procedures to be set in motion. Once you have begun, do not falter or hold back. Let everyone concerned know that adequate opportunities for reform have already been given. Follow the required procedures completely.

In the event that your company, school, or group refuses to help, you have recourse to the law. Approach an attorney and/or psychological counselor. The latter may be needed since you're bound to be under undue stress, and the counselor can be called in as an expert witness if the matter comes to trial. (But be advised that the counselor might be required to turn over his written records of his sessions with you.) As a rule, if a company sees that you are serious about suing them over this matter, they'll usually offer to settle, get rid of the offender, pay you compensation, or some combination of these actions. At that point it's up to you and your advisers to decide what action to take.

In some cases, sexual harassment arrives from someone in your personal life. For example, a man you once dated and decided not to see again may begin calling you and hanging up or sending you ambiguous, unsigned letters. It can be even worse if he signs the letters, fantasizing that you're in love with him. Or someone you used to date or even live with may accost you on the street and threaten you about your seeing anyone else. This is *stalking*, the worst kind of sexual harassment. Stalkers are driven by their own twisted fixation and there's little you can do or say to alter their obsession. Anything you say—even public utterances or writings—will be misinterpreted to contain a secret message for the stalker. In this situation, the *last thing* you should do is confront him. Stalkers consider their victim their personal property to dispose of however they deem fit, and the result of a confrontation may not be pretty.

If you are being stalked, you may have to change your phone number and get a new, unpublished one. You may also have to change your habits so he is less able to follow you. In extreme cases, you may even have to change your place of residence. If you know him, you will probably have to file a court order against him, making it a crime for him to come any closer than a specified distance. If he has threatened your life, you may ask the police to tap your phone to help stop him. In larger American cities with celebrity populations such as New York and Los Angeles, stalking is a felony crime and is treated gravely indeed. The Stalking Division of both cities is located within the Homicide Division of their police departments. A frightening fact: Stalking can end in rape, torture, and murder. One of the authors of this book was stalked across the length of the United States during book tours for several years by a person he barely knew, and when he relocated, a local Stalking Division did all the legwork, taking care that he was living in a gated community where the man could not find him. They also ensured that his address and phone number would not be made available to anyone who requested it no matter whom they claimed to be. Even so there's always a possibility that a dedicated stalker can somehow connect with the PD or FBI and still track down his victim.

Whether it's stalking or sexual harassment, always keep in mind that you are *not* guilty of anything and that you *do* have recourse to the law. Also keep in mind that sexual harassment can show up in a wide assortment of forms. Probably the most fascinating male/male sex harassment suit in recent years concerned a youngish, slightly built, and attractive straight male working on an oil rig in the Gulf of Mexico who was sexually harassed by two to four other straight males whenever he was in the shower and sometimes when he was in his room. He accused them of holding him while the others touched and grabbed him and simulated gay sex with him. The victim naturally came to fear being at the least manhandled and at the worst raped. Yet neither his supervisor nor his boss nor his company would do anything to alter the other men's behavior. Oddly enough, as a result of his lawsuit, while the oil company and his bosses ended up paying fines and compensation, the men actually doing the harassing were neither fined nor fired. Presumably they're still at work on the oil rig, either awaiting another attractive man to victimize or already busily harassing one.

Sexually Transmitted Diseases

Sex is the spice that makes life exciting. That excitement, however, may come at a price, in the form of sexually transmitted diseases (STDs). Whether you're young and still going through your slut phase, or are tricking outside a long-term relationship, you may have to pay the piper for all that fun. It would be hard to find a sexually active gay man who's never had to see his physician for an STD, either something pesky such as crabs or more serious such as hepatitis.

As a gay man it is essential that you have a basic knowledge of STDs so that you can recognize the symptoms in you and in your sexual partners. If you discover symptoms that may be STD-related, it's your responsibility to insist on being given the correct diagnostic tests and treatment by your physician (see *Finding a Physician*). But you have another responsibility: to notify your sex partners about your infection. Not doing so is a sign of childishness and hostility.

At one time we used to talk about venereal diseases, those that directly affected the genitals, such as gonorrhea and syphilis. (The term *venereal* came from Venus, the Roman goddess of love.) But we have a more sophisticated understanding of disease today, and doctors generally divide them into bacterial, viral, and parasitical (what we call larger critters). We'll follow that classification below.

Since AIDS is covered in a different section, we're not going to discuss it here (see *HIV Disease*).

Bacterial STDs

Bacteria are everywhere in the world around us and are believed to live in the most hostile environments—beneath the sea at the Mid-Atlantic Ridge, where hot lava geysers out of the earth at boiling temperatures, under antarctic ice, within dust molecules in the upper atmosphere, and even inside rock miles deep beneath the earth. Some biologists believe that bacteria constitute the largest and oldest body of life on earth. It's impossible to avoid bacteria in daily life, and some bacteria are needed by the body to function, in your digestive tract for example, where they help digest food. Bacteria reproduce by themselves and only a relatively few (given their enormous number) are harmful to humans. Your blood generally produces white blood cells to fight off hostile bacterial invaders. Some potent ones, however, gang up and get the upper hand; that's when you get sick. Among the most common sexually transmitted bacteria are:

Gonorrhea. Commonly called the clap, after Mother Clap, who ran a bawdy house for homosexual men in Holborn, a section of London. Thirty to forty men a night were entertained there until one day in 1726, she was charged with keeping a "sodomitical house." (The term *homosexual* wasn't coined until 1869.) The poor lady was fined, pilloried, and sentenced to two years of hard labor. We don't know if she survived.

Clap is a major health problem in gay men. About 15 percent of men who get gonorrhea in the penis *do not* develop symptoms, and even those who do may not see them for two weeks. That makes detection difficult. Carriers without symptoms *can* transmit the disease without knowing it. Therefore, men who practice unsafe sex should have a routine STD checkup every six months (every three months if you're still being a slut), which means an anal, penile, and throat smear, and a urinalysis for clap (and a blood test for syphilis while you're at it). A blood test alone will not diagnose gonorrhea. Even if you have regular checkups, you can unwittingly infect an awful lot of people before you discover you have the clap. Called *Neisseria gonorrhoeae* (a gram-negative diplococcus, for those who care), the bacteria prefer a warm, moist environment like your cock, rectum, and throat.

You can get clap in the cock by getting a blow job from someone whose mouth is infected—or you can get it in the mouth or throat by sucking someone with an infected dick. Symptoms normally appear between twenty-four hours and five days after exposure. The chief symptoms are a discharge of thick, creamy pus and burning during urination. The pus is produced when bacteria invade the cells that line the urethra (the canal that carries urine). By milking down your cock, you can see the earliest signs of pus. You should also check your underwear; the dried pus will make the pouch of your underwear stiff. Some sexually active gay men *never* undress with a trick with the lights off. They quietly take down the trick's underwear in the light (in a sexy way) and check his dick for a discharge. If they find it, the trick goes packing. He shouldn't be having sex while he's infectious. This procedure needn't be clinical—use your imagination! If, however, you delay treatment, the infection will spread up the urethra and into your prostate—which will really fuck you up.

You can develop the clap in the ass if someone with gonorrhea fucks you without a condom. Symptoms are usually slower to show up in the rectum (if they develop at all), and detection is certain only if your doctor looks at a smear under a microscope or cultures the bacteria in a laboratory. The symptoms you might notice are rectal fullness (feeling as if you have to crap), pain, frequent farting, rectal bleeding, hemorrhoids, pus or blood in the stool, diarrhea, constipation, and sometimes an inability to piss. This urinary retention is brought about when bladder nerves are infected by gonorrhea. (The symptoms don't necessarily mean you have gonorrhea. Only a test can determine this.) But be forewarned: You may not have symptoms at all, or you can have clap in both your cock and your ass, but because you can feel the symptoms in your cock more clearly, you might not notice what's happening in your butt.

If your doctor is heterosexual or unfamiliar with gay health problems, get over your shyness and tell him that you need to be regularly tested in the rectum. Don't be reticent about asking for an anal smear. Some straight physicians are embarrassed about asking. If your doctor refuses to do an anal smear, walk out, don't pay the bill, and get a new doctor.

Gay men also contract gonorrhea in the throat. Symptoms are often absent, but when present are a sore throat, a cough, respiratory congestion, and other coldlike disturbances. Sometimes the glands under the jaw swell. Clap in the throat is less frequent than clap in the penis and anus, but then again it depends upon your sexual behavior—what you do and with whom.

Gonorrhea should be treated immediately. If it is not treated, the acute symptoms will go away after about six months, but the disease may lead to arthritis, pericarditis (inflammation of the sac around the heart), or emphysema. *Medical authorities have also learned that men with clap are at an increased risk for getting infected (and infecting others) with HIV.*

Your physician, of course, must confirm all these suggestions. He alone can prescribe treatment, though you should insist that he take a "cure culture" after treatment. That means testing you again for the disease to be certain that you are cured.

Don't even think about telling your lover (should you infect him) that you picked up the clap (or any of the following STDs) from kissing an "old flame," sitting on a toilet seat at work, using a "dirty" towel at the gym, or drinking from a "greasy" water cup. This kind of bacteria needs a constant supply of carbon dioxide and die seconds after exposure to air. In any event, your boyfriend won't believe your bullshit and you'll be correctly accused of both tricking *and* lying. This will cost you at least ten sessions of couple therapy, lectures about double betrayal, and a bill of particulars about your tawdry behavior going back to childhood. Pony up to your infidelity, take your punishment, and don't lie.

Syphilis The first recorded outbreak of the disease appeared in 1494 among French soldiers stationed in Naples. At that time the mortality rate was virtually 100 percent. Everyone in Europe blamed it on everyone else. The Italians called it the French disease, while the French called it the Neapolitan disease. When it arrived in Turkey, the Turks called it the Christian disease. And the Chinese called it the Portuguese disease. Everyone finally agreed to blame it on Columbus, whose men, it is said, brought it from the New World after being contaminated by the Carib Indians. There's some recent historical evidence that suggests that Columbus and his men got a bad rap. Syphilis may already have been in the Old World.

Treponema pallidum is the name of a corkscrew-shaped bacteria called a spirochete that literally burrows through your skin and into the bloodstream. It is most usually transmitted through anal sex, although a much smaller percentage has been known to get it through oral sex. The first symptom of syphilis is a red sore called a chancre (about the size of a pea), though this sore does not always appear. The skin breaks open to reveal the chancre, which may soon be covered by a yellow or gray scab. It is painless and does not easily bleed, although it may be painful in the butt. Syphilis is *highly contagious* at this stage. Left untreated, the chancre heals by itself in a few weeks; unfortunately, the disease continues to develop. This is the time to get to the doctor because, while syphilis is less common than gonorrhea, it's more serious.

The sore, if it appears, can show up as early as ten days after sexual contact but ordinarily occurs about three weeks after infection. Aside from it there are no symptoms, except that lymph nodes often become tender, inflamed, and enlarged to the size of grapes.

Secondary syphilis starts about four to six weeks after the initial infection. A rash, which does not necessarily itch, breaks out (usually all over the body); it can even appear on the palms and the soles of your feet. The patient has a general feeling of ill health—headaches, nausea, loss of appetite, and fever. Hair sometimes falls out. (Luckily it grows back.) The person is highly contagious; he can transmit syphilis through all the mucous membranes, including those of the mouth and anus. The second set of symptoms will also disappear within a few weeks, but then the illness enters a third, more dangerous stage.

For several years the untreated disease will be latent in the body. There will probably not be symptoms, though a sore may appear at the site of the original infection after a year or two. Once a year has passed, the patient is no longer infectious. Some advanced cases will move on to tertiary syphilis. There are three kinds: One, benign, is characterized by the development of large lesions in and on the body; the second, *cardiovascular syphilis*, often ends in death from heart failure. The third kind, *general paresis*, leads to the deterioration of the central nervous system and psychosis. This stage is usually reached ten to twenty years after the initial infection. Fortunately, with the discovery of penicillin in 1943, there are few cases of tertiary syphilis.

Although syphilis can be cured easily if it's caught in its early stages, probably more than fifty thousand gay men contract syphilis each year. A blood test for syphilis is usually negative during the first four or five weeks of the infection, but it then turns positive. Blood tests are not always reliable for early syphilis infection, so if you have disturbing symptoms, have a second test even if the results of the first were negative. The treatment for early syphilis is a large dose of penicillin, though other antibiotics are used for people allergic to this drug. And don't forget follow-up blood tests. The presence of the HIV usually complicates the treatment of syphilis (see *HIV Disease*).

Prostatitis and Urethritis Prostatitis is a bacterial infection of the prostate gland that may result in its becoming enlarged or inflamed. The prostate is a gland lying next to the urethra. It squirts a fluid into the urethra when you come that mixes with sperm traveling up from your balls (see *Male Sexual Response*). Strictly speaking, prostatitis is not a problem that is sexually transmitted, but sometimes bacteria that enter the urethral canal during anal sex can work their way into the prostate and cause infection. Symptoms of prostatitis are burning in the urethra during urination and more frequent urination than usual. An erection is not painful, but sometimes ejaculation hurts. Pain is occasionally felt in or behind the balls, and once in a while specks of blood show up in the semen or urine. Inflammation of the prostate gland can also be a side effect of penile gonorrhea. A more frequent cause, however, is occasional bursts of sexual activity followed by regular periods of inactivity. Yet another cause is delayed ejaculation ("blue balls"). If you have an enlarged prostate, your doctor may recommend that you not get fucked until the swelling is reduced. To compensate for avoiding sex, he may suggest that you jerk off frequently, which may help your prostate condition.

The major cause of nongonococcal urethritis (an inflammation not caused by gonorrhea of the cells that line the urethra) is *chlamydia*. Chlamydia is the number one STD among heterosexuals, and so it can be spread to those gays who have sex with straight men. It's far less common in the gay community. About 60 percent of all the cases of an inflamed urethral canal are called nonspecific urethritis (NSU), which merely means that doctors don't know what the hell is causing it. It may be caused by chlamydia. The incubation period is one to five weeks. Chlamydia is hard to culture, so most doctors will treat it if they find white blood cells in your discharge. The primary symptoms of this very contagious disease are burning of the urethra during urination, and a discharge (usually clear). Vigorous sexual activity (such as fucking a trick like there's no tomorrow) can also cause abrasion of the penis that may lead to urethritis. Perfumed soaps and bubble baths can also cause urethral irritations. If you have a discharge of any sort, see your doctor and alert your partner.

Epididymitis The epididymis is a set of coiled tubes toward the back of and above each of your balls that store sperm. You can feel them easily with your hands. Urethritis, if not treated, may spread down to the epididymides and infect them. They become tender and swollen. If still not treated, the infection will redden your scrotum and infect your balls. You will have frequent discharges, painful pissing, and your balls will swell and hurt like hell.

Viral STDs

Unlike bacteria, a virus cannot reproduce by itself; it must invade a living cell to multiply. When a virus enters your body, generally through a break or pore opening in your skin, it moves in quickly. Your immune system creates T cells to attack it, but men with compromised immune systems may not be able to produce enough T cells to kill the virus. Therefore, AIDS patients may be either more susceptible to viral infections and/or suffer a more serious illness.

Hepatitis. This serious liver disease is widespread in the gay community. It is communicated in many ways—by kissing, by contact with any of the mucous membranes, by eating infected shellfish, by rimming (fecal/oral transmission), by infected semen (introduced orally or anally), and through transfusions of infected blood. There are several types of hepatitis: infectious (now called Type A); serum (Type B); and Type C, which is similar to Type B. Symptomatically they are all similar. Type B is the one that is spread sexually, but they are all highly contagious.

If you have hepatitis, you must be careful not to infect other household members. No kissing—of any kind. Keep separate dishes and wash them thoroughly. Since hepatitis is transmitted by feces (shit), you should wash your hands after every bowel movement.

The virus infects the liver. The early symptoms resemble the flu—severe muscle aches and pains, fatigue, fever, nausea, and at times vomiting. Sometimes a rash breaks out as well. Soon these symptoms disappear and you become extremely fatigued. Your urine turns mahogany brown and your shit becomes gray-white. Smokers lose their taste for cigarettes. Nausea and nearly complete loss of appetite occur; then your eyeballs and skin turn yellow (this is called jaundice). By this time, the worst is over, although you certainly won't look or feel your best. You may even have trouble getting out of bed.

Hepatitis A is generally spread by feces that enter your mouth either through rimming someone or through food you eat if a food preparer hasn't washed his hands properly after crapping. Shellfish can pick up the virus in contaminated water. Salads are a common transmitter if washed in contaminated water. The incubation period is two to six weeks, and during this time you are infectious. The disease runs its course by two months, and your liver generally recovers completely. But alcoholics, whose liver may already be damaged, may have a more difficult time with the disease; cirrhosis may occur.

Hepatitis Types B and C are similar. Type B is often called the gay hepatitis because it is often contracted while tricking, particularly in gay men who are fond of rimming. The incubation period for Types B and C is three weeks to ninety days. Hepatitis B and C can be lethal in HIV patients. Statistics also show that 90 percent of AIDS patients who contract hepatitis will become *chronic* sufferers.

There is no cure for hepatitis, just supportive treatment. You must seek a doctor's care, and he will probably suggest plenty of rest, eating a bland diet rich in vitamins, and during the acute stage, eliminating all fats (otherwise you'll become nauseated). He may also want to give you a shot of gamma globulin as a booster. *Cut out liquor and recreational drugs for at least six months after you regain your health or you'll have a relapse, which may be worse than the original disease.* Don't make the mistake of thinking that you are cured of the disease when your eye color returns to normal. Take a multiple vitamin daily. In the past, complete bed rest was recommended during the acute stage, but evidence now suggests that moderate exercise is preferable. Discuss this with your physician first. Don't go to the gym without his permission. You will not be able to work for weeks, and during this period you will sleep more hours than you're awake. Only in exceptionally severe cases is there reason to be hospitalized; home care is normally adequate. Your lover, roommate, or friends will have to run errands for you. Don't be a hero; ask for help.

There is now an effective vaccine for hepatitis A and B, but not for C. If you are sexually active, get the vaccination. Don't put it off. You can get hepatitis more than once, and a relapse is possible. It is a very serious disease.

Herpes. Herpes infections are caused by the same virus that causes cold sores. Its source is the herpes zoster virus, which causes the childhood disease chicken pox and the adult disease known as shingles. In sexually active gay men, herpes generally appears in the form of small, clear sores usually seen on the penis, especially just under the foreskin, though they may show up anywhere on the body, including the face.

Herpes simplex can be transmitted only during sex. Blow jobs, rimming, or merely rubbing your cock against a trick's ass can transmit it. The incubation period is from two to twenty days, although some cases are asymptomatic for as long as four years. The herpes virus invades the skin, and a burning sensation occurs within a week. A couple of days later, you'll notice a cluster of small blisters. You are highly contagious at this point. If you touch the blisters, wash your hands, because you can spread it to other parts of your body.

Afterward the virus enters a "latent phase," in which it goes into hiding, remaining dormant until it is triggered again. Once herpes goes away, it can come back again suddenly. Subsequent outbreaks are completely unpredictable.

There is no cure for herpes. There are treatments, based on the drug Zovirax, that can reduce its effect or shorten the time of the outbreak. Don't have sex while you have these sores, even with a condom, because the condom may not cover all of the sores. You may not be inclined to have sex anyway because the sores often make fucking painful.

AIDS makes herpes a more serious disease. Kaposi's sarcoma (KS) may be caused by a herpes virus called HHV8.

Venereal Warts. Venereal warts are caused by the human papillomavirus (HPV), transmitted during sex. It's as common as herpes and, like it, can recur. It's estimated that half of HIV-negative men and almost all HIV-positive men carry it. A partner fucking you without a condom or simply rubbing his cock against your ass can transmit it. Dildos and other sex toys can also carry the virus. You can develop a venereal wart on your asshole, ass cheeks, penis, and scrotum—the whole pubic area. Your hands are likely to carry the virus from one part of your body to another, although you will not develop symptoms on your hands themselves.

Warts are not usually painful, but they can become irritated and make fucking uncomfortable. Appearing as clusters of small, rough granules, they can easily be seen and felt, especially on your asshole or perineum (the skin between your asshole and your balls). They are clusters of small, rough growths. If they are inside your ass, you'll feel pain, itching, and bleeding after crapping or getting fucked. The incubation period for venereal warts varies from one month to many months.

If you and a regular lover or partner both have warts, do not resume sex until you *both* have been cured, or the contagious nature of the warts will lead to continued reinfecting. Lasers are now used to treat warts.

Larger Critters

Crabs. These little devils (*Pediculosis pubis*) are lice that are picked up during sex, either by contact with an infected man's pubic hair or by using infected sheets and towels. Frottage (pussy bumping) is enough to spread them (see *Frottage*). They are relatively harmless, though they itch like hell, especially at night. They grow chiefly in the pubic hair, but they have also been found under the arms, around the chest, around the crotch, and between the cheeks of your ass. If ignored, over time they have even been known to go exploring southward from hair to hair on the legs all the way down to the knees. Some idiotic gay men wait until they settle down in their eyebrows or beard. Crabs are different from head lice that nest only on the scalp. (How crabs and head lice know in which direction to march is a mystery.)

You can see crabs if you look hard enough. They are dark in color and usually live at the base of the hair follicle. You may catch some if you run a fine comb through your pubic hair—they mostly hang upon hair follicles and clutch dead skin—but they're not gorgeous to look at. You may also notice little blood spots on your underwear.

The best treatments are liquid preparations called A-200 and Rid, which can be bought in drugstores without a prescription. Your physician, however, may want to prescribe a more powerful treatment called Kwell. All medications come with careful instructions regarding their use. Wash your clothing (including the clothing you wore for the past couple of days), towels, sheets, and underwear in very hot water. Be sure to tell your sex partners to treat themselves for crabs, or you'll be reinfecting one another for months. Fortunately, crabs do not carry disease.

Parasites. The gay community has been heavily hit by sexually transmitted parasites, which cause gastrointestinal health problems. Doctors should check gay patients routinely for parasites, especially if the patients have bowel complaints.

Two kinds of parasites have become common among gays (and in many straights): *Entamoeba histolytica* and *Giardia lamblia*. Many people who travel to foreign destinations return home with these pests, which entered their bodies through contaminated food and water. Both varieties produce similar symptoms, which can range from no outward signs at all to violent dysentery. In between these extremes are such symptoms as soft stools, abdominal cramps, unusually smelly stools, gas, fatigue, fever and chills, loss of appetite, nausea, occasional vomiting, and a feeling of general malaise.

Parasites are one of the hazards of rimming, but there are many other intermediate and hard-to-discern methods of transmission (see *Rimming*). For instance, parasites can be transmitted by sucking someone's cock during anonymous sex: Your partner may have been fucking someone with parasites just before he met you. Hands are frequent carriers of parasites, particularly when they haven't been properly washed after shitting.

Diagnosis is difficult unless you go to a trained parasitologist or your doctor works with a lab technician who knows what to look for. Tropical disease centers are particularly knowledgeable about parasites. Usually a test is made upon a bit of fecal matter. The parasitologist can simply extract a bit of feces from the anus with a Q-tip, put it on a slide, and examine it under the microscope. A wet-stool test, however, is sometimes necessary in hard-to-detect cases. There are effective medications to rid the body of parasites. Treatment lasts from a couple of weeks to a few months. Don't have sex until your doctor okays it.

Scabies. Scabies are common among gay men. They are tiny parasites (actually mites called *Sarcoptes scabiei*) that live just below the surface of the skin, usually around the wrists, but often on the ankles, near the groin, and under the arms. They are itchy, especially at night. They are transmitted by skin contact, but can also be picked up from sheets and towels. If not treated, they will not produce dangerous symptoms, but they will drive you crazy. The preferred treatment is Kwell lotion, which must be prescribed by your doctor. Scabies are highly contagious.

Sex with Animals

Sex with animals seems to have been much more common throughout history than many of us would suspect. In the Western world, it was labeled sodomy by the church and the courts—a category that also included masturbation, anal intercourse, oral-genital contact, and coitus interruptus (pulling out before you come)—and punished harshly. The most famous case in America was that of Thomas Granger, a teenager who lived in Plymouth Colony in 1642. The unfortunate (and horny) boy confessed to and was found guilty of buggery (fucking) with a mare, a cow, two goats, five sheep, two calves, and a turkey (don't ask!). Now that's what you call a sexual appetite! Sex historian Vern Bullough tells us, "Though there was some difficulty in identifying the sheep so unnaturally used, mixed as they were with the flock, somehow five were selected to be executed along with the other animals, and they were burned in a great pit." Young Granger himself was also executed. The peculiarity of burning animals for sodomy was understandable since the Puritans believed that animals, like people, were responsible for their behavior.

The Chinese were constantly accused of having "love affairs with geese." Both Sir Richard Burton (the English explorer) and Paolo Mantegazza (an Italian anthropologist) accused them of fucking geese and wringing their necks at the moment of ejaculation so as "to get the pleasurable benefit of the anal sphincter's last spasms in the victim." French farmers were said to do the same; they claimed to have learned the sex practice from the English. And sex with animals is probably the only thing never blamed on the Italians.

One supposes life on the average farm was lonely much of the time. Shepherds tending their flocks day after boring day must have done a certain amount of jerking off in the fields. No surprise if, over time, they started fucking the sheep they were caring for. Only the most sexually repressed would blame them, though admittedly we city boys snicker about farm boys fucking the livestock. Or are we just jealous?

There doesn't seem to be a lot of sex with animals these days, although perhaps it's merely closeted. We suspect the incidence of animal sex is lower than it's ever been because of so much mechanization on the farm, the population shift to urban centers, and the replacement of family farms with corporate ones.

Moralists condemn sex with animals as disgusting, immoral, and generally horrible. Fortunately it's no longer a crime in a great many places, and nowhere in the United States is it a capital crime. We disagree with the moralists. Lots of children have looked at and played with the genitals of their pet cats and dogs, and we've heard of more than one who has masturbated his pet dog. A sexual partner of one of the authors had a large and likable Great Dane who sometimes attempted to get involved in their twosomes. Only after many complaints did the trick admit he'd trained the dog to have sex with him. The cowardly author failed to make this a three-way. Like other inexperienced city dwellers, we may not so readily fathom the mechanics of cow, sheep, or horse fucking, but see no reason to condemn it out of hand. We hope it doesn't become the *only* sexual contact in a man's life.

Frederick the Great took a practical attitude. During an important battle, he observed a soldier he recognized, fettered in irons. "Why is that excellent soldier in irons?" he asked of the officer in charge. "For bestiality with his horse" was the reply. "Fool," said Frederick the Great, "don't put him in irons, put him in the infantry."

* * *

Sex with Straight Men

It's not unusual for gay men just coming out to fall in love with straight men. It may be another student at school, a work colleague, or a man at the gym. It often happens because the gay man hasn't yet integrated himself into the gay community and the only men around are straight. This usually changes as the gay man moves on in life, begins to participate in gay activities, and meets and has sex with other gay men. In this sense, falling in love with straight men is a phase and part of the process of coming out.

But other gay men never emerge out of this phase, and remain attracted *only* to straight men. They become infatuated with these men as symbols of masculinity and attempt to seduce them into sexual situations. In the worst cases, they also express repulsion toward gay men, claiming homosexuals are feminine, weak, and inadequate.

There is a typical pattern to this behavior. The gay man concentrates on a straight man and campaigns hard to become his friend. Special favors (perhaps gifts) and anticipation of the straight man's needs follow, all designed to make the gay man indispensable. Inevitably, because of sexual fantasies and frustration, the gay man ends up obsessed with the straight man, and like many obsessions, it can consume his life.

Sex rarely occurs for an obvious reason: Straight men are attracted to women. If sex does occur between the two men, it's usually because the straight man is drunk or high, and reciprocity is not expected. After sex, the straight man often rebels by becoming distant. The gay man ends up as depressed and lonely as before.

How do we explain this self-destructive pattern? We believe it is one of the strongest forms of homophobia. Remember, homophobia maintains a sharp division between male and female behavior (see *Homophobia*). A gay man desiring only straight men believes he lacks real masculinity. Being with a straight man allows him to stand beneath the man's umbrella of virility, partake of his strength, and become whole again. In this scenario, other gay men are simply poor reflections of his own failure as a man, and so to be scorned.

Society's homophobia created these gay men, many of whom were taunted as sissies in childhood and watched "real boys" receive the praise and acceptance of both children and adults. The gay boys came to believe all the bad things others said about them, and in time—and this is most important—they became their own accuser.

Getting out of this straight-men-only pattern is difficult. Becoming more involved in gay activities, particularly political groups, can help the gay man face his prejudice and come to terms with his underlying depression. Once he is surrounded by gay men, he may learn to distinguish what truly constitutes masculinity and how it differs from the superficial version he has constructed.

Many gay men have relationships with straight men that do not fit into this pattern. Often the other man is a bisexual. In other cases he is a gay man who either by choice or involuntarily fell into straight instead of gay life. Some wed their childhood sweetheart when they were too young to figure out they were gay and are now enmeshed in marriage, with children and obligations. Some of these men knew they were gay but wanted a married life with children anyway. Unlike the straight man who allows himself to be adored by a gay man and may tolerate occasional sex, these "straight" men are active sex hunters, going after gay men for sexual and emotional gratification. The relationship between a gay man and such a "straight" man can be as fulfilling or unfulfilling as any other gay relationship: They can be lovers, fuck buddies, or anything in between.

Around the world, especially in many Asian, Arabic, and Southern European countries with strong conservative traditions, it's not unusual to find many more or less socially accepted relationships between a gay man and a straight man—and the straight man's family. Often the gay man is the "uncle" or benefactor of the (usually younger) married man and his family, and the wife and in-laws turn a blind eye to the sexual relationship because of whatever financial advantage or added status they derive from the alliance with a gay man.

Shaving

The sudden appearance of pubic and body hair, along with other changes accompanying puberty, such as the deepening of the voice and the surge of sexual desire, is surely the most dramatic event in the life of boys. Yet, paradoxically, because things like body hair quickly come to seem so natural, and sexual longings quickly become so all-encompassing in our imagination, it's often close to impossible for adult men to recall how their body looked and felt before they passed through the great hormonal divide.

Of all the changes that occur at puberty, only the presence of body hair is changeable. Maybe it's for this reason that some men like to recapture their boyishness by shaving their body.

The first thing you'll discover when you shave your crotch, your chest, your armpits, or your legs is a deliciously heightened sensitivity. Every inch of your newly mown skin will sing as thigh rubs thigh or pant leg, balls rub against underwear, or chest rubs against shirt. Your whole body will be much more sensitive against your sheets. The intensified sensation you'll experience might feel something like the focused, heightened awareness of bodily sensations some guys say so-called sex-enhancing drugs induce. But remember, as body hair begins to grow back, it will itch quite a lot. Only those with the most refined and peculiar sensibilities will enjoy that feeling for long.

Shaving your body will make your skin smoother and will tend to make you look more boyish, feminine, or androgynous. This is not everybody's idea of a good time, of course, but it will be a big turn-on to some. Today's porn stars, male models, and younger film actors almost all do it, making it a popular current trend. Admiring yourself in a mirror or stroking your smooth, shorn skin (or having your partner do it) may excite your sexual imagination and heighten masturbatory pleasure.

A man might prefer to be hairless for many reasons. You might want to offer your lover a new thrill. You might want to attract a new type—men who prefer smooth, boyish bodies. For other guys, a preference for smooth skin beneath them may simply be aesthetic or tied to unfathomable preconscious associations; Eros often leads us to prefer certain appearances and activities. So if you feel more fuckable with the kind of elegant legs that would look good in nylons, go ahead, enjoy the fantasy. Of course, this whole section is unfathomable to bears, who insist on growing more, not less, hair (see *Bears*).

The actual mechanics of shaving are easy. If you are fairly limber, most of your body (except your back) is within reach. When you get to your balls, you will have to make your wrinkled skin taut by holding on to the base of the sack and pulling the skin tight.

Shaved heads have become fashionable in gay life, especially so among the S/M set, and many men have learned to keep their head shaved (see *Sadomasochism*). The first time it is usually done by a barber, who will demonstrate how you can do it yourself.

For many men, shaving—especially shaving the crotch—has become a prelude to, even a part of, sex with their partner. The act connotes trust, intimacy, and a special bond between the men not available otherwise.

Allowing someone else to shave you, whether your balls or your whole body, may bring you in touch with little-boy fantasies (see *Daddy/Son Fantasies*). If you are going to be shaving someone else, remember you're likely to draw a little blood, and if there is any doubt in your mind about the health of the person you're playing with, wear latex gloves. It's also a good idea to use disposable razors. Don't forget there's a lot more surface area on the body than on the face; and on some hairy guys the skin is overgrown with a lush jungle. You don't want to run out of razors when half his crotch is shaved. As far as we know, asymmetrical or random-pattern shaving has not yet made it into fashionable gay consciousness.

If instead of shaving you'd rather use chemical depilatories to remove hair, go ahead. But follow the instructions and don't ever use depilatories on or around your asshole, because they burn like hell.

. . .

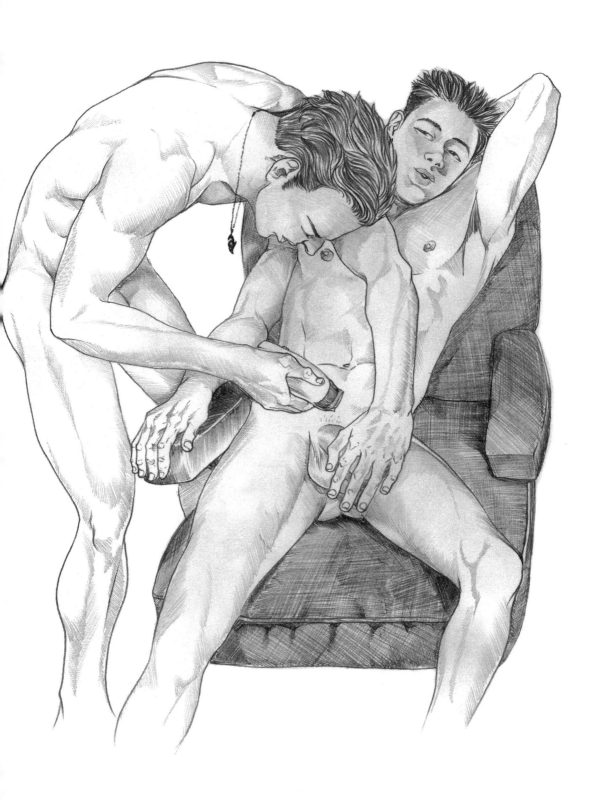

Side by Side

This is a comfortable and peaceful position for fucking. Both men lie on their side, one with his back to the other (spoonlike). The man behind lubricates a finger and opens up his partner's asshole with patience and tenderness. When the muscles are fully relaxed, he slowly pushes his cock in. It is one of the easiest positions for a novice to be fucked in. The penetration of the cock up his asshole is not as deep as in several other positions (see *Face-to-Face; Sitting on It*); he is not as immobile as when he is lying flat on his stomach. Nor is his own cock inaccessible. In fact, the man doing the fucking can easily wrap his arms around his partner and masturbate and fondle him.

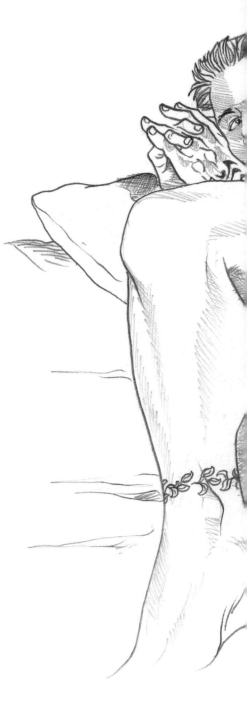

Sit on My Face

This polite imperative, offering comfort and pleasure, is hard to resist. Gay men spend a lot of time working on their buns at the gym and buying just the right pants to show them off. Gay men's tongues have also learned to explore these exotic regions. From the grasslands of the armpits down to the subtropical balls is as far a journey as some tongues used to take. But nowadays the adventurous tongue's trip around the world would be incomplete without a visit to that tropical rain forest of the body—

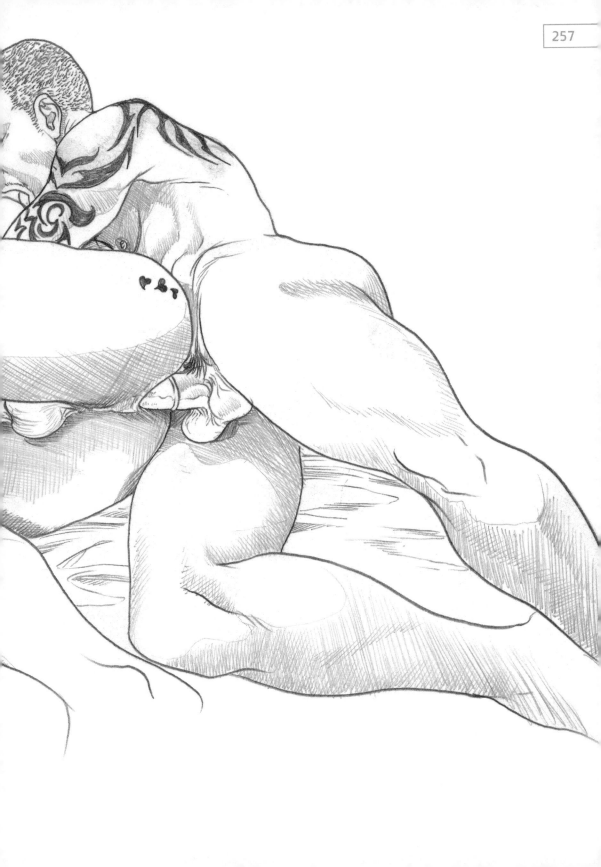

that land of perpetual moisture, tangled vegetation, and exotic smells: the asshole and environs.

As the eminent English poet W. H. Auden said:

I've often thought that I would like
To be the saddle on a bike.

Whether you are the sitter or the seat, it's a delicate and intimate maneuver. Get into position gradually, taking into account each other's weight, size, and flexibility, or else the man on the bottom will find his eyes, nose, and his mouth squeezed and sealed shut. If you just plop down, the partner beneath you will writhe hysterically, fearing imminent asphyxiation, while your ass will feel as if it is being attacked by gnawing rodents escaping from a trap. For some men, the thrill of the experience lies in submission to the weight and smell and oxygen-blocking properties of their partner's body. For others, the turn-on is in inflicting humiliation as their bottom becomes literally their ass-kisser.

But for many, there is something tender and intimate and delicate about the pleasure of this trip. Before he actually sits on your face, try this. Put him on his back with his legs over his head. Make sure your face is wet with saliva. Close your eyes and mouth, and rub your face in one long motion from the small of his back, up his crack, all the way across his rectum, and up over his balls. With a little patience you will be able to end up with your head upside down on his belly and your mouth on his dick.

Have him straddle your chest on his knees, facing your feet, while he lowers his buns over your face. In this position you can keep one hand on his belly and cock, and one hand on his ass to steady his weight, while he can reach your cock with his hands and his mouth. You'll have tantalizing glimpses up his tensed, straining back as your tongue and lips and teeth dart around. If he moves up a bit and sits on your forehead, he can rub his buns hard on your brow while you lick his balls. Or, if you want a better view, have him turn around and straddle your head. In this position, you get a wonderful worm's-eye view of his head thrown back, and of his erection rising in the foreground against a backdrop of belly and chest. Nibble, suck, and bite gently, and don't forget to wet his balls thoroughly with your saliva.

For many men, the smells down under are the chief thrill. Rank and dank odors from the interior mix with the smell of soap, clean or dirty underwear, talcum powder, and sweat. The kaleidoscope of odors will vary depending upon what he's been up to. For some, the smell of a man fresh from a three-piece suit and the air-conditioned executive suite is the only way to go. Others prefer the riper odor of a man fresh out of his jogging or exercise clothes. More delicate palates prefer the experience right after a shower with plenty of soap and warm water.

Let's stop and remember that rimming is sensational but potentially dangerous (see *Rimming; Safe Sex; Sexually Transmitted Diseases*). Fortunately, there is lots of

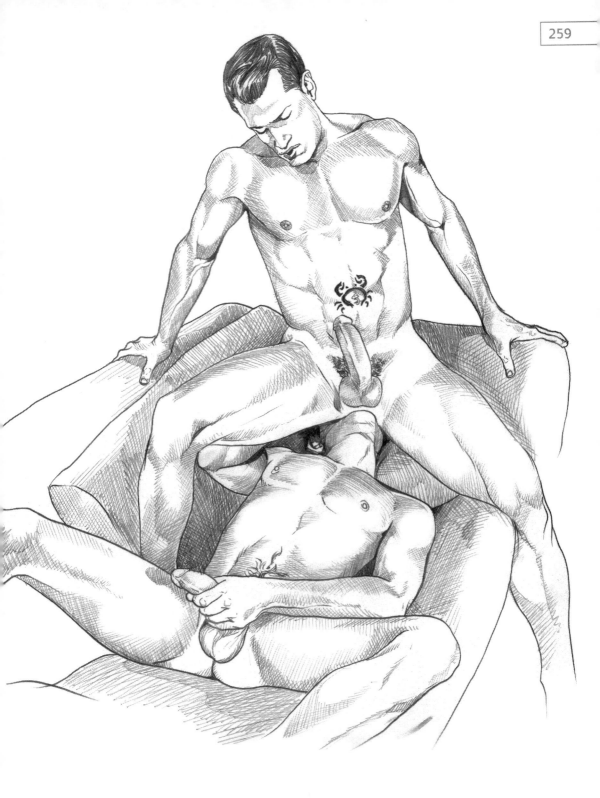

wild territory down there besides the asshole on the flip side of the lap. Poke around and explore, once you get comfortable.

Some men take particular delight in the royal road between the asshole and the base of the penis at the back of the balls, and in the underground cord that carries the throbbing of a hard dick deep within the body. (You can feel this cord if you press upward with your fingers between your anus and your balls while you squeeze your asshole closed.)

So get into the saddle—or be the saddle. As Andrew Holleran has a character say in his gay novel *Dancer from the Dance*, "My face seats five, my honey pot's on fire."

Sitting on It

Sitting on a cock is a reversal of the more common "missionary position." Here, the man being fucked is in complete control, which can be highly reassuring, especially if he's new to gay sex (see *First Time*). That's because he determines the rate of initial entry, the depth of penetration, and the speed and force of fucking. This position reduces anxiety in someone who equates getting fucked with discomfort and passivity. The man getting fucked can ride the cock to his heart's content and can bend down and kiss his partner whenever he chooses. He's taking what he wants in the way he wants it.

For the man doing the fucking, this position can be both relaxing and highly arousing. He can lie back and do nothing but watch the torso and shoulders and face of his partner. He can see his cock sliding in and out of those buns. Or he can take a more active role, urging his lover on, jerking him off, even learning forward to suck his cock. For those men who can remain at a high "plateau" of sexual excitement while fucking, often without coming at all, this is a perfect position, as they can pleasure their lover without having the pressure of coming themselves.

A few technical notes on this position. Straddle your partner and kneel facing him. The penis needs to be vertical. If it isn't, the man on top should fondle or suck it until it is hard. The man on top may have to place the sole of one foot on the mattress and rise a bit to get the cock completely inside him.

Rock forward and backward toward your partner's feet and feel his cock inside, rubbing against your prostate (see *Male Sexual Response*). Experienced men have expert control over their rectal muscles and can loosen or tighten their grip on a cock at will; they can use their assholes to grasp just the head of the cock, flexing the sphincter until their partner is ready to come.

This position can also be performed on a cocktail table, on the edge of a dinner

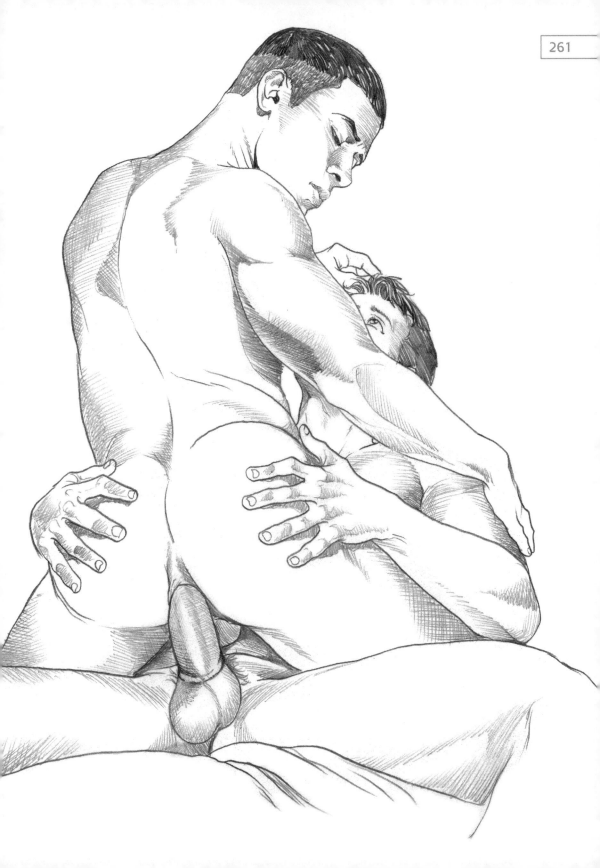

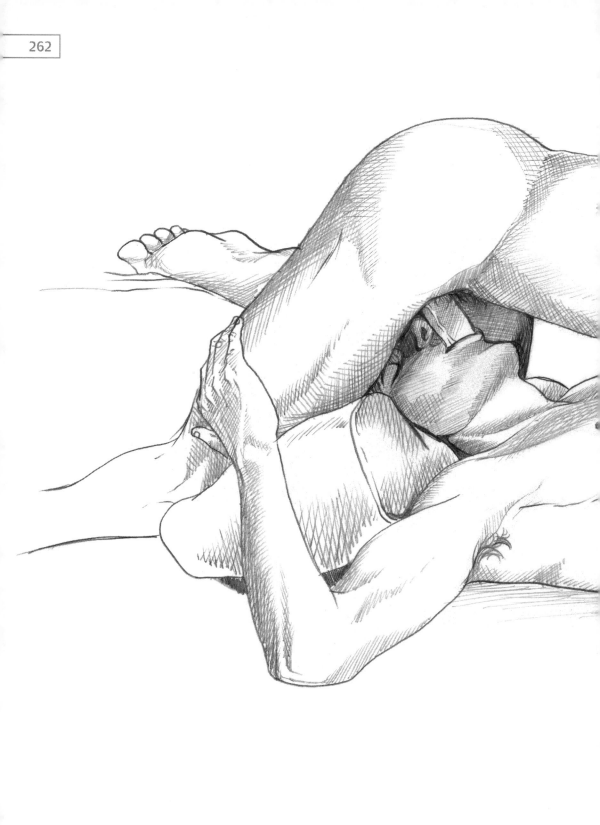

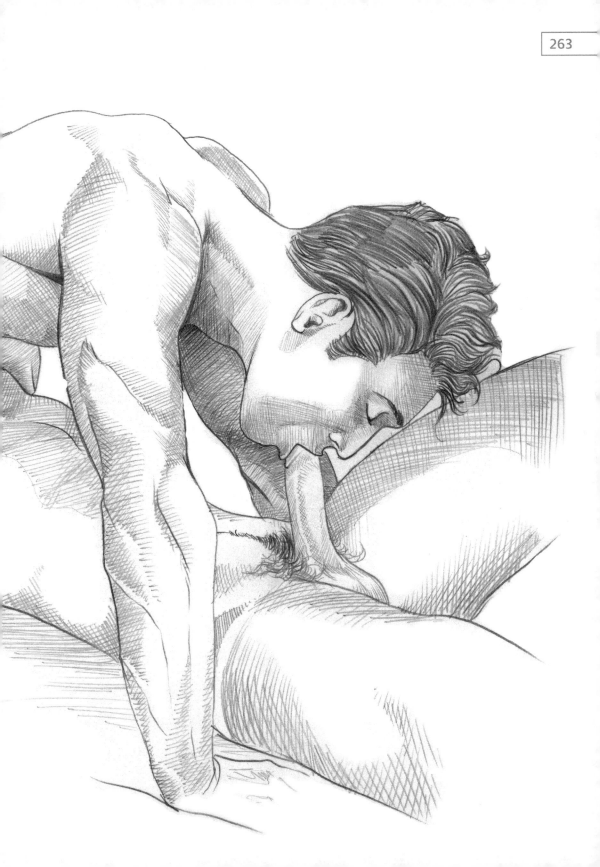

table, and even in a roomy armchair. In these cases, first make sure these objects are solid, flat on the floor, and not liable to tip over. The man on top can face either toward or away from his partner, or he can spiral himself on the cock without getting off. This latter position allows him to then lie flat on top of his lover and thus get fucked spoon fashion (see *Side by Side*).

Some tops don't like this position, or like it only briefly. They object because it makes them feel powerless. Other men dislike being fucked when on top because they equate being fucked with being dominated, covered, controlled. Others simply regard the position as unaesthetic.

Sixty-Nining

So called because 69 is the figure formed by the bodies of two men when they are in bed, facing each other, sucking each other's cock. It also has variations. If one partner is very strong, for example, he can stand and hold his partner upside down, so his mate's legs are over his shoulders. Others prefer a less athletic method, such as lying flat on their backs, feet to head, with only their upper torsos, necks, and heads twisted to reach the cock.

There used to be a joke that sixty-nining is what Princeton boys like to do since it's so *fair*. And the fairness, the equality, is both the most exciting and pleasant aspect of this position and also the main reason for complaint. What most people complain about is how difficult it is to concentrate both on the pleasure of sucking cock and being sucked, since both delights are simultaneously offered. The problem is an embarrassment of riches. For others, this problem is more than offset by sixty-nining's distinct charms. If someone's doing you, you may become so carried away with ecstasy that you long for more. As a result of your own excitement you tend to attend more excitedly to the sexual object in your possession, his cock, sucking it even more vigorously, until he responds with equal vigor, and you increase your abandon, and he increases his abandon, etc. There is total reciprocity, and the result can be truly terrific, bone-crunching, simultaneous (or nearly so) orgasms.

Sixty-nining is also a simple way to show someone whose cock you're sucking that you also want to be sucked. If he also happens to be young or inexperienced, fearful or embarrassed, you can use this position to present your cock to him without forcing him into doing anything he's not ready for (see *First Time*). Since you can arrange it so that you're not looking directly at him (until you wish to), you leave him even more free to decide to try to suck cock for the first time, without guilt or the sense of being watched.

Many gays admit that gradual sixty-nining was how they became more involved in active oral sex and finally in reciprocal intercourse. Another aspect to sixty-nining is that it leads to or allows easy access to your partner's asshole and so can lead to rimming (see *Rimming and Felching; Safe Sex*).

Some men swear by sixty-nining; it not only begins their gay sex experience, but can become their favorite position.

Sleazy Sex

Prenatally housed and nurtured within an organic stew, we spend a good deal of our infant life being wiped, washed, and generally brought up to hygienic snuff. As toddlers, we enjoy getting dirty in mud, but the powers that be still swoop down and scrub us up as though our souls depended on soap and water and carefully ironed outfits.

The teenage boy is implored by family, friends, and advertisers to swab the deck of his body lest he be wrecked on the reef of social ostracism. A swamplike whiff from his pits will sink romance; a ravaging horde of piratical bacteria in his mouth will march him off the plank to drown in a sea of embarrassment. Better to brush, scrub, gargle, and spray than to exude the faintest hint of body odor.

Yet despite all this—or maybe because of it—some men never lose the little-boy love of making a mess and reveling in it. Perhaps sleazy sex is a person's contrariness rebelling against the modern American obsession with antisepsis. Whether we realize it consciously or not, we are influenced by pheromones—irrepressible bodily scents creeping from head to toe, from crotch to nose. New studies show that men's sweat, for instance, is usually a strong turn-off to women, unless they are ovulating; in which case, it's a powerful aphrodisiac. For many gay men, sweat is always an intense attractant, and men not particularly into sleaze admit that ripe, unwashed armpits in a crowded room draw them like flies to honey.

There is sleaze and sleaze. Much of it is fun and safe. Some guys like to wear a jockstrap or underwear or exercise pants encrusted with dried sweat, come, and urine and find the odor more redolent of passion and masculinity than an expensive after-shave. Dried and exposed to air, these bodily secretions are considered safe by most doctors, at least as far as HIV is concerned, since the virus soon perishes on contact with air.

For other men, sleaze is more of a fashion statement. For them, torn, dirty jeans, mud-caked boots, and shirts stained with sweat at the armpits all scream hardworking, shit-kicking, rock-hard masculinity stripped of social pretense and Mama's middle-class morality. For some, automotive grease or the grime of construction-worker clothing is the sign of authentic machismo.

For others, it's not so much the bodies involved; their passion is enhanced when sleazy is enacted in role playing, calling themselves and their partners "pigs," and having sex in especially sleazy environments: automobile shops, warehouses, fields, or construction sites. The activity may be plain old sucking and fucking, but played out in abandoned warehouses or back alleys, between truckers' garages or even inside closed-for-the-night construction sites, the scene becomes fraught with the fascination of dirt and decay—what the French call *nostalgie de la boue*. For some men, the sour scent of sperm and sweat and urine in an enclosed and airless film-viewing booth, a closetlike space, or an underground room is sweetness indeed.

We should not overlook the psychological element in all these scenes. Hamlet says, "There is nothing either good or bad but thinking makes it so," and the same goes for sleaze. Something as innocuous as two days of stubble on a jaw can be read several ways. For some it's simply a prelude to possible beard burn, while for others it's a crotch-quivering symbol of sleaze and sloth. For still others it is sophisticated Italian fashion right out of *Uomo*. Still others will tell you it once was sleazy, then was fashionable, and now that it's featured on every good-looking male on every television commercial, it's just out-of-date.

Deeper, messier levels of sleaze involve men having sex while playing with their own or each other's urine and feces (see *Water Sports; Scat*). Whatever you do is fine so long as you're prepared to clean up thoroughly afterward.

A final note about sleaze: Let's not confuse medicine and morality, or safety and symbols. If you're practicing safe sex, you are getting the same protection whether you're smeared with STP motor oil in some filthy, slippery garage or you're in your own home. By the same token, dangerous practices are dangerous even in the privacy of your own bedroom, even if it has been dusted, vacuumed, and "air-freshened" with completely artificial "natural" scents (see *Dangerous Sex*).

Spanking

There are many ways to heighten sensations during sex play. One old favorite is an occasional slap on the ass. It's a good contrast to gentler, more tender touching and, for some men, is a real turn-on while getting fucked.

Don't assume that every partner likes it: Find out. Let's say you're having sex with someone new. You're lying down and he's sucking your cock. After a minute or so, give a sharp slap to his ass—just hard enough to be a surprise, yet not painful. He'll react to it one way or another. If he doesn't object, give him another slap. By this time, he'll either be moaning in pleasure or pushing your hand away, saying, "Stop." Or he may stop sex altogether while giving you a lecture about "not liking that kinky stuff" (see *Kinky Sex; Sleazy Sex*). Another variation for slapping is to have your partner lying on his stomach while you slap his ass. But slapping is most prevalent during sex when two men are fucking.

If you're the one who likes an occasional slap, don't be shy about letting your partner know. Depending upon the situation, you might ask him, or guide him, taking his open hand and slapping yourself with it until he gets the picture and takes over.

Most men who like a little ass slapping integrate it into the full menu of sex. For others, spanking may be the full meal. The spanking scene often (but not always) occurs within a "daddy" fantasy of punishing or rewarding a boy (see *Daddy/Son Fantasies*). Another popular spanking fantasy is the frat-house scenario. In this fantasy, the sex partners act out scenes where one is the freshman, pledging the fraternity, who is

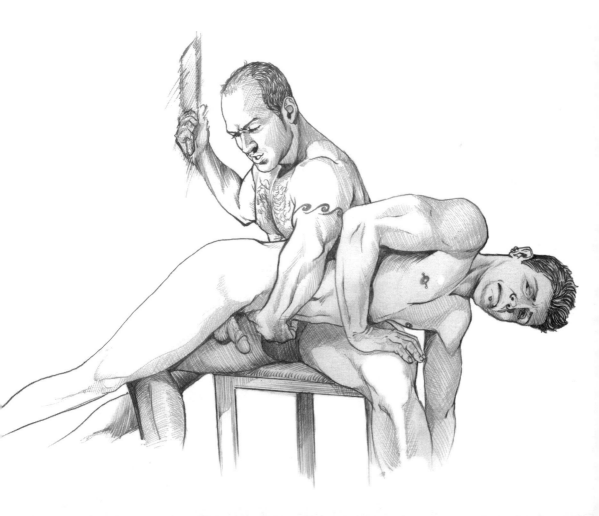

spanked, paddled, and sometimes forced into sexually servicing the frat-house senior, all as part of the accepted hazing ritual. A variety of porn videos, as well as magazines and newsletters, is devoted to spanking, and increasingly, a variety of Web sites (see *On-line Cruising*).

Spirituality

By spirituality, we don't mean séances to contact the spirit world or Ouija boards, but how we perceive reality on a higher level than the world immediately obtainable by the senses. It is a definition kept purposely vague to be large and inclusive, because that is how spirituality seems to work in gay life. Even during the wildest and sexiest days in the pre-AIDS 1970s, gay men sought answers beyond the here and now, and many found them in a variety of institutions either derived from existing religions or patterned after them. Many men used to arrive home from all-night dance, drug, and sex sprees at dawn on Sunday mornings only to immediately change clothing and go to church. Many still do.

During the earliest days of gay liberation, when it was difficult to find any Christians at all who would support homosexuals, several non-Christian groups opened themselves up to gay worshipers. These included Nichiren, a sect of Japanese Buddhism, with "chanting" for health and happiness. Buddhism does not condemn homosexuality at all, and this particular sect has been especially welcoming to gays.

Another group, Santería, is a composite of African voodoo and Roman Catholicism, which not only welcomes gays but already possesses as one of its guardians the transsexual Saint Barbara, who is assigned to especially care for gays. Santería has been specifically attractive to Latino gays who feel excluded by Roman Catholicism.

Hinduism possesses a pantheon of many different gods, all of whom in some way represent a single God, Brahmin, who literally breathes existence into being. Among Brahmin's manifestations are gods who have well-known histories of same-sex love and others who easily change gender (as well as color).

For those gay men raised as Christians looking for more familiar religious affiliations, two long-established denominations, Quakers (or Society of Friends) and Unitarians, do not discriminate and have become progressively more open to gay men.

Most other Christian congregations have some exclusionary practices toward gays. These can be mild, as in the case of Anglicans and U.S. Episcopalians, or extremely severe, as in the case of Roman Catholicism and most Baptist and Evangelical congregations.

Because of the great desire of many gay men who have been raised religiously to remain in some contact with their church, but who have found themselves driven away (see *Sex Phobia*), gay ministers and the devout have formed their own gay congregations of varied legitimacy, most notably the Metropolitan Community Church and Integrity (for Protestants) and Dignity (for Catholics). In some cities, these gay churches have quite large, influential, and active congregations. And gay Jews aren't excluded either: One can find gay synagogues, such as Beth Simchat Torah in New York's Greenwich Village. In addition, internationally respected religious figures are an important component of gay life. Gay men such as author Malcolm Boyd (*Are You Running with Me, Jesus?*), an Episcopalian bishop, and Mel White, formerly associated with the bigoted Reverend Jerry Falwell, are two who come to mind.

If you are gay and have been involuntarily separated from your religion upon coming out, finding a way to include spirituality in your life may not be as simple as it once was, but it does now involve a very grown-up quality: You get to choose. To scope out what's available, and what other gay men have done in similar situations, it may be worthwhile to check out books like Mark Thompson's *Gay Spirituality* (HarperCollins), Brian Bouldrey's wonderfully inclusive anthology, *Wrestling with the Angel: Faith and Religion in the Lives of Gay Men* (Back Bay), and *Gay Karma*, volumes 1 and 2 (Gay Sunshine Press), writings by gay men following Eastern religions. And there are always gay bookstores, many of which have surprisingly well-stocked religion sections (see Appendix).

Suicide

Self-destruction can occur whenever a person feels helpless, love-less, hopeless—and thoroughly defeated by life. In gay life we are most prone to suicidal thoughts at three times. If you do not fall into one of these, read on anyway, as there is useful information here for everyone.

First among the three are when we are gay teenagers. The Centers for Disease Control (CDC) has studied adolescent suicide extensively and arrived at a truly gut-wrenching statistic: fully one-third of all teenagers who kill themselves are gay.

It's not difficult to understand the prevalence of gay-teen suicide. Being gay at this age can be traumatic in our society (see *Teenagers*). Middle-school and high-school counselors can be as unconsciously homophobic as the general population. Their main aim is getting the teen to succeed in school life, and this often means conforming and being less openly gay. It is well documented how obsessed with conforming students are, and how unthinkingly homophobic. The slur most heard on school grounds is "Faggot!"—applied almost indiscriminately. Many school adults and teachers are indifferent, overworked, or themselves homophobic—no help to the gay teen. And too often gay teenagers return home to another hostile environment. It can be an overwhelming pressure cooker of negative day-to-day experience. Depression and emotional explosions are only to be expected, and these sometimes end in suicide.

The CDC notes three danger signs of a teenager especially at risk of committing suicide. First, if he is gay-identified from preadolescence and has faced bigotry, ostracism, and violence from early on in life. Second, if he is effeminate, there's the additional burden of harassment and bullying. Third, if he gets crushes on other boys and constantly encounters rejection. Straight boys can usually talk to their peers about unrequited love. This isn't usually an option for gay teens. Another danger, not listed by the CDC, commonly found in private, military, and other gender-segregated schools, is when a gay teen is forced to become a sex slave to a group of other students. These factors can add up to a lethal combination on impressionable youths. Most gay teens run into so much bigotry that it only deepens their sense of being different and their feeling of helplessness. And even when a gay teenager does find a lover, the two may feel so alone and harassed that they form and carry out a suicide pact.

Recently, laws against gay harassment by anyone on school grounds have been passed—most notably by the state of California—and teachers are increasingly receiving training about how to spot and stop such harassment. But it remains a small Band-Aid on a large problem and, while welcome, is too late for many kids.

Some gay men (and lesbians, too, naturally) who have received a fatal prognosis or are either seropositive or showing symptoms of HIV disease may contemplate suicide (see *HIV Disease*). At first, it's only a vague thought, but later, if serious illnesses invade the body, they may wonder at what point life becomes more painful than death. Some of us who get very ill are more upset by our increased dependence upon lovers, friends, or family than by the actual illness. Because so many gays have been forced to work hard at making their own life apart from family and background, this extra blow can seem unnecessarily intense. The prouder the man, the more uncomfortable it may be for him to feel like a burden. Such men may consider suicide to preserve their sense of personal dignity. It's as if they are saying, "I'm the one who's going to make the important decisions about my life, not this illness, and not doctors." The thinking behind this decision to take control is that it will make them psychologically stronger, if only for a short time.

Older gays are another group who may be at risk for suicide. While research shows that older gay men are generally quite happy with their lives, this is a time when increasing isolation can lead to thoughts of suicide. Some men have always been isolated and without close friends or lovers, and with advancing age and infirmity, they feel all the more lonely. Many self-styled "independent" gay men, proud of their self-reliance, or dependent upon their sexual encounters for a sense of self-worth, are most prone to deepening depression as they age. As their few acquaintances die or move away, and especially—in our age-phobic gay community—as their sexual attraction wanes, their self-esteem can plummet. Unless they find other reasons to live, they can become suicidal.

What should you do if you are contemplating suicide? Talking about these feelings with a trusted friend or lover can restore some emotional attachments. If you discuss the problem with someone close, suicide can become both less terrifying and less likely, though it remains an option. Sometimes, people feel timid and incompetent when a friend or lover comes to them to talk about suicide. The best advice in such a case is to talk openly with your friend about his fantasies of self-destruction and express your own feelings about it. Don't be afraid that you'll say the wrong thing or that you'll push him over the edge. You won't. Only he can decide that for himself. Someone close to a person with HIV disease should contact a local AIDS service organization, or if needed, a therapist can be consulted who can treat depression.

If you don't have a close friend to discuss your suicidal feelings with or if you are a gay teen who is considering suicide, call your local lesbian/gay hot line or teen-runaway hot line (look it up in the telephone book). Older gay men would do well to look into groups like Senior Action in a Gay Environment (SAGE), the oldest and largest service organization for gay and lesbian seniors. They have affiliates throughout the country (see Appendix). Additional hot lines offer nonjudgmental assistance to anyone in need, regardless of age. Look in your local telephone book for a suicide hot line. Operators are trained and willing to talk to you and to help you. Many gay community centers often have their own therapist on staff and emergency hot lines. There are also lesbian/gay Web sites that can refer you to someone who will talk with you.

Tearooms and Back Rooms

T*earoom* is the slang term used by gays for any public toilet where men engage in sex. In French-speaking and other European regions, they are more descriptively known as pissoirs. In England and countries influenced by British terminology, tearooms are called cottages and frequenting them is referred to as cottaging. Regulars of these sites are known as tearoom queens or cottagers, the latter a useful term when abroad (see *Travel*). Every town seems to have at least one "notorious" tearoom—at the bus station, at a rest stop on the highway, in the public library, at a subway stop, in the student union.

Pay toilets with single or multiple stalls are preferred, since the rattle of the coin in the outside door slot serves as a warning to the men already inside the toilet and gives them time to pull up their pants before someone (especially a policeman) walks in.

The etiquette of tearoom sex is elaborate. Two men stand side by side at a urinal. Each gets a hard-on. If no one else is around, they reach for each other. If other people are present and are just standing around, they are presumably gay and sympathetic.

Cruising from one toilet stall to another has its own rituals. In some cases, small holes have been pierced through the partitions (sometimes even through a slab of marble. When? Using what tools? It's a mystery). One man looks through the hole and sees another playing with himself. One may stand to give a better view of his erect cock. Then the process is reversed. In some tearooms the hole is large enough to stick a cock through. Such "glory holes" are used for masturbation, giving and receiving blow jobs, even rimming and fucking. If there are no holes in the partition, the men may instead begin to "tap-dance." Jack taps with his shoe. Bill taps back. Jack inches his shoe toward Bill's; then Bill's shoe moves in Jack's direction. Eventually shoes touch. Bill reaches under the partition and Jack squats so Bill can grab his cock. Bill feels Jack up. Finally Jack shoves as far as possible under the partition and Bill sucks him off, or vice versa. Or one man passes the other a note, possibly scribbled on toilet paper: "Do you have a place? Do you have time? What do you like? What do you look like? Are you hairy? Hung? What are you into?" The questionnaires can rival the U.S. army's for details requested.

Tearooms can be dangerous. Policemen, either in uniform or more frequently in plainclothes, keep tabs on them and sometimes videotape or observe the activities from concealed vantage points. The police in some towns entrap gays by initiating sex, flashing a badge just as the man is about to go down on the officer (or just after he's finished sucking the cop off).

Most municipalities have laws against public sex, so you're never safe in a tearoom and you're especially vulnerable if you're inexperienced, horny, and therefore not tuned in to danger signals you might ordinarily notice. One sign: You start fooling around with a guy whose heart is pounding and who can't get an erection; he might be anxious, or he might be about to rob you. Often hoodlums and petty thugs corner a gay man after soliciting him in a tearoom, rob him, and beat him up. If you have any doubt at all, move away, zip up, and get out.

Because of their ubiquity in gay life, tearooms have been the subject of sociological studies, some of which are quite enlightening. Read *Tearoom Trade* by Laud Humphreys. Many of the habitués of tearooms are "straight" married or closeted gay men who, to hide their homosexuality, will not be seen in a public gay bar, club, or restaurant (see *Married Men*). The age range, depending on the specific tearoom, can be anywhere from the teens to the seventies.

The sexual reciprocation in tearooms is as often on a chain basis as it is one-to-one. That is to say, Mark sucks off Bill, who leaves. Terry, who was perhaps watching that encounter, then sucks off Mark, who leaves, and so on. Three-ways and orgies are also not uncommon in tearooms (see *Three-Ways*).

The most active tearooms—after work, during lunch—usually develop "monitors," men who do nothing sexually, but watch other men have sex. They stand at the entry and monitor those approaching; they warn of a policeman, teen thugs, or anyone suspicious. Before the public toilets were closed, elaborately detailed maps of the New York City subway system were prepared by tearoom mavens, complete with comments on the best times to visit and the kind of people to be found there. Some even specifically named men who might be met at any of the hundreds of station johns in the system. We assume similar ones exist for other American and international undergrounds.

In the United States, back rooms are the dark places in gay bars or clubs where men have sex. Back rooms were the liberated gay male's answer to tearooms in the late sixties through the eighties, but because of health reasons, they are far less common today, except in Europe, where they continue to be found in many cities. These rooms are so dark you can scarcely see whom you're fucking or sucking. On the other hand, they can be awfully democratic since they eliminate many prejudices based on looks, age, and race (see *Racism*). If you meet someone terrific in a back room, you can always whisper an invitation to come home, though you may be in for a surprise (pleasant or otherwise) when you see him in the light.

Back rooms are much less hazardous than tearooms. There's virtually no chance that the police will bust you or that a mugger will beat you up. But pickpockets routinely lift wallets in the obscurity of back rooms, and the places can be breeding grounds for disease (see *Sexually Transmitted Diseases*). Be sure to leave your money, identification, and credit cards at home, or hide them in the bottom of your shoes. Unfortunately, like sex clubs, back rooms are fast becoming unsafe environments (see *Sex Clubs*).

Teenagers

Called a "genius" by a flatterer, the great scientist Albert Einstein replied, "Everyone's a genius—until sex comes along." For boys, sexual feelings can begin as early as age seven, although for most the age is generally twelve to fourteen, and even older for late bloomers. Being a teenage boy means hard-ons when you least want them, such as having a boner when the teacher calls you to the blackboard (how do they always know?). A particular person, a flash of bare skin, a spoken name, a sentence in a book, even a piece of music, can trigger the often mysterious psychological and physical responses that cause erections. When the trigger is another boy, or a man, many boys figure out they're gay.

The junior-high and high-school locker room is usually a place of danger for erection-prone teenage gay boys, as they're surrounded by other naked boys showering and involved in horseplay such as slapping one another's ass. The gay boy, while entranced by the riches that surround him, may have feelings of fear about getting a hard-on and the ensuing ridicule of his classmates.

Because we grow up in a heterosexual society, in which all socialization is geared around straight love and sex, coming out as a gay teenager can take a long time and be difficult, sometimes painful. However, if you have supportive parents, or a confident, relaxed attitude about your identity, then in this day and age, coming out can be easy, even fun (see *Coming Out*). Thanks to two decades of gay liberation, gay teenagers can come out (some in high school), experiment with sex, and even find reciprocal sex with a lover (see *Gay Liberation; Gay Politics*). Some gay teens now join after-school gay clubs, where they meet other gay kids and start to develop a teenage social network. A few large cities have all-gay schools, such as the various branches of the Harvey Milk School and the Hetrick Martin Institute (212-674-2400). Gay teens can date, have sex, and fall in love. They can discuss dating problems with best friends who may be another gay boy, lesbian, straight girl, even a straight boy. Taking your boyfriend to the school prom may still be a problem. A few schools will allow it, but most of the time it will cause controversy. And because of how gays are being positively portrayed on TV series, many straight teens are beginning to be a bit more relaxed about homosexuality.

Out gay teens are the lucky ones. But for every teenager who is more or less out, six

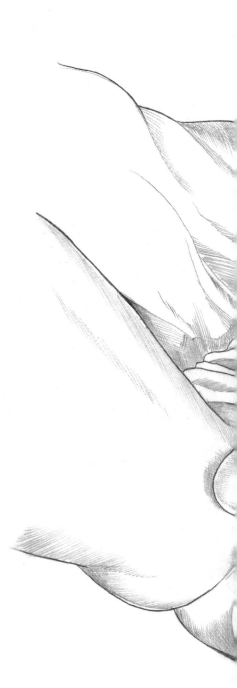

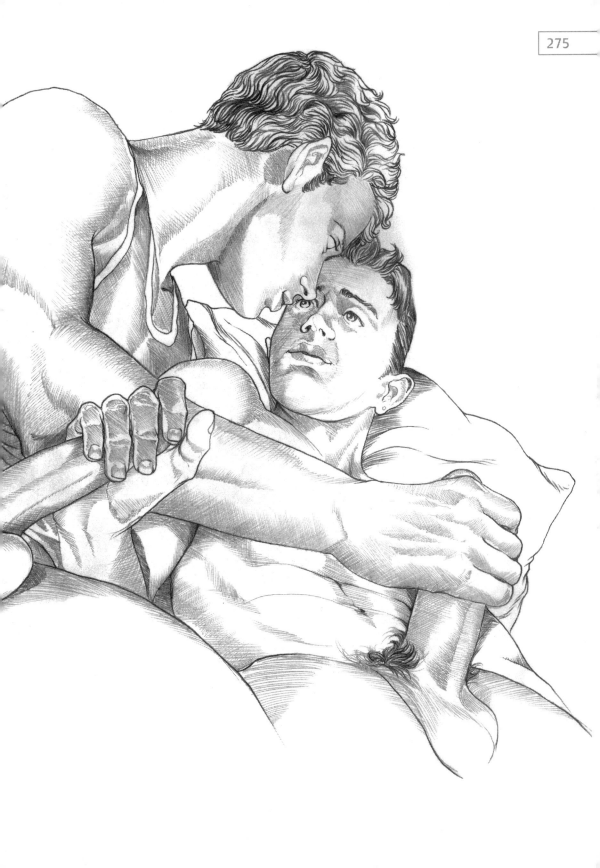

others are still in the closet. They fear their parents' rejection, and being tormented at school (see *Parents*).

Parents can be a hassle. By now, pretty much every adult knows about AIDS, so obviously you must expect them to be concerned for your health. If you're out to them, you might get them gay-positive books. You'll find Web sites for Insightout Books and A Different Light. They'll have many books useful to your parents—and you, too (see Appendix).

Even if your family is okay with you being gay, you'll have to learn to negotiate many situations in your school and community. A major one can arise when you first fall in love with another boy. The object of your affection may be gay, straight, or (an apparently swelling category) not yet decided on his sexuality. If he's gay and he returns your interest or affection, great! All you have to deal with is the usual difficulty of two kids trying to get together. We recommend you go slowly and attempt to exercise some caution as you whirl through the sex acts in this book. Most boys begin with touching, jerking off, and blow jobs. But you might also begin with kissing, licking, and nibbling, together with body rubbing or frottage (dressed or naked). Fucking is generally (but not always) the last. As you gain sexual experience, you'll have to recognize the dangers in the world of sexual plenty. You can always get laid if you know the right places to go to, but you'd better learn about STDs (see *Sexually Transmitted Diseases*; *HIV Disease*). If you get an STD, get it treated ASAP. If you wait too long, it might cause permanent damage in your body.

If the boy you are interested in is straight, it's a bit more complicated—though not impossible. Some boys will feel disgusted or upset the second you suggest sex with them. Apologize and put distance between you. Act toward him as if it never happened. If you must, jerk off to fantasies about him—but leave him alone.

Some straight boys, however, like to experiment sexually. With these guys, you may get limited access—perhaps you can only jerk them off, or they're willing to engage in mutual masturbation or blow jobs. We don't think it a good idea for you to get involved with these straight kids. The sex usually isn't reciprocal (you merely service him), and too often you're not finding someone who could love you (see *Pleasure Trap*; *Dangerous Sex*). Also he's likely to dump you once he gets a girlfriend.

Feeling that you're all alone and totally different from people around you can be really upsetting when you're young. But some gay teens find comfort and companionship with other boys and girls in school who also do not fit in with the majority for nonsexual reasons: the math and science geeks, the poets, the intellectuals, the *artistes*. They tend to hang out together and can usually be found in clubs or after-school activities: theater, newspaper, geology club, school magazine, or yearbook. Seek out their company even if you have no interest in journalism, old musicals, or rock climbing. It may not be the group you wanted to belong to, but it *is* a group and it will afford some solace, and you may end up being surprised by friendships and even lifelong relationships that can develop. At the very least, you'll have someone to hang with and to bitch with about parents and school. Everyone needs that.

Many gay teens have discovered Internet sex sites. There are places to learn about gay sex, but usually not what gay life is about. There are hazards to jerking off to pictures on the Net, especially if you're not out to your parents. For example, your Internet browser keeps a history of the Web sites you've surfed, and your parents—or anyone else—could easily access them. It's a good idea to learn to erase any evidence of visiting such Web sites. The Internet can be a wonderful place for isolated teens to form a community and meet other like-minded gay teens and gay men. However, there are well-documented hazards to this as well. You could meet someone who exploits others, either sexually or financially. If you decide to meet someone in person, we advise you to meet first in some public place such as a coffee shop or restaurant. Get a chance to size him up. On the other hand, don't be surprised if adult gay men avoid you like the plague. It's because you're jailbait.

E-mail is a perfect means of conversing with other gay teenagers. You may be able to develop a group of buddies to provide mutual support, not to mention warnings about other guys, homophobes, and potentially dangerous places.

Yes, there are places where gays cruise in even the most sparsely populated areas (see *Cruising*). These may include the library men's room or a particular park, shopping mall, or department-store dressing room or rest room in the nearby town (see *Tearooms and Back Rooms*). For many gay teens this may be your first chance to see or encounter gay sex, and for many it may be the only chance before leaving home for college or your career. Be cautious if you find yourself in these places. There is a risk of being entrapped and arrested by the police, and if you are not safe, you could be infected with STDs.

You may find an adult is sexually or romantically interested in you. If the adult is your parents' friend, your teacher, Scout leader, pastor, or other religious or community leader, the situation can quickly become far too complex for you to handle. You may feel forced to do what he wants (see *Early Abuse*). Or, because of his legal jeopardy, you may discover that you have the power to force the man to do whatever *you* want. Both are bad ideas. We live in a time and place where adult-teenage sex is harshly punished. Understand that under the law, as a teenager, you cannot give legal consent to have sex with an adult, even if you want to. The age of consent varies by state, but it's usually anywhere from sixteen to eighteen. If an adult is discovered having sex with you, he will be charged with statutory rape and may be imprisoned for up to twenty years. We think this is good enough reason to limit your sex to people your own age, but it's only one reason.

Another problem arises if you're a gay teen and effeminate (see *Effeminacy*). School bullying and harassment are inevitable and can be daily. This problem can be worse when teachers and other adults ignore how bad bullying can get; some people foolishly believe such harassment will "toughen you up." If everyone—including your parents—disregards your justified fears about antigay harassment at school, we strongly suggest you contact any gay hot line (call information), the local police, and/or state or federal child-welfare authorities. Some states (such as California) and municipalities have laws on the books specifically to combat harassment in school because of sexuality—go to your dean of students or principal (see *Sexual Harassment*). Their legal systems will support and represent you, even if no one else does. Whether or not they do, you can probably find a gay-friendly attorney willing to help you pro bono (i.e., for the public good—meaning free). You may press battery charges against your bully, or if your school is ignoring the problem, you may institute a suit against your school principal for endangering your life. It's refreshing how taking out an official assault charge on someone or threatening a lawsuit has a way of ending bullying.

Probably the worst scenario is the hopefully unlikely but all too common one of a gay teen being rejected by his parents. Gays represent an overly large portion of teen runaways. If you've been kicked out and you're headed toward a big city, you're in real trouble, unless you know an adult or family member who can put you up. Older and smarter people will prey upon you, try to manipulate you into drug use, prostitution, and crime. Your health is at risk, and so may be your life. Your best bet in this case is to *immediately* locate a program that helps runaway kids like yourself. In Los Angeles and San Francisco, for example, GLASS, the Gay & Lesbian Adolescent Social Service, has multiple group residences, as well as health, educational, and vocational programs for kids who've been abandoned by or forced to flee their family. Begun in New York City, Covenant House is now in seven other U.S. cities. Their phone is 800-999-9999. Another good resource is the National Runaway Switchboard at 800-621-4000, 24/7.

None of these agencies is perfect and they're always understaffed and underfunded, but they can literally save your life and get you on the road to becoming a well-adjusted gay adult. Invest that quarter dollar and call your local gay hot line or the local lesbian/gay community center for help (see Appendix).

Tenderness

Some men just want sex, but most want more—we want tenderness. At times our sexual desires feel like nothing more than an itch that needs to be scratched, and no tenderness is involved. When tenderness *is* involved, sex is not an isolated event, but the continuation of a long, lively communication.

Tenderness is based on such a dialogue. Although tenderness can be gentle, it need not be. If you are attentive and responsive to your partner's sexual needs, even when he needs to be treated roughly, then you are tender. Whether the touch is soft or tough, tenderness is expressed when you evaluate the needs of your partner and then meet them—and when you allow him to meet yours. Reciprocity is especially important when expressing tenderness; talking, touching, and holding are its means of communication (see *Touching and Holding*).

If you are cold and indifferent to your partner, or if you can establish a narrow, mechanical sexual program for your encounters with him, one that disregards his moods and taste for variety, then you are not being tender. And if you refuse to express your own sexual needs and insist on only servicing his, then you are also open to being accused of a lack of tenderness (see *Pleasure Trap*).

Tenderness requires that you understand the rhythm of sexual passion—that you indulge in foreplay, that you pick up signals, that you accommodate yourself to your partner's predilections, and that after sex you assure him of your affection. Newcomers to sex can learn the various positions easily enough; what requires more patience is the acquisition of tenderness. It comes only with experience and self-examination.

Three-Ways

A three-way is like adding spice to home cooking by throwing in a new flavor.

It can also be satisfying when the participants have just met. The best three-ways occur when all members are sexually versatile (see *Versatility*).

A man in the proper mood can get his face and ass fucked simultaneously. Or he can kneel and suck both his buddies simultaneously while they stand and kiss. One man can fuck a second lying on his back, and while fucking he can also suck a third who's standing or kneeling. Or the two doing the fucking can simultaneously suck off the third, who at the same time may be opposite them in bed, kissing, caressing, and even sucking the genitals of one or both of them.

Some men are able to get fucked by two cocks at once. One man may like to watch his lover fucking someone else, especially if he can't get fucked by his lover himself, or if he finds getting fucked more exciting an idea than a reality. Another may like to fuck and get fucked simultaneously, once he'd gotten the pelvic motions coordinated.

Three-ways aren't always problem-free. It's not unusual for one participant to become jealous or to feel left out. Some lovers think a three-way would be nifty, but when it comes to execution, one of them turns possessive and brooding (see *Jealousy, Envy, and Possessiveness*). If three strangers are involved, two may hit it off so well they want to be alone, and the third feels abandoned. If three-ways are the only sex lovers do anymore, they could fall into a pat routine, mechanical in its action (pairs have been known to call "play numbers," like gridiron quarterbacks, signifying, say, that it's time for all to suck now).

If all goes well, however, a three-way can be exhilarating and surprisingly intimate. After three men have explored every possible sensual aspect and sexual potentiality of one another's body in every conceivable combination, they often lie around and talk for hours, suffused with a warm glow. Nor is it unusual for them to go on-line and enroll a few more to join them (see *Sex Parties; On-line Cruising*). At times, three-ways seem so natural one has to wonder why lovers don't come in threes more often.

The answer is that once love and romance have been added to the pot, the simple three-way becomes the far more complex triangle. While love triangles are responsible for much of the world's great literature and opera (not to mention most daily gossip), triangles require the utmost of intelligence, affection, common sense, and selflessness to pull off. Even then few triangles last over time without major adjustments in all three lovers' minds and lives.

One unexpected positive sidelight of three-ways is that it's a lot easier to get your partner to wear a condom than if it's only two of you. The subtle and not so subtle pressures men use on each other when they're a couple usually fall by the wayside in the more practical triad.

• • •

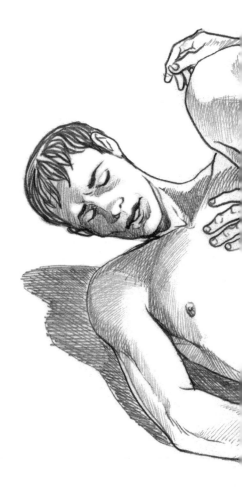

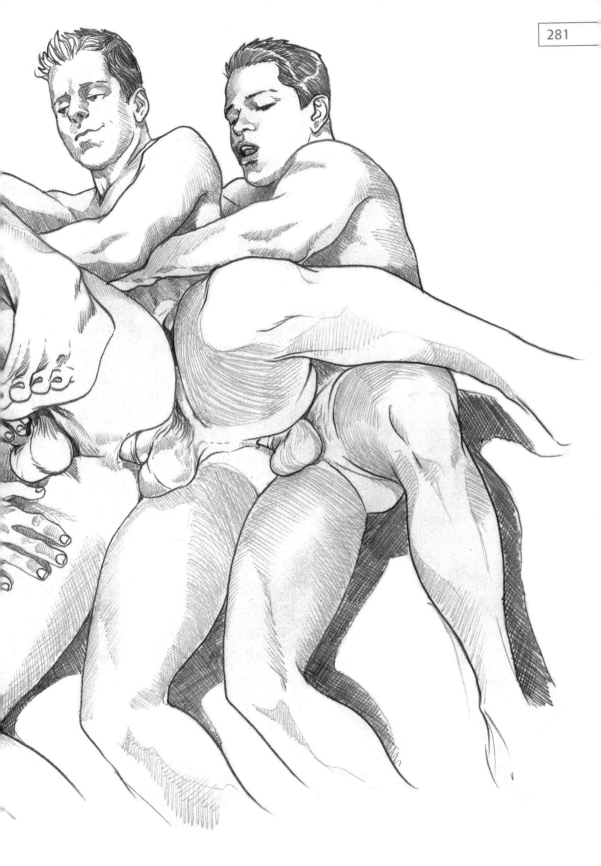

Top

Being known as a top can be helpful in meeting potential sex partners (see *Bottom*). People not interested in being bottoms automatically eliminate themselves, while those interested let it be known. It's also useful when placing ads or meeting someone on-line (see *Sex Ads*; *Profiles*; *On-line Cruising*) to let people know your sexual preference from the start. Being a top does not mean that you're more desirable than a bottom. It also doesn't mean that you must rigidly remain in that role or that you can't get fucked if you like. Assuming you practice safe sex, feel free to alternate as a top or a bottom according to the situation or your partner (see *Versatility*).

There are differences, though, between tops and bottoms. The top, for example, would seem to be the protector, the controller, the one who does the bulk of the leading and guiding, the one who takes on the responsibilities.

Ironically, before the gay liberation movement, when gays were far more closeted than today, roles like top and bottom were more rigid because gay men felt required to assume invariable roles. In a sense, it was a mirror of heterosexual role playing, the bottom assuming a more femalelike persona, while the top was the man (see *Gay Liberation*). Terms like *butch* and *femme* were commonly used by American gay men to describe themselves, right up through the 1960s. One still hears these terms used by a few gay men and lesbians, and of course, it also explains the use of the pronoun *she* to refer to another gay man.

Memoirs of and interviews with gays who flourished in earlier decades make those distinctions clear. As a rule, femmes lived more or less openly gay lives. They dressed in "womanish" slacks and fluffy mohair sweaters; their hair was cut in gender-ambiguous styles. They often wore makeup. And they paid dearly for this freedom: They were discriminated against severely, even by other gays (see *Effeminacy*). They worked in specifically gay occupations such as hairdressing, theatrical costuming, and interior decoration, or in low-paying jobs inside the tiny gay ghettos of New York and San Francisco as stage dancers, waiters, and shop clerks.

By contrast, the butch gay could be in any profession, from sanitation man to company CEO, since he was passing for straight. He never allowed himself a "feminine" word or action, except when disinhibited by liquor or drugs, and only in the most secure gay company. Unlike the femme, he had the freedom to live and work wherever he chose.

The American public of the first half of this century only recognized femmes as gay, never butches. But femmes also used this instant recognition. They could have "straight" male admirers and boyfriends—especially if they were themselves rich, powerful, or beautiful, or if they were in glamorous show business fields such as the cinema and music.

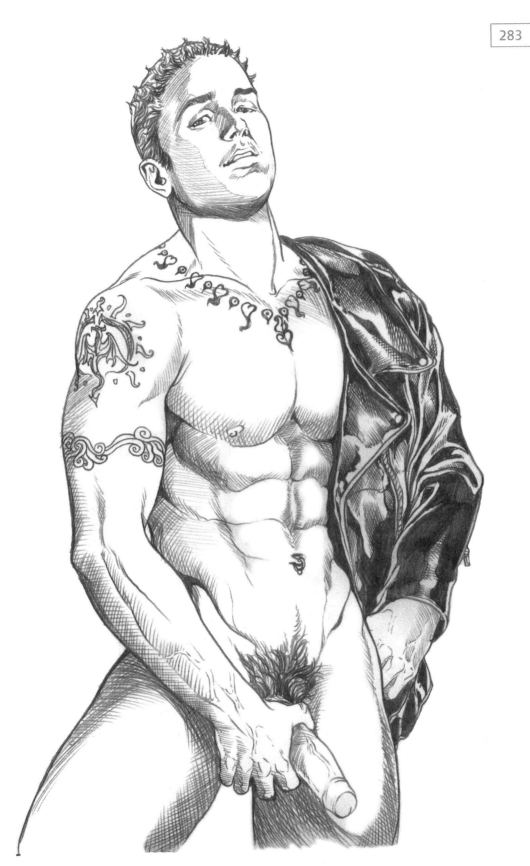

Those gay men who came out around the time of the Stonewall riots wanted to lock away butch and femme role playing into the closet of history forever. The gay liberationists' point was that all gays, no matter what their specific sexual behavior, were men. As a result of the surprising success of the gay movement, butch gays became free to try new roles, while effeminate gays found themselves politically passé. Yet it's interesting to note that political correctness hasn't changed the fact that gay men have sexual preferences even today, even among those just coming out, totally unaware of gay history, suggesting that something more deeply human is involved in these choices. The terms *top* and *bottom* no longer convey a heterosexual dichotomy of husband and wife, as *butch* and *femme* did. Even so, while some men easily move from one to the other, most gay men prefer one over the other. We assume that it's perfectly normal to be either solidly top or bottom.

Touching and Holding

Of all the means of communication, touch is by far the most sensitive. Through touch the child learns either to trust or mistrust other people around him, and consequently touch and trust become intimately related.

Some of us become elegant in speech, charmers who use our verbal facility to hide our feelings as often as to express them. Other men, less competent verbally, fine-tune their hands and know how to please other men sexually. Lucky for us to find a lover skilled at both.

The problem with touch is that it often conveys the truth about one's feelings, rather than the lie one may be telling. In other words, people "read" touch more accurately than speech.

Touch as a communicator of our feelings has a number of components. Softness conveys closeness, but hardness expresses anger or resentment. The speed of our touch is another obvious indicator. A quick cuddle or massage is tantamount to saying, "Let's get this over with because I'd rather do something else." How many fingers one uses while touching is also important. We all know that the tips of our fingers are the most sensitive areas, and using them—all of them—expresses our desire to remain in contact with our partner.

At times we use touch like a lie-detector test. The hand may be touching and caressing us, but we notice our lover's arm fully extended and the rest of his body far away. Physical distance during touch may express conflicts in people's feelings toward each other. Commonly, while a man's words are affectionate, his touching expresses his ambivalence about his partner or the relationship.

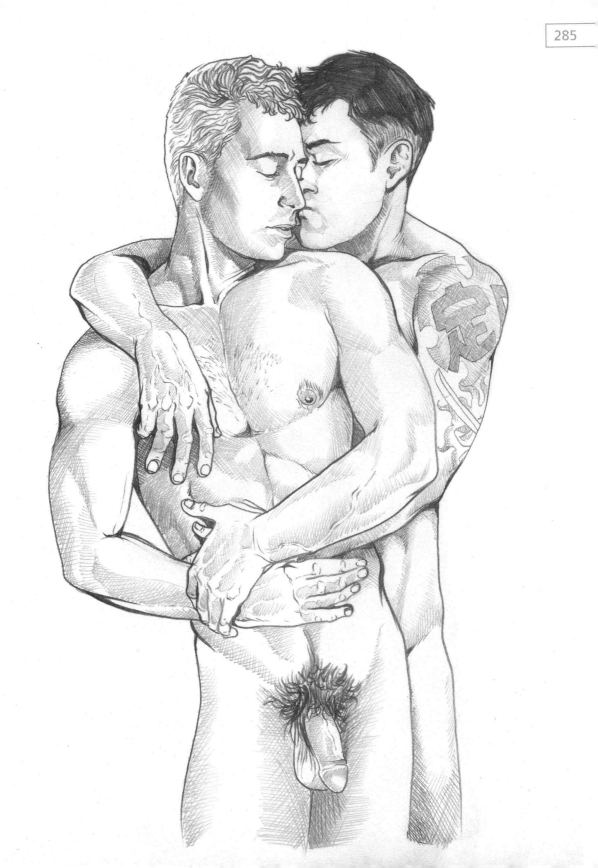

Touch becomes more varied when our lover is willing to touch with his tongue and mouth and we do the same to him. Part of the fun of being lovers is to explore with hand, tongue, and mouth every inch of your partner's skin, and to find the special spots that encourage him to squirm with pleasure.

Occasionally we find a lover who pleases us completely. He's usually a man in whom one finds a congruence of words and touch. Whether for just a night or for a lifetime, we feel safe in his arms. While we can't all meet that standard, we can learn to become better at touch, and at communicating in general.

Here's a good touching exercise to do with a partner:

You'll need a long stretch of uninterrupted time, so turn on your answering machine. Take showers, and clear your minds of work or other outside activities. Let's say you're going to pleasure your partner first. He should get naked and lie on his back. You have a choice of starting at his head and working down to his toes, or the other way around. Your goal is to gently caress every square inch of his skin. If you're starting at his feet, caress every toe, the soles of his feet, the sides, and work your way up the foot slowly. Sometimes you'll just use a few fingers, sometimes a whole hand, and when appropriate, both hands. Use your imagination. Play with his hair and lightly pinch his skin if you wish. Use your tongue and mouth whenever and wherever you want. Except—you are not to give him a blow job. No orgasms! Otherwise you'll interrupt the exercise midway. Naturally he'll have a hard-on. Let it be. Feel free to stop and play at any interesting spot, say his belly button or the hair just below it, his nipples or earlobes. Touch them, lick them, suck them—and at some point touch and lick at the same time.

When you've finished one side of his body, turn him over and slowly and gently do the other side. Pay particular attention to his butt. Nibble or lick or chew on his ass cheeks (see *Nibbling and Biting; Licking*). Spread his cheeks and rub your nose around the crack. Wet all the hair by drenching the area with saliva, but don't do any rimming. If the area around his butt hole isn't your cup of tea, then skip it (see *Rimming and Felching*).

If you're the one being touched, your only responsibility is to lie there and enjoy it. Ironically, that's a problem for lots of men, because we're so used to being in control that passivity can make us anxious. If one kind of touch is uncomfortable, tell him so (see *Massage*).

People who are HIV-positive or who have AIDS or other serious illnesses also need to be touched (see *HIV Disease*). In fact, their need is even greater than it is for the rest of us, because they may fear being abandoned by friends and family. The touching exercise described above can and should be done with them, as there are no physical dangers to it. Some gay men fear physical closeness with a sick friend, for a variety of reasons. The first is obviously fear of infection. It's a natural, primitive fear of being harmed, even though the person knows that the virus isn't transmitted that way. Some refrain from contact because they're afraid a sick friend may become dependent upon them. Some men simply feel incompetent to express their warmth and compassion with a friend. Yet those who touch, hug, and cuddle with their friends invariably leave feeling enriched by the experience, while the ill friends become energized, feeling cared for by a world that may slowly be slipping from their grasp.

Trade

Men who either are or pretend to be straight will sometimes allow a gay man to suck them off. These men are called *trade*. The word may be confusing when first heard since it suggests reciprocity, but sometimes the exchange that is being spoken of is the payment that hustlers receive for the use of their body (see *Hustlers*).

In gay slang, *trade* crops up in many contexts. "Just let me do you for trade," one gay might say, half-humorously, to another who has rejected him. Translation: "You don't have to do anything except lie back and let me blow you."

Someone unquestionably straight is called *rough trade*. Hustlers are known as *commercial trade*. Both terms connote danger. Two constants emerge: He who is trade plays the straight role, and the sex is geared to his climax, not to mutual orgasm.

Why does the concept of trade persist long after Stonewall and gay liberation? Is it that the gay man who habitually gives the blow jobs hates his homosexuality and prefers to identify with a "real man"? Or is the man who's trade afraid of losing his masculine image and becoming a "faggot," and thus his pose is a defense?

Possibly. Perhaps for the gay man, self-abasement before an ostensibly heterosexual man may have come to seem deeply erotic, or the gay man may be sexually conditioned to humiliation. Hostility intermingled with sexual excitement may motivate both: The trade feels contempt for the faggot servicing him and the faggot feels contempt for the straight man whose heterosexuality is so easily bypassed (see *Sex with Straight Men*). This contempt felt by gay men for their trade comes out in the old adage "Today's trade is tomorrow's competition." As with many adages, this one has a kernel of truth to it.

Yet another widespread usage of *trade* describes a teenager or young man who is experimenting with his homosexuality, or bisexuality, and who wishes to experience as much as possible with little change to his self-image. Being "trade" he can do this, associate with gays, learn about gay life, and discover what will be required of him socially as well as sexually should he come out.

Like many mid-twentieth-century slang terms, this one is quickly becoming passé.

Transgender

The term *transgender* includes both transvestites and transsexuals. Though these two groups have often been confused, they are quite distinct, although they've joined forces for political purposes, as a legitimate part of the gay liberation movement. Transvestites are men who dress up as women, while transsexuals are people who have decided to physically alter their bodies in order to conform to their mental and emotional identity. Perhaps half, maybe more, of all transvestites are heterosexuals with no sexual interest in other men.

Homosexual transvestites are also called drag queens, a term that can be used with either respect or contempt. Drag queens, in turn, often call other men "butch" or "butch queens." Until quite recently, gay transvestites have been both poorly understood and mistreated by most of the male population; not only have they had to endure the jeers of straights but also the put-downs of other gays. In the last two decades or so, however, public awareness of drag queens has startlingly increased, beginning in New York City's East Village with its annual Wigstock Festival, a celebration devoted to drag acts and drag in general. The mainstream success continued in the 1990s with the likes of talented drag queens such as Lady Bunny, Coco Peru, Eileen Dover, and most widely known, RuPaul. Unfortunately, Wigstock came to an end after it moved to Greenwich Village because of rowdy straight people and financial mismanagement.

Gay transvestites cross-dress for many different reasons. Some dress as men in public and wear drag only at home or during private parties. Others lead a double life and wear a male costume on the job and female attire at all other times. Some transvestites are so accomplished in their dress and manner that they live publicly as a woman 24/7 without detection. Some are so convincing, they have succeeded undetected in trades usually reserved for women. La Putassa was a famous drag model of the eighties whose picture graced many fashion ads. One Rio de Janeiro beauty named Roberto/Roberta was even Miss Brazil in the Miss Universe contest.

A central event in drag culture in many cities are annual balls, a tradition going back a century and noted in gay histories, including George Chauncey's *Gay New York*. Many transvestites spend an entire year and a small fortune designing and assembling their gown for this occasion. The costumes can be miracles of invention: One year the winner of a New Orleans Mardi Gras contest was carried to the judge's stand in a gilded cage, which at the climactic moment sprang open, releasing hundreds of birds—and the drag artist in a fantasy of feathers. An excellent, prizewinning film about drags and drag balls, *Paris Is Burning*, examines this life, especially among African-American and third world drag queens, with great style, verve, humor, understanding, and sometimes sadness.

Transvestism bears little relationship to actual sexual behavior or to problems with gender assignment. Some gay transvestites can be surprisingly aggressive in sex or quite versatile, fucking, being fucked, or both (see *Versatility*). To be sure, others refer to themselves as women and employ the feminine pronoun in talking about themselves and other transvestites as wives, both socially and sexually, with "butch" husbands. Some transvestites are ultraconventional, even morally uptight; others may be sex workers (see *Hustlers*). Although occasionally a gay transvestite may long to have a sex change, most are happy having it both ways.

Because of how roughly they've been treated, drag queens can be very tough, particularly those from a working-class background. It was drag queens, along with street hustlers, who began the riots at the Stonewall Inn in 1969 (see *Gay Liberation*). Immediately afterward the TVs (as they sometimes refer to themselves) formed STAR (Street Transvestite Activist Revolutionaries), one of the gutsiest gay political organizations in New York City. Transvestites are justifiably resentful they are not given credit for their contribution to the gay liberation movement by gay men, many of whom consider drag an embarrassment to the gay struggle. We opine that this prejudice is a form of homophobia on the part of masculine gays who don't want to be associated with feminine behavior.

Transvestism is hardly new. There have been a number of important transvestites throughout history. "Monsieur," the brother of Louis XIV of France, was considered the best general in the army even though he was a transvestite who wore drag underneath his chain mail. He often complained that the smoke of battle messed up his makeup. Joan of Arc was accused, tried, and burned at the stake for wearing men's clothes, a serious crime in those days. Magnus Hirschfeld, a pioneer of sex research in Germany before World War II, was thought to be a transvestite. These and other examples demonstrate the continuity of transvestism in history. Of course one cannot know how many transvestites of yesteryear might have preferred a sex change, since the procedure was unavailable then.

In more recent times, during the 1970s, the gender-fuck movement was popular. A twist on transvestism, men would dress in women's clothes while sporting beards, mustaches, and other obvious symbols of masculinity. Gender-fuck was especially active on the West Coast. Gender-fucks enjoyed muddying the conventional distinctions between the sexes, both for its shock value and for political reasons.

In contrast, transsexuals are men or women (either gay or straight) who believe they must surgically change their physical body and identity to that of the other sex. They have an unshakable conviction (sometimes begun in earliest childhood) that fate played some dreadful prank on them by bringing them into the world as the incorrect sex. They sometimes feel like feminine dryads trapped within masculine bark; they long to be released. Several medical centers, both in the United States and abroad, have helped these people make the transition from one sex to the other.

Because it is socially, emotionally, and physically complex, and the surgical procedure irreversible, the process can take years to complete. First the client is given an extensive psychological examination. He/she probably begins counseling or psychotherapy at the same time to deal with the emotional aspects of gender reassignment. A man's beard is removed through electrolysis, and he receives injections of female hormones (which he must continue for the rest of his life). The hormones cause breasts to swell, hair to acquire a new luster, skin to become softer, and hips to enlarge and become curvaceous. Women taking male hormones experience a different set of physical changes. They lose extra pads of body fat, and hair grows where it never had before.

Some transsexuals decide to go no further than this. But most request the final stage of treatment, surgical reassignment. For a born male this means that the scrotum is removed as well as most of the penis. Portions of the latter—the sensitive glans, the urethra, and a certain amount of muscle—are retained to surgically form the clitoris and inner wall of the new vagina. Other changes include cosmetic facial surgery intended to soften and demasculinize the appearance. The Adam's apple, for instance, is surgically made smaller, and other secondary sex characteristics are softened. For a woman the operations include double mastectomy, hysterectomy to remove childbearing organs, the surgical reshaping of the clitoris to form a penis, and the reshaping of the vagina into a scrotum. Other cosmetic surgeries for facial changes and for chest expansion are often included. If all goes well, the sexually reassigned man, now a woman, or woman, now a man, should look and respond sexually like the other sex. In fact, quite a few male transsexuals are married and their husbands remain unaware of their born gender. The secret is sometimes disclosed only when the question of bearing children arises—transsexuals are incapable of it.

The entire reassignment procedure, from the initial consultation to the final operation, is financially and psychologically expensive. Medical insurance will not pay for the treatments, and considerable absences from work can be expected. Psychological treatment is likely to continue even after the procedure is finished. Problems may include reestablishing relationships with family members and friends, and accepting the emotional difficulties that reassignment brings.

Unfortunately, some gay men do not accept transsexualism as a bona fide life choice. They believe that transsexuals suffer from a form of internalized homophobia, so extreme that they're willing to sacrifice their genitalia, an awesome thought to most gay men, who identify with theirs. Transsexuals (and transvestites) are, therefore, a sexual minority within a minority.

Inevitably, the question arises, What causes all this gender confusion? There was a great deal of research after World War II into the nature of hermaphrodites, infants born with both male and female genitalia. The scientists of the day believed that gender identity was determined by socialization, specifically by parental influence. If parents brought up the baby as a girl, it would become an adult woman; if as a boy, an adult man.

A famous case purportedly proving this was that of identical male twins born in Toronto. An accident occurred during circumcision with one of the boys, and his penis was burned so severely that doctors opted to complete a sexual reassignment. The other one was unaffected physically. The parents consulted the esteemed professionals of the day and were told to raise the twin without a penis as a girl, the idea being that "she" would easily adopt a female gender identity, while "her" brother would adopt a male gender identity. A book was written about the case: *As Nature Made Him: The Boy Who Was Raised as a Girl*, by John Colapinto.

As we now know, it didn't work. "Brenda" (her female name) wasn't like other girls—she even stood up at the urinal—and was so convinced that she was the wrong gender that by her late teens she demanded surgical reassignment back to male. This has now happened, and Brendan says he's far happier.

The many cases in the sex literature like Brenda's are convincing evidence that our sense of being a man or a woman is controlled more by genetics than by socialization. This is not necessarily the politically correct view these days. Many people still believe that our "gender" identity is socially conditioned. While that's admirable from an egalitarian sense, research into hormone production in the uterus has provided further evidence of the genetic connection. We believe that the evidence of a genetic link is irrefutable; however, we also believe that, regardless of the causes, whether social or biological, differences need to be respected.

Some Interesting Historical Transgenders

Henry III of France (1551–1589) dressed in women's clothes and had gay lovers, whom he called his *mignons*. He used makeup and earrings and dressed as an Amazon.

Abbé de Choisy (1644–1724) was trained by his mother to wear women's clothes. He pretended to marry a girl who was dressed as a boy. When he moved out of Paris, he took the name of the Comtesse de Barres, pretended to be a widow, and founded a school to teach young women to be ladies.

Chevalier d'Eon de Beaumont (1728–1810) joined the service of Louis XV and served as a dragoon in the Russian court. He then joined the secret service in London, where he argued with the French ambassador, who, in retribution, denounced d'Eon as a hermaphrodite. Members of the French court bet on which sex he was and planned to kidnap him to settle the question. He confessed his true identity to the king and was allowed to return to France under the condition that he either wear women's dress or give up his pension. He agreed. Later, d'Eon went back to England, where he gave fencing lessons dressed as a woman. He died in poverty in 1810 and was found to be a perfectly formed man. He was supposedly the model for the Barber of Seville.

You can read about historical transgenders in *The Mysteries of Sex: Women Who Posed as Men* by C. J. S. Thompson.

Travel

One of the great benefits and joys for gays traveling to other countries is that they are certain to find other gay men. For some this means making new friends, while for others, it means fresh fields in which to trick, slut around, or find a partner. American gay men enjoy unprecedented access to gay life on every continent except for Antarctica (and we're not sure of that). With a proliferation of gay guides specifically for gay men traveling abroad, as well as several excellent gay travel bureaus, you are limited only by the amounts of free time, money, and curiosity you have (see Appendix).

Of course foreign travel was always part of some gay men's lives. "Finishing" or "polishing" oneself via the European tour has been an important rite in many British and American men's lives. For some famous gay artists, such as the novelist Henry James, the painter John Singer Sargent, the playwright/composer Noël Coward, the journalist Norman Douglas, or the writer Paul Bowles, the discovery of ultrasophisticated gay life elsewhere generally meant remaining where one landed and seldom returning home. As a result, many other gay men heard of and came to wish to visit these foreign places.

But one didn't have to be wealthy or talented to enjoy the benefits of travel. Throughout the last century, but especially during World War II, gay men from small farming communities, big-city ghettos, and medium-sized industrial centers all over America traveled extensively through service in the armed forces. Many scholars consider those servicemen's travel experiences one of the driving causes behind the founding of such gay organizations back home as the Mattachine Society (see *Gay Liberation*). Having found established gay society abroad, and having seen how large their own numbers were, many American gay servicemen felt driven to continue to associate with other gays, and to found their own versions of the gay clubs, bars, restaurants, salons, and theaters they had experienced while "on leave."

In the 1960s, with the advent of discounted jet travel, large numbers of American college students began to spend summers abroad in Europe, North Africa, and the Far East. Many of these students found their experiences with foreign gay cultures to be sexually liberating, even life-altering. This same generation of gays that kicked gay politics into high gear also widely expanded international travel among gay men (see *Gay Politics*).

Today, a brief glance into any *Spartacus* or *Damron Guide* (among others now available) is all you need to recognize that dozens of lodgings, bars, restaurants, bookstores, and other retail stores in most major foreign cities cater specifically to gay travelers. No matter what you do in the way of sightseeing, sports, or other activities, you can be among gay people most or all of the time. Well-known and much loved destinations for gay travelers in Europe include Barcelona, Spain, and its gay beach at Sitges; Amsterdam in the Netherlands; Berlin, Munich, and Hamburg in Germany; Milan, Florence, and Rome in Italy; Paris, Marseille, and the Riviera in France; London, Manchester, Dublin, Ireland, and Edinburgh in Great Britain; Copenhagen, Denmark; and Prague, in the Czech Republic. The most visited cities in Asia and the Pacific area remain Manila in the Philippines; Sydney and Melbourne, Australia; Tokyo and Kyoto, Japan; Bangkok, Thailand; and Kathmandu, Nepal. Other cities that draw gay men specifically seeking the exotic yet familiar include Cape Town, South Africa; Marrakech and Casablanca, Morocco; Cairo and Alexandria, Egypt; Tel Aviv, Israel; Beirut, Lebanon; Istanbul, Turkey; and Athens, Rhodes, and Mykonos in Greece.

Being a gay man abroad means that, in a sense, you are representing your country. Like most gay travelers, the authors have discovered the upsides and downsides of this. Many foreign gays will have prejudices about you based on what they have read, heard, or viewed on TV and in films. In Tokyo, for example, where foreigners (*gaijin*) are usually barely tolerated, all gay Americans are seen as "rice queens"—i.e., desperately seeking Japanese men, until proven otherwise. In Hamburg, on the other hand, gay Americans are believed to be spectacularly well versed in the uses of the most up-to-date S/M equipment. Unless you correct the misimpression, what you thought would be a romantic night with maybe a little vanilla sex may turn out to be filled with whips, chains, and stockades. In much of Southeast Asia, whether you want a young man for the night or not, several will be available; whereas in some European cities you may be avoided like the plague—indeed considered an AIDS carrier—unless you have your HIV-negative blood tests on you at the time to contradict this. While traveling, some people will ask you to defend your nation's politics, culture, and history.

Each country, city, and ethnic group has its own culture (despite the alleged internationalized wonders of the "new globalism"), and before you travel to a new country, we suggest you try to learn something about its culture, if only so you won't do or say something offensive. One of the great benefits of gay travel groups is that their tour leaders can help you get acclimated. A few guidebooks can offer this kind of assistance. However, they won't detail much beyond that a particular bar caters to younger men or that a "cottage" (tearoom) in a particular Yorkshire moor is "considered dangerous."

There are travel books about most countries for gay travelers by gay people, as well as Internet sites, and even a few up-to-date anthologies with excerpts about many places by well-known authors, such as *Gay Travels* (Whereabout Press, San Francisco), which can help enormously. Fodors now has gay travel guides. Many foreign cities and towns have gay community centers, most of which are willing to assist gay tourists. The same goes for travel information centers, and hotel concierges around the world are noted for their savoir faire—and their confidential recommendations for gay travelers. Before the Iron Curtain fell in Eastern Europe, one of the authors, adrift for the night in Budapest, Hungary, went looking for a gay bar, and lacking any leads, he asked for assistance from a multilingual taxi driver. The author was told that no such thing existed, but he was directed—and driven to—the men's rest room in the basement of the city's Communist headquarters, where the cabbie assured him he'd find sexual action in a completely safe environment because, "after all, who would dare arrest a Party official?" This recommendation proved totally accurate, although the author never checked for Party ID during the ensuing orgy.

While you can have a terrific time traveling, there are also terrible times to be had if you are not properly prepared. If you have extraordinary health problems, if you have special mobility issues, if you need particular mechanisms to get around, you may not find these available to you, nor may you find your own equipment readily accepted at foreign airports, train stations, bus depots, or seaports. Inquire ahead. Accommodations may be more difficult or easier than you thought.

Meeting people while traveling can be more exciting and also more difficult than doing so at home. Foreigners' different look and accent may significantly heighten their allure, and you may end up having the best time of your life. But keep in mind, even if you speak his language or the person you meet seems fluent in yours, you may not know some unspoken rules of conduct. One of the authors met a terrific man at a Berlin sauna. After a wonderful sex session, he asked for the man's phone number and was rejected. Only sex, never romance, he was told, ever resulted from encounters at saunas. Maybe, just maybe, the fellow hinted, he would be at a particular gay restaurant the following weekend where they could meet and perhaps exchange phone numbers.

Keep in mind that as a tourist you make a vulnerable target for the unscrupulous. Act with caution, common sense, and courtesy, or you could put your money, your health, even your life, at risk. The Chinese, among the greatest of world travelers for millennia, suggest travelers keep in mind at all times that they are strangers in a strange land, and dependent upon strangers (see *Etiquette*).

Tricking

At some periods in a gay man's life, he feels like having a lot of sex with many different guys. Generally, although not always, these periods come right after a young man has accepted his homosexuality or when he has broken out of a difficult, lingering, bad relationship. It can happen when you leave home for college, leave college for work, move to a new town, take a new job, come into money, or lose a parent who never approved of your gay life. It could even happen if you're fired from your job or if you lose an important social position. You find yourself with time on your hands; you feel frustrated or, more often, simply feel an extra surge of libido. In short, you become a horny bastard.

The word *tricking* comes from prostitutes' slang *turning a trick*, which signifies having sex with a paying client, known as the trick or john. Making such a date is called turning a trick. In gay life we've shortened it to *tricking*.

Gays adopted the term possibly because they associated with prostitutes. Since the sexual revolution of the sixties and seventies, several new terms have come into usage with less of the accompanying stigma of the word *trick*.

For example, *one-night stand*, used by gays and straights alike, signifies that two people who just met plan to spend a limited time together, during which they'll have sex. If this occurs at one of the two partners' homes, the encounter is not expected to last beyond the next morning. As likely, one partner will leave after sex, perhaps after having exchanged phone numbers and promises to call. Implicit in the idea of the one-night stand is that if the pair like each other enough, they'll spend a second night together or a third, perhaps more.

A great deal has been written about how shallow and vapid one-night stands are, how geared to the "consumer society"—just "fast-food sex"—and all of these criticisms seem apt. On the other hand, if people are not looking for commitment, and they'd like to have sex with many people, and they are healthy, prudent, and safe, why not trick around? Who's being hurt?

Probably no one. Which is probably why the term *trick*, with its pejorative connotations, has widely been replaced by the terms *dating* and *dating around*. This may seem like a contradiction, since when people are seeing each other consistently, they are generally said to be dating. But this new term does answer the question "Are you dating anyone?" with a less negative response than a simple no. Instead you say, "I'm dating around."

Whether tricking or having one-night stands or dating around, the person doing it gets to spend time with a variety of people and to learn how to handle himself in a variety of sexual situations. Perhaps he wants to taste many different physical types from chubby to Adonis, from effeminate queen to biker leatherman, from milk-skinned blond to ebony-skinned African-American (see *Types*). What better way to carry on your own Study of Man? Or the man might want to experiment with different sexual roles (see *Versatility; Role Playing; Sadomasochism*).

And tricks or dates can turn into fuck buddies, lovers, friends, business associates, customers (see *Fuck Buddies; Couples*). Many older gays swear that in the years they were tricking around they formed a social network for the rest of their life and learned how to handle themselves socially.

That's the good part. On the other hand, you can hurt yourself dating around if (1) you can't stop yourself; (2) you've met someone you like a lot but you won't see him a second or third time because there might be someone even better out there; or (3) you've begun a relationship with someone, but as soon as difficulties arise, you quickly bow out, telling yourself, "I don't need this hassle: I can have sex whenever I want."

Once dating around becomes obsessive behavior out of which you gain less and less pleasure, then it's hurting you.

Until then, be safe, be careful, and enjoy yourself (see *Cruising; Promiscuity; Safe Sex; Seduction*).

Types

We often forget that most people have definitely preferred physical types. The African-American guy you're so hot for may have turned you down because you're white; study him a few nights and you'll probably notice he only leaves with other blacks. The cowboy who turned you down probably did so because you're dark and tall; observe, and you will doubtless see he's always got a small, fey-looking blond in tow. The cultivated balletomane, with whom you discussed Mark Morris and Twyla Tharp's latest with such pleasure, more than likely didn't go home with you because he's only turned on by monosyllabic, Neanderthal-looking guys with twenty-four-inch necks.

Spare yourself grief: Recognize that you are not the universal solvent, no matter how attractive you may be. No one is. Even your assets may work against you: Your perfect features and bulging biceps may intimidate men who feel more comfortable with ordinary looks. Conversely, what you may label your flaws may constitute your chief appeal to others: Your beard grew in bicolored, black and ginger, which you consider a tragedy, but it may be irresistible to some men, especially to those who like "bears" (see *Bears*).

There's another dimension to the subject of types—how do you avoid being type-cast? Sexual proclivities seldom conform to appearance. A small, cuddly young man may like to dominate others in bed. A muscular, oversize guy may tire of having his smaller, slimmer tricks demand that he ravish them. A slender Asian may not always want to play the shy geisha; a man in his sixties may not like to play daddy all the time. If you find yourself trapped by other's stereotypes about you, the best move you can make is to state your desires explicitly. On the other hand you've got to be willing to stop dressing and behaving in a way that arouses stereotypical—and in your case false—expectations. If you look like a cute kid and dress the part, you may succeed in getting lots of attention. If you depart from this look, you may be less popular. No matter. What's the use of awakening desire in others if it's the wrong desire? Gather your courage and butch up your act to make it true to your sexual personality. Even if you are less of a hit on the streets or in the bars, it's more than likely you'll meet the exact cute kid you want, and whom everyone used to think you were.

Another aspect to types is that they can get in the way of beginning new relationships. You may only go out with short, stocky Mediterranean guys with dark seraglio eyes, but now find you've met a lanky, blue-eyed WASP who won't leave you alone and who seems strangely more simpatico—and even attractive—than your usual type. You have to break your rigid type mold to find out if this man is a potential romance, maybe life mate. Your sexual repertoire may enlarge if you date out of your type (see *Versatility*). That would make a positive change in your life. Combining sexual and social versatility opens us up to more intimate relationships.

Then there's the question of race (see *Racism*). Even the most intelligent and liberal among us harbor unconscious fears and hatreds, which may have been years in the making by those around us stupider and more bigoted; these can strongly influence our selection of sex partners. Be aware and remain open. Try dating someone the exact opposite of your usual type. You could be pleasantly surprised. You might never again have a type.

Uniforms

If you've ever been struck by a particularly sexy highway patrolman or the smoke-blackened face of a fireman or a hunky drill sergeant marine, you already know how much what a man is wearing can increase his allure. That's especially true if he has on clothing not found in everyone's wardrobe, and even more so if what he's wearing stands for masculinity in action, heroism, or authority.

Many gay men are naturally drawn to good-looking men in uniform because of the extra machismo to be found in the image of a soldier or sailor or police officer, with its promise of free-flying testosterone and the sexual pleasures to be received from such a surfeit of hormones. But it's also true that some gay men get off on other uniforms, not usually thought of as particularly macho. Some guys go for the bus-driver look, especially if he's wearing the uniform of a Trailways or Greyhound bus driver, while others drool over chefs or go ape for doctors in surgery or emergency-related clothing like loose-fitting "scrubs." Train conductors' and auto or airport garage mechanics' garb can also be turn-ons. And for a few, the outfit worn by your plumber or the man who checks your electric meter can also be sexy.

Obviously, what's going on here—like much of our sexuality, which is centered in our mind first, then in our body—is more than meets the eye. Besides the evident turn-on due to clothing, other, less apparent turn-ons are happening in the subconscious or unconscious. And sometimes it's fully conscious. The trick who arrives with a yellow construction or Con Edison helmet is telling you, "This is my fantasy today. Help me play it out." With the increase in casual wear at the workplace among men, some guys have discovered that they are turned on by what few of us consider an erotic, or in fact any kind of, uniform, i.e., the stockbroker, banker, yuppie executive look, complete with shining black Johnston & Murphy wing-tip shoes, clocked socks, and the double-striped tie. As you can see, anything that can be worn can become eroticized enough to be a uniform.

Even so, there are the old favorites—policeman, fireman, soldier—and whenever gay men's uniform parties are given, these are the ones that dominate—and thrill. For some guys, there's an extra charge to getting fucked by a highway patrolman with his tight jodhpurs and high leather boots; while for others the idea of "thanking" a brave firefighter from a position on your knees, mouth wide open, is the ultimate sexual high. Scenes involving men in uniform make some of the best playacting, porn videos, and masturbation fantasies. And what would be truly humiliating or upsetting in real life for many gay men (being forced to suck off a cop or risk being thrown in jail) takes on a much lighter-hearted, scintillating coloring when it happens at a sex party or at home (see *Sex Parties*).

Some bars, clubs, and restaurants either cater to guys in uniform or have regular "uniform nights." If you're interested in seeing how this clothing on a gay man affects you, take a look. It's a lot safer and easier than trying it with a man whose sexuality you do not know and with whom you may end up in trouble. Many couples participate in uniform sex, whether they're into S/M or vanilla. Usually one of the two is the cop or

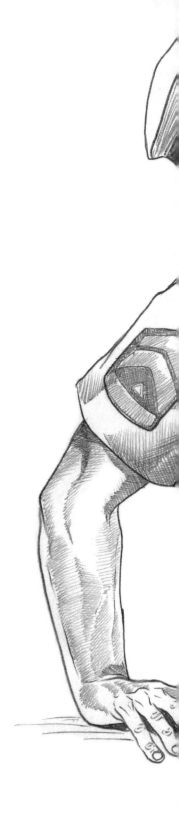

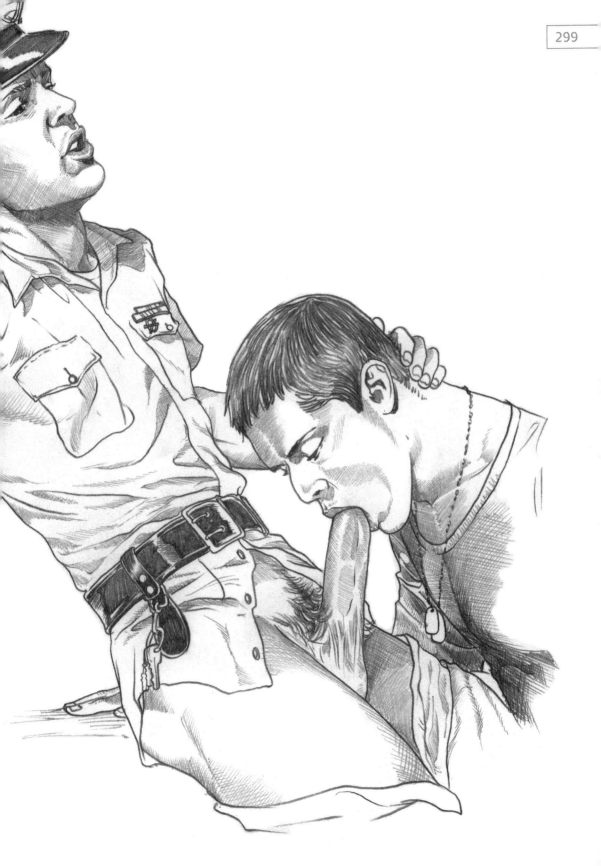

marine sergeant in full regalia, while the other member of the couple wears civvies or a less full version of the outfit.

One reason for the discrepancy is that inequality (an agreed-upon power differential) is needed in any such encounter: It's the essence of the sexual charge. Of course, another reason is that a good, full, real-looking uniform can be pricey. Buying one at your local gay leather shop or Pleasure Chest could set you back several hundred dollars. On the other hand, many gays can find discounted prices on the same items if they can locate a clothing shop next to their city's or state's policemen's, firemen's, or servicemen's training center. These shops furnish men in uniform for a living and will have the most authentic gear. The staff will also show you how to wear it properly.

Be advised, however, that in many counties, municipalities, and states you cannot wear a weapon of any kind with the uniform, as that constitutes "impersonating an officer," a serious misdemeanor or even a felony. Also keep in mind that parading around the streets in a military or police department uniform—even without a weapon—on any day other than Halloween can constitute a crime. Get local ordinances on the matter.

Vanilla Sex

Like the ice cream of the same name, it's both popular and plain. Used by some in a merely descriptive way, and by others pejoratively, *vanilla* refers to sexual fantasies and actions that are among the most socially approved both by gays and straights. An emphasis on kissing and affection, and a healthy dose of sucking and fucking, are the basic repertoire of those into vanilla. They like hygienic bodies clad in freshly laundered clothes (especially underwear) and view with undisguised suspicion those gay men whose dress, accoutrements, and behavior are darker, less savory, and obviously kinky (see *Sleazy Sex*; *Kinky Sex*; *Sadomasochism*).

Someone whose sexual behavior is said to be vanilla may still prefer to be a top or a bottom, or to be versatile, switching roles depending upon his feelings at the time and toward his partner (see *Versatility*). But he's not into the sleazier styles of lovemaking; he avoids heavy sexual smells, sex toys (except for dildos), S/M, fetishes, kinky fantasy scenes, spanking, or piercing (except for *an* earring). Clothes make the man, it is said, and men into vanilla advertise it prominently with preppy and yuppie-style clothes.

Just occasionally someone vanilla makes a mistake and goes home with a man who turns out to be kinky, even though he was dressed like a Swarthmore postgrad. If you're the vanilla gay, it will do no good to accuse him of false advertising. State your sexual limits, and if he tries to make you feel guilty or to pressure you into an uncomfortable scene, simply refuse. If need be, get out of his house or ask him to leave yours (see *Saying No*).

Versatility

Sexual versatility is one of the assets and pleasures of gay life. One is not required to be only a top or a bottom, or only vanilla (see *Vanilla*). Many gay men are capable of changing their sexual role depending upon the sexual circumstances or the physical characteristics of their sexual partner.

For instance, a gay man may prefer to be a top when his partner is younger or slight of build, while preferring to get fucked by an older man, or someone he perceives as very butch (see *Types*). He might also, by altering his own role to suit his partner's, be the perfect complement to another man who is a dyed-in-the-wool top or bottom. Some men also think of themselves as having both male and female characteristics; when feeling male, they want to fuck, while wanting to get fucked when they're feeling female. For whatever reason, the sexually flexible man has opened his body for pleasure.

Versatile is one of the key words found in profiles on Internet gay sex sites (see *Profiles*). It opens up a greater range of potential partners and sexual activities than would otherwise be possible. As such, it's a distinct advantage.

There is only one potential problem in this heavenly state of affairs. While it's okay to please another man's sexual desires, it's not okay to ignore your own. If your sexual behavior is oriented *only* toward pleasing your partner, you'll make it impossible for him to know how to please you (see *Pleasure Trap*). This is never a problem for a trick, but it will become troublesome in a long-lasting love relationship.

• • •

Water Sports

Not boating or skiing off the back of a motor launch, but guys pissing on each other or drinking each other's piss is water sports. Another term for pissing or being pissed on is *golden shower*, and the person who prefers this activity to all others in sex is often called a golden-shower queen. Giving and receiving enemas is another if less common aspect of water sports (see *Kinky Sex*).

Drinking piss is not harmful, unless pathogenic bacteria are in the urine. It can be harmful if you have a compromised immune system because of a disease like cancer or HIV. Only a small percentage of gay men go for water sports regularly. Indeed, few gay men are attracted by them at all. Nevertheless, the appeal isn't hard to fathom; those who enjoy it explain it this way: You can usually come only twice or three times a night, but you can piss dozens of times. Even so, few enjoy drinking highly concentrated toxic urine retained in the body for many hours. But if guys drink a lot of fluids, their urine will be plentiful and not bitter. Pissing of any sort is unlikely to be a way to start off an evening. But sometimes two men will get together for a long session of cocksucking, and once they can no longer have orgasms or produce come, they'll move into water sports.

The Internet is a great place to find men into water sports. There are also regular "meetings" of men into it.

For the slave in an S/M scene, being pissed on or drinking his master's piss is a form of humiliation he enjoys. The piss is

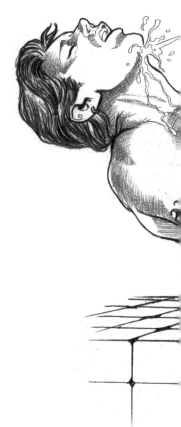

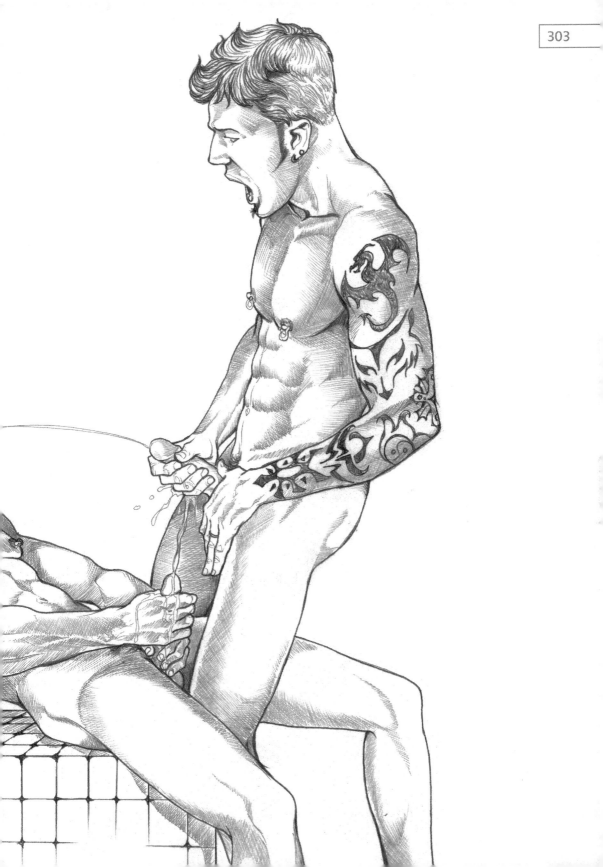

seen as a gift from the master's body. For vanilla gays offended by S/M, this seems too kinky, but there is an erotic logic to it.

Regarding enemas: To some the idea of having a sex partner administer an enema is exciting. The sensation of a liquid being repeatedly and forcefully squirted inside their ass could feel like being fucked over and over and then literally flooded with come. Guys into enemas have their own favorite sizes, shapes, and even forms of enema tube to be inserted inside them, as well as favorite liquids to be squirted, from the simplest—warm water—to coffee, soft drinks, their partner's piss, even expensive wines. However, using alcoholic drinks in large enough quantities (no one knows how large) can lead to death as alcohol is quickly absorbed. Also be advised that excessive flushing of the colon may damage it.

Webcams

Webcams are a technological innovation and a boon for gay men who get off on being exhibitionists, as well as for their coconspirators, the voyeurs. What could be more exciting (for some) than knowing that some naked gay men are jerking off while watching us jerk off on the computer screen, all in real time?

Aren't all men voyeurs? That appears to be the foundation for the appeal of all porn. It's likely that many of us wish we could be exhibitionists as well, flaunting a hard body, a big dick, a fabulous six-pack abdomen, and an ass to die for. At least on a superficial level, we could then feel desired by other admiring men. The problem is that most of us are normal, not at the top of the attractiveness curve—and a sterling personality, good sense of humor, and the capacity for intimate relationships simply aren't currency on the Internet.

Gay men mainly use the Webcam for sexual purposes. Some charge a monthly fee to watch them perform. There are also commercial sites: "Watch college freshmen jerk off and fuck each other in the shower—only $12 a month." Of course most of the time you're watching them, you'll only see an empty bed and wrinkled sheets because even exhibitionists have to go to work or to school or whatever it is that they do when not playing with themselves.

If you decide to put the spotlight on yourself, you may consider connecting it to a Web site (see *Web Site*). That will give your admirers more information about you. We think that's a mistake. Admirers have a habit of calling at any hour of the day or night, and some could turn out to be loonies who might stalk you (see *Sex-*

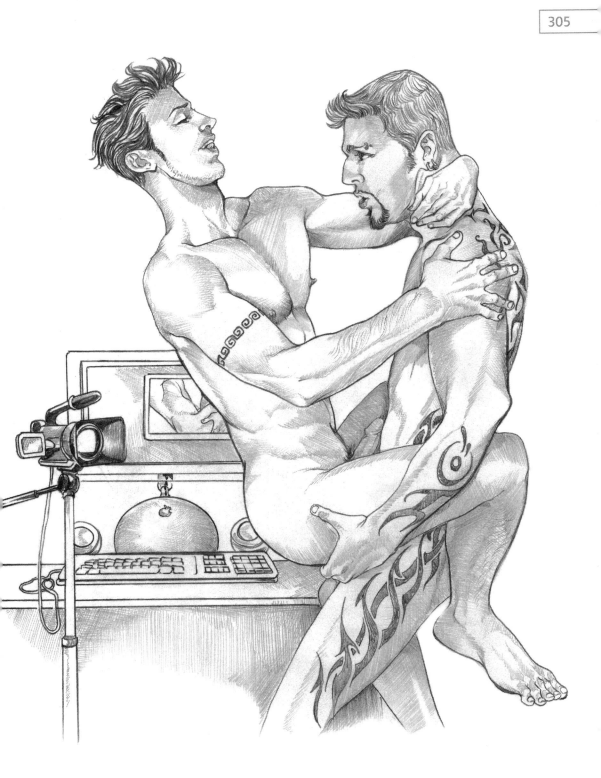

ual Harassment). We also suggest you *not* use your real name since resourceful men will do the detective work and get your phone number. If someone who has watched you sends an e-mail, and you like what he has to say (or his picture), you can choose to respond.

Web Site

There are usually two different kinds of Web sites in gay life today: one a "vanilla" site, built to appeal to your family and straight friends, containing whatever will bring smiles to your family's face. You may want to include a bio, such as where you grew up, maybe accompanied by your baby pictures and/or what you looked like at various stages of your life. Since the Internet is so visual, place many other photos of you and your family on your Web site, and if you've already come out, photos of your gay friends. If you have a lover, you might consider doing a joint Web page with him. You might want to have links on your site to other family members, gay friends, and to gay service organizations. If you have a good sense of design, you might consider dressing it up with elaborate graphics. But, remember, your vanilla site should be squeaky-clean.

The other Web site, by contrast, should run from being risqué to raunchy as hell—no holds barred. Naked pictures of you, some with a hard-on, pictures of you having sex, naked pictures of other men—all are acceptable, if you're willing to be that exhibitionist (see *Exhibitionism and Voyeurism*). You may decide to include a video hookup, known as a Webcam, focused on you while you're naked, jacking off or doing anything else you want others to see—in "real time" (see *Webcams*). The Webcam can be an integral part of your Web page. An alternative is to use "streaming videos," which are like decal-sized little films, placed in an archive, and these can also be used on the vanilla Web page. Computer nerds often introduce animation on their sex sites to simulate fucking and blow jobs. The links you choose for this site should be to other sex sites, but choose free ones, please, unless you're advertising your own or someone else's on-line business. Assuming you have a profile on one or more gay sex sites, be sure you link your sex Web site to them (see *Profiles*). If you're proud of the goods, let people see what you've got.

Both your vanilla and sex sites can be fun and creative. As computer technology advances, the sophistication of Web-page design is sure to develop. One caution, however: Be careful that you do not mix up your vanilla and sex e-mail and Web-page addresses. Your Thanksgiving visit home might end up being memorable in ways you hadn't planned for if your family and neighbors have inadvertently witnessed you being an energetic bottom on their home computer screens.

Wills

The ancient Egyptians were well prepared for death. They filled their tombs with furniture, food, jewelry, and all the things they thought would be needed in the afterlife. They believed they could "take it with them," an odd belief to us Westerners, with our heads filled with the fear of death and remorse over sin. Most of us not only believe that we can't take it with us, many of us worry about where we're going in our afterlife.

Thinking about wills is understandably distasteful to many men because they don't like to think about dying. While giving lip service to the idea that we're all going to perish one way or another, we all secretly believe we're immortal, and so we put off confronting death; to do so we use one or more rationalizations. The most common is "I don't have any money or property." You might not be a Bill Gates, but you would be surprised at how many things of value you possess. It might be worthwhile to go through your house and list what you own. Do this before making out a will, and along the way you might decide what to leave to various friends and family.

Even so, a will is not entirely about money and things. It's also about how you want to be remembered by family and friends. After all, it will probably be the only document that speaks for you after death, and that's especially important to gay people because we're seldom protected by the law. Your wishes about your property, including items with sentimental value, and about the disposal of your body, may not be respected if you don't have a will.

The AIDS crisis brought home to gay men the importance of will making. Some parents are sympathetic to their gay son and welcome his partner into the family. Other parents, however, have little compassion or warmth, and they see their son's homosexuality as nothing but a blight upon their own reputations (see *Parents*). Still other parents are downright spiteful, selfish people who refuse to visit a son ill with AIDS, cancer, or any other life-threatening illness or to have contact with their son's partner. Most gay men know their family situation quite well, whether they admit it to others or not, and so they need to protect both themselves and their heirs, especially a lover or children, against parents like these. That's another function of a will.

When drawing up a will—whether you are using an attorney or doing it yourself using a kit available for just such a use—you will need the following information:

1. A list of your valuables, including money, property, and stocks.

2. A list of your sentimental items.

3. Exactly how you want your body disposed of.

4. If you have minor children, who their guardians will be.

5. Whom you want as executor of your estate.

Many gay men don't think these matters through well enough and name heirs but assign a hostile parent or family member as executor of the will. Their excuse is that the family member will "make trouble" otherwise. But they ought to know that by doing this they are as good as letting the hostile family member walk off with their estate, leaving lover, child, or friend little or nothing.

In addition to the list above, quite a few gay men have made special provisions in their will. Holding a memorial service to celebrate one's life is one example. The will usually appoints a lover or friend to organize the service (it might even be a party), and the estate provides the money to pay for it. This should clearly be stated in the will, which should also name those who are to do the work, and you should state the amount of money you wish to spend out of your estate.

You may want to discuss your will with your parents or family, but only if you have a good relationship with them. You might even want them to have a copy of the will. By doing so, you'll put them on notice about your wishes, but this in no way guarantees they will follow them. If you have a lover, you may want him to join in this discussion. It's also common for gay men who feel rejected by their primary family to think of their closest friends as their new family (see *Gay Families*). They may look to these new family members when appointing executors and designating heirs. It may be wise to tell your parents or siblings that a friend or your lover or someone else you name will be your executor and that you've discussed your wishes with him or her in detail. On the other hand, if your parents disapprove of your gay life and are certain to cause problems after your death, be careful about disclosing too much information (or even any).

These are questions that should be discussed with an attorney. The lawyer is professionally bound to defend the will against any depredations. It's by no means foolproof: One example is of a will in which a man of Jewish faith stipulated that he be cremated—which goes against that religion's teaching—and his ashes be strewn at a designated spot. The body was burned all right, but the ashes were then buried in a family plot.

Some gay men cannot afford even basic attorney's fees, and for them there are books such as *How to Write a Will*, containing the appropriate forms and information. Remember that all wills must be signed and witnessed before a notary public to remain in force.

Can parents or siblings contest your will? Yes. Any will can be contested, but most of the time the will you wrote will stand up in court. The question is, do you want to worry your heirs or make them go through hassles and additional legal fees? Traditionally a will can be contested in three ways:

1. It was improperly executed. Handwritten and quirky wills usually fall into this category. Any attorney who deals often with gay people will know how to write the will to conform to state law. And books on the subject are helpful.

2. It was the result of undue influence. This used to be a favorite way for parents to contest a will by a gay son who left all or the bulk of his estate to a lover. The argument—no longer accepted in courts—is that the lover seduced the man and made him homosexual.

3. The gay man was incompetent to make out the will. This argument can be raised when a person is mentally or physically incapable of understanding the components of the will. In other words, make out your will when you're still in good contact with your mental faculties. Don't wait until you're senile or have Alzheimer's or dementia or are in a coma.

Also note that when a person dies within a certain time after making a will—even a perfectly legitimate will—the state or municipal court (or an estate court) may hold it up for a thorough examination of the circumstances of the death. The time varies from state to state, but is usually under a year.

Your will is not the only way to protect a lover, children, and friends. Other methods to do so that you ought to look into include insurance policies making them beneficiaries, bank accounts in their name, joint holdings of property that automatically go to the survivor, and putting money into noncontestable funds, trust funds, or living trusts (see *Insurance*). Lovers need to discuss their joint holdings and, in the discussion with legal advisers, arrange to protect themselves (and their children) in the event that one of them dies.

Be aware that any large property that you own only in your name and that you wish to will to someone else after your death will force your estate into a process called probate. This is literally "proving" the will; that is, your ownership of the property, its value, and all other aspects of your will. Houses, condos, cars, and bank accounts generally force probate, which can take from months to a year. Books have been written showing how to avoid this process. If avoiding probate is a concern for you and your legatees, you might want to make a bequest while you're still alive or sell the property.

Also keep in mind that if you have a large estate, while you are alive, you can legally make gifts of up to $10,000 per person, per year, to family members, including those who are adopted. While they will have to pay income taxes on these gifts, this can substantially reduce heavy estate taxes once you are gone.

Many people confuse a will with a living will, which is a legal instrument that protects your wishes *before* you die (see *Living Wills*).

* * *

Wrestling

Many homosexuals like to wrestle before or even during sex—for some it's a virtual substitute for sex. Whereas some men like to know from the outset the role they will play during a particular sexual encounter, others are only truly excited when there's a struggle to determine who will be "top man," which is tantamount to saying who will do the fucking and who will get fucked. Luckily, people have different tastes, and while winning may be thrilling, in wrestling, defeat can be pleasurable.

The pleasure is not only one of vying for position. It comes from the sensuality of two strong male bodies engaging in strenuous physical exertion: Back muscles flare, biceps bulge, sweat flows, buttocks become rigid with strain. For some men the prevailing flat hardness of flesh, the rigid musculature, and the long, exposed bones that so totally contrast the male body to the female is the real turn-on. Allied (perhaps) to memories of adolescent or juvenile roughhouse play, such physical combativeness and competition with its underlying threat of real harm and the possibility of total subjugation can become the ultimate aphrodisiac.

For more than a few, this interest in wrestling may have evolved out of their adolescence when, for many gay youths, the closest they could come—or allow themselves to come—to physical contact with another youth was through wrestling, in either its spontaneous sense of "just fooling around" with another guy on the grass, or more formally in school gyms and/or at the many intra- and interstate competitions.

Some given to wrestling have well-equipped game rooms with professional mats. The main difference between professional and sexual bouts, however, is that the latter are almost always done in the nude or at most in jockstraps. Often wrestlers oil their bodies. Climax is sometimes achieved through fucking and sucking, though some wrestlers like to end up in a clench—jerking off. Wrestling can also be integrated into S/M sessions, with the difference that the master is chosen not in advance but in action, right there on the mat.

Many wrestling Web sites are welcoming to gays. You'll also find gay wrestling clubs that meet periodically in many cities. A recent novel about adolescent wrestlers, *PINS* by Jim Provenzano (Myrmidude Press), deals with this arena in a sympathetic and knowledgeable manner.

APPENDIX

National Organizations

National Gay and Lesbian Task Force
(NGLTF)
1700 Kalorama Road, NW
Washington, D.C. 20009
(202) 332-6483
www.ngltf.org

Gay & Lesbian Alliance Against Defamation
(GLAAD)
248 West 35th Street, 8th Floor
New York, NY 10001
(212) 629-3322
and
5422 Wilshire Blvd, #1500
Los Angeles, CA 90048
(323) 933-2241
(There is also a San Francisco office)
www.glaad.org

American Civil Liberties Union
Lesbian and Gay Rights Project
125 Broad Street
New York, NY 10004
(212) 549-2627
www.aclu.org

The Centers for Disease Control and
Prevention
1600 Clifton Road
Atlanta, GA 30333
(404) 639-3311
www.cdc.gov

Federation of Parents, Families and Friends of
Lesbians and Gays, Inc. (PFLAG)
1726 M Street, NW
Suite 400
Washington, D.C. 20036
(202) 467-8180
www.pflag.org

Gay & Lesbian National Hotline
PMB #296
2261 Market Street
San Francisco, CA 94114
(888) 843-4564
www.glnh.org

Gayellow Pages™
Renaissance House
P.O. Box 533
Village Station
New York, NY 10014
(212) 674-0120
(This is the most complete compendium of gay
services and businesses published today.)
www.gayellowpages.com

Metropolitan Community Churches
8704 Santa Monica Blvd.
West Hollywood, CA 90069
www.ufmcc.org

Gay History and Politics

Bayer, Ronald. *Homosexuality and American
Psychiatry: The Politics of Diagnosis.* New Jersey: Princeton University Press, 1987.

Berube, Allan. *Coming Out Under Fire: The History of Gay Men and Women in World War II.* New York: Plume, 1991.

Chauncey, George. *Gay New York: Gender, Urban Culture, and the Making of the Gay Male World, 1890–1940.* New York: Basic Books, 1994.

Clendinen, Dudley, and Adam Nagourney. *Out for Good: The Struggle to Build a Gay Rights Movement in America.* New York: Simon & Schuster, 1999.

Loughery, John. *The Other Side of Silence: Men's Lives and Gay Identities—A Twentieth-Century History.* New York: Owl Books, 1999.

Marcus, Eric. *Making Gay History: The Half-Century Fight for Lesbian and Gay Equal Rights.* New York: Perennial, 2002.

Thompson, Mark, ed. *Long Road to Freedom: The Advocate History of the Gay and Lesbian Movement.* New York: St. Martin's Press, 1995.

ONE Institute & Archives
909 West Adams Blvd.
Los Angeles, CA 90007
(213) 741-0094
www.oneinstitute.org

Gay History Project
The Lesbian, Gay, Bisexual & Transgender Community Services Center
(see Gay Community Centers)

Gay History Com
www.gayhistory.com

Coming Out

McNaught, Brian. *Now That I'm Out What Do I Do?* New York: Stonewall Inn Editions, 1998.

Merla, Patrick, ed. *Boys Like Us: Gay Writers Tell Their Coming Out Stories.* New York: Avon, 1996.

Signorile, Michelangelo. *Outing Yourself.* New York: Fireside, 1996.

National Coming Out Project,
Human Rights Campaign
919 18th Street Suite 800, NW
Washington, D.C. 20006
(202) 628-4160
www.ncod@hrc.org

Teenagers

Bass, Ella, and Kate Kaufman. *Free Your Mind: The Book for Gay, Lesbian and Bisexual Youth—And Their Allies.* Canada: HarperCollins, 1996.

DeCrescenzo, Teresa, ed. *Helping Gay and Lesbian Youth: New Policies, New Programs, New Practice.* New York: Haworth Press, 1994.

Heron, Ann. *Two Teenagers in Twenty: Writings by Gay and Lesbian Youth.* Los Angeles: Alyson Publications, 1995.

Fairchild, Betty, and Nancy Hayward. *Now That You Know: A Parent's Guide to Understanding Their Gay and Lesbian Children.* New York: Harcourt Brace, 1998.

Relationships

Barzon, Betty. *The Intimacy Dance: A Guide to Long-Term Success in Gay and Lesbian Relationships.* New York: Plume, 1997.

George, Kenneth D. *Mr. Right Is Out There: The Gay Man's Guide to Finding and Maintaining Love.* Los Angeles: Alyson Publications, 2000.

Marcus, Eric. *The Male Couple's Guide to Living Together: What Gay Men Should Know About Living with Each Other and Coping in the Straight World*. New York: HarperCollins, 1988.

Silverstein, Charles. *Man to Man: Gay Couples in America*. New York: William Morrow, 1981.

Partners Task Force for Gay & Lesbian Couples
Box 9685
Seattle, WA 98109-0685
(206) 935-1206
www.buddybuddy.com

Health

Goldstone, Stephen E. *The Ins and Outs of Gay Sex: A Medical Handbook for Men*. New York: Dell, 1999.

Morin, Jack. *Anal Pleasure and Health: A Guide for Men and Women, 3rd Edition*. San Francisco: Down There Press, 1998.

Wolfe, Daniel. *Men Like Us: The GMHC Complete Guide to Gay Men's Sexual, Physical, and Emotional Well-Being*. New York: Ballantine Books, 2000.

(Many of the health centers listed below also offer psychological counseling, or have referral lists of licensed psychotherapists. Some of them are associated with medical schools and/or hospitals.)

Gay & Lesbian Medical Association
459 Fulton Street
Suite 107
San Francisco, CA 94102
(415) 255-4547
www.glma.org

Callen/Lorde Community Health Center
356 West 18th Street
New York, NY 10011
(212) 271-7200
www.callen-lorde.org

Fenway Community Health
7 Haviland Street
Boston, MA 02115
(617) 267-0900
www.fchc.org

Whitman-Walker Clinic
1407 S Street, NW
Washington, D.C. 20009
(202) 797-3500
www.wwc.org

Howard Brown Health Center
4025 North Sheridan Road
Chicago, IL 60613
(773) 388-1600
www.howardbrown.org

Montrose Clinic
215 Westheimer
Houston, TX 77006
(713) 830-3000
www.montrose-clinic.org

Jeffrey Goodman Clinic
(see Los Angeles Gay and Lesbian Center)

The following Web site is indispensable for quick, reliable gay health information on the Internet. They also maintain a list of gay-friendly medical and psychological providers.
www.gayhealth.com

Gay Counseling Centers

Institute for Human Identity
322 Eighth Avenue
Suite 802
New York, NY 10001
(212) 243-2830
www.IHI-therapycenter.org

Counseling Center of Milwaukee
2038 North Bartlett Avenue
Milwaukee, WI 53202
(414) 271-4610
e-mail:Shelter@execpc.com

Persad Center
5150 Penn Avenue
Pittsburgh, PA 15224
(412) 441-9786

Lambda Center
4228 Wisconsin Avenue, NW
Washington, D.C. 20016
(202) 885-5794

Montrose Counseling Center
701 Richmond Avenue
Houston, TX 77006
(713) 529-0037
www.montrosecounselingcenter.org

HIV Disease

Powell, Josh. *AIDS and HIV-Related Diseases: An Educational Guide for Professionals and the Public.* New York: Perseus Press, 1996.

Rotello, Gabriel. *Sexual Ecology: AIDS and the Destiny of Gay Men.* New York: Dutton, 1997.

Signorile, Michelangelo. *Life Outside. The Signorile Report on Gay Men: Sex, Drugs, Muscles, and the Passages of Life.* New York: HarperCollins, 1997.

White, Edmund, ed. *Loss Within Loss: Artists in the Age of AIDS.* Madison: University of Wisconsin Press, 2001.

AIDS Treatment and Information Centers

(Many of the centers listed below also offer psychological counseling. If it does not, they will refer you to the nearest gay counseling center. Some of them also publish helpful newsletters of the latest research about HIV and AIDS. A more complete list by state and city can be found in the *Gayellow Pages*.)

AIDS Action Committee of Massachusetts
131 Clarendon Street
Boston, MA 02116
(617) 437-6200
www.aac.org

AIDS Project Los Angeles
3550 Wilshire Blvd.
Suite 300
Los Angeles, CA 90010
(213) 201-1600
www.apla.org

Gay Men's Health Crisis
The Tisch Building
119 West 24th Street
New York, NY 10011
(212) 807-6655
www.gmhc.org

Lifelong AIDS Alliance
1002 East Seneca Street
Seattle, WA 98122
(206) 329-6923
www.lifelongaidsalliance.org

Project Inform
1965 Market Street
San Francisco, CA 92103
(415) 558-8669
www.projectinform.org

San Francisco AIDS Foundation
995 Market Street
San Francisco, CA 94103
(415) 487-3000
www.sfaf.org

Whitman-Walker Clinic
1407 S Street, NW
Washington, D.C. 20009
(202) 797-3500
www.wwc.org

Gay Community Centers

National Association of Lesbian, Gay, Bisexual & Transgender Community Centers. (This is an association of 130 community centers around the country. Some of the oldest are listed below.)
www.lgbtcenters.org

The Lesbian, Gay, Bisexual & Transgender Community Center
208 West 13th Street
New York, NY 10011
(212) 620-7310
www.gaycenter.org

San Francisco Lesbian, Gay, Bisexual & Transgender Community Center
1800 Market Street
San Francisco, CA 94102
(415) 865-5555
www.sfcenter.org

Gay & Lesbian Community Service Center of Orange County
12832 Garden Grove Blvd.
Suite A
Garden Grove, CA 92843
(714) 534-0862
www.thecenteroc.org

L.A. Gay & Lesbian Center
1625 North Schrader Blvd.
Los Angeles, CA 90028
(323) 993-7400
www.laglc.org

John Thomas Gay & Lesbian Community Center
2701 Reagan Street
Dallas, TX 75219
(214) 528-9254
www.resourcecenterdallas.org

Gay Bookstores

There are many gay bookstores in the country. Most of them are listed in the following two Web sites. The *Gayellow Pages* lists them by state and city. Gay books are also available on-line. The bookstores listed below are the largest and oldest in the country.

www.bookweb.org

www.stonewallinn.com

A Different Light
489 Castro Street
San Francisco, CA 94114
(415) 431-0891
and
8853 Santa Monica Blvd.
West Hollywood, CA 90069
(310) 854-6601
www.adifferentlightbookstore.com

Oscar Wilde Bookshop
15 Christopher Street
New York, NY 10014
(212) 255-8097
www.oscarwildebooks.com

Giovanni's Room
345 South 12th Street
Philadelphia, PA 19107
(215) 923-2960
www.giovannisroom.com

Crossroads Market & Bookstore
3930 Cedar Springs
Dallas, TX 75219
(214) 521-8919

Lobo Bookshop & Café
3939 Montrose Blvd.
Houston, TX 77006
(713) 522-1132
www.lobobookshop.com

Calamus Bookstore
92B South Street
Boston, MA 02111
(617) 338-1931
www.calamusbooks.com

A Different Drummer Books
1294-C S Coast Highway
Laguna Beach, CA
(949) 497-6699

Glad Day Bookshop
598A Yonge Street
Toronto, Canada M4Y1Z3
(416) 961-4161
www.abebooks.com/home/gdbookshop

Lambda Rising
39 Baltimore Avenue
Rehoboth Beach, DE 19971
(302) 227-6969
and
1625 Connecticut Avenue, NW
Washington, D.C. 20009
(202) 462-6969
and
241 West Chase Street
Baltimore, MD 21201
(410) 234-0069
Gay book club on the Internet
www.insightoutbooks.com

Out of Print Gay Books
Bolerium Books
2141 Mission Street
Suite 300
San Francisco, CA 94110
(800) 326-6353
www.bolerium.com

Transgender

Colapinto, John. *As Nature Made Him: The Boy Who Was Raised as a Girl.* New York: HarperCollins, 2000.

Feinberg, Leslie. *Transgender Warriors: Making History from Joan of Arc to RuPaul.* Boston: Beacon Press, 1997.

Jones, Aphrodite. *All She Wanted.* New York: Simon & Schuster, 1996.

Psychology

Cabaj, Robert P., and Terry S. Stein. *Textbook of Homosexuality and Mental Health.* Washington, D.C.: American Psychiatric Press, Incorporated, 1996.

Isay, Richard A. *Becoming Gay: The Journey to Self-Acceptance.* New York: Henry Holt, 1997.

Silverstein, Charles. *Gays, Lesbians and Their Therapists: Studies in Psychotherapy.* New York: W.W. Norton, 1991.

Homophobia

Berzon, Betty. *Setting Them Straight: You Can Do Something About Bigotry and Homophobia in Your Life.* New York: Penguin, 1999.

Fone, Byrne. *Homophobia: A History.* New York: Picador USA, 2001.

Signorile, Michelangelo. *Queer in America.* New York: Random House, 1992.

Legal

Curry, Hayden, and Denis Clifford. *A Legal Guide for Lesbian and Gay Couples.* Nolo Press, 2002.

Haman, Edward A. *How to Write Your Own Living Will.* Illinois: Sourcebooks, 2000.

Lambda Legal
120 Wall Street
Suite 1500
New York, NY 10005-3904
(212) 809-8585

(Also see their Western, Midwest, and Southern Regional Offices)
www.lambdalegal.org

Gay & Lesbian Advocates & Defenders
294 Washington Street
Suite 301
Boston, MA 02108
(617) 426-1350
www.glad.org

The National Journal of Sexual Orientations Law
(on-line law journal)
www.ibiblio.org/gaylaw

Employment

McNaught, Brian. *On Being Gay, Gay Issues in the Workplace*. New York: St. Martin's Press, 1989.

Zuckerman, Amy J., and George F. Simmons. *Sexual Orientation in the Workplace: Gay Men, Lesbians, Bisexuals and Heterosexuals Working Together*. California: Sage Publications, 1995.

Gay and Lesbian Workplace Issues
www.unm.edu/~oeounm/glrights.htm

Aging

Berger, Raymond M. *Gay and Gray: The Older Homosexual Man*. New York: Haworth Press, 1995.

Ellis, Alan L., ed. *Gay Men at Mid-Life: Age Before Beauty*. Binghamton: Harrington Park, 2001.

Quam, Jean. *Social Services for Senior Gay Men and Lesbians*. New York: Haworth Press, 1997.

Senior Action in a Gay Environment (SAGE)
305 Seventh Avenue, 16th Floor
New York, NY 10001
(212) 741-2247
www.sageusa.org

Prime Timers Worldwide
P.O. Box 436
Manchaca, TX 78652
(512) 282-2861
www.primetimersww.org

Pride Senior Network
132 West 22nd St., 4th Floor
New York, NY 10011
(212) 675-1936
www.pridesenior.org

Gay and Lesbian Association of Retiring Persons
10940 Wilshire Blvd.
Suite 1600
Los Angeles, CA 90024
(310) 966-1500
www.gaylesbianretiring.org

Racism and Ethnicity

Brandt, Eric. *Dangerous Liaisons—Blacks, Gays, and the Struggle for Equality*. New York: The New Press, 1999.

Gay Men of African Descent (GMAD)
103 East 125th Street
Suite 503
New York, NY 10035
(212) 828-1697
www.gmad.org

The National Latina/o Lesbian, Gay, Bisexual & Transgender Organization (LLEGO)
1420 K Street, NW
Suite 200
Washington, D.C. 20005
(202) 408-5380
www.llego.org

National Native American AIDS Prevention Center (NNAAPC)
436 14th Street, Suite 1020
Oakland, CA 946120
(510) 444-2051
www.nnaapc.org

Religion and Spirituality

Bouldrey, Brian, ed. *Wrestling with the Angel: Faith and Religion in the Lives of Gay Men.* New York: Riverhead Books, 1995.

Helminiak, Daniel A. *What the Bible Really Says About Homosexuality*: Millennium Edition. New Mexico: Alamo Square Press, 2000.

Leyland, Winston, ed. *Queer Dharma: Voices of Gay Buddhists.* California: Gay Sunshine Press, 1998.

Integrity (Episcopalian)
1718 M Street, NW
PM Box 48
Washington, D.C. 20036
(800) 462-9498
www.integrityusa.org

Lutherans Concerned/North America
2466 Sharondale Drive
Atlanta, GA 30305
www.lcna.org

The World Congress of Gay, Lesbian, Bisexual, and Transgender Jews
Keshlt Ga'avah
Box 23379
Washington, D.C. 20026
(202) 452-7424
www.glbtjews.org

Dignity/USA (Roman Catholic)
1500 Massachusetts Avenue
Suite 11
Washington, D.C. 20005
(202) 861-0017
www.dignityusa.org

The Gay Arts

Bergman, David, ed. *The Violet Quill Reader: The Emergence of Gay Writing After Stonewall.* New York: St. Martin's Press, 1994.

Capsuto, Steven. *Alternate Channels: The Uncensored Story of Gay and Lesbian Images on Radio and Television.* New York: Ballantine, 2000.

Curtin, Kaier, ed. *We Can Always Call Them Bulgarians.* Boston: Alyson Publications, 1987.

Russo, Vito. *The Celluloid Closet: Homosexuality and the Movies.* New York: HarperCollins, 1987.

Lambda Literary Foundation
(Publisher of *The James White Review* and *Lambda Book Report*)
1217 11th Street, NW
Washington, D.C. 20001
(202) 682-0952
www.lambdalit.org

The Gay & Lesbian Review Worldwide
Box 180300
Boston, MA 02118
(617) 421-0082
www.glreview.com

Blithe House Quarterly of Gay Fiction
Lodestar Quarterly (on-line journal)
www.lodestarquarterly.com

Travel Guides

The Damron Men's Travel Guide
www.damron.com

Spartacus International Gay Guide
No Web site. (see Gay Bookstores)

Gay and Lesbian Europe
Frommer's Guides
www.frommers.com

Fodors Gay Travel Guides
www.fodors.com

Odysseus International Guide
www.odyusa.com

Purple Roofs
(for Gay/Lesbian Travel Accommodations)
www.purpleroofs.com

S&M

Townsend, Larry. *The Leatherman's Handbook*. California: LT Publications, 2000.

Preston, John. *In Search of a Master*. Secaucus: Meadowland Books, 1989.

Preston, John, ed. *Flesh and the Word: An Anthology of Gay Erotic Writing*. New York: Plume, 1992.

Thompson, Mark, ed. *Leather Folk: Radical Sex, People, Politics, and Practice*. Los Angeles: Alyson Publications, 2001.

Bears

Kampf, Ray, ed. *The Bear Handbook: A Comprehensive Guide for Those Who Are Husky, Hairy, and Homosexual, and Those Who Love 'Em*. Harrington Park, 2000.

Suresha, Ron J., ed. *Bears on Bears: Interviews and Discussions*. Los Angeles: Alyson Publications, 2002.

Bears of San Francisco
2215R Market Street #266
San Francisco, CA 94114
(415) 541-5000
www.bosf.org

Metrobears New York
P.O. Box 1802
New York, NY 10185
(212) 460-1845
www.metrobears.org

Bear History Project
www.bearhistory.com

Bears Mailing List
www.queernet.org/bml

DR. CHARLES SILVERSTEIN is a licensed psychologist in private practice in New York City. He also serves as a clinical instructor in the Department of Psychiatry at New York University Medical College and as a supervisor of therapists at the Institute for Human Identity, a nonprofit gay counseling center. He is best known for his presentation before the Nomenclature Committee of the American Psychiatric Association that led to the removal of homosexuality as a mental illness from their *Diagnostic and Statistical Manual*. He founded two nonprofit gay counseling centers and was the founding editor of the *Journal of Homosexuality*. He has made significant contributions to the psychological literature concerning homosexuality, and these may be read on his Web page www.doctorsilverstein.com.

FELICE PICANO's first book was a finalist for the PEN/Hemingway Award. Since then he has published twenty volumes of fiction, poetry, and memoirs. Considered a founder of modern gay literature along with other members of the Violet Quill Club, Picano founded two publishing companies: SeaHorse Press and Gay Presses of New York. Among his award-winning books are the novels *Like People in History*, *The Book of Lies*, and *Onyx*. Picano's plays—*Immortal*, an adaptation of his novella *An Asian Minor*, *One O'Clock Jump*, and the comedy-thriller *The Bombay Trunk*—are regularly performed. He lives in Los Angeles, where he's adapting his novel *Late in the Season* into a film. See FelicePicano.com.

JOSEPH PHILLIPS is a fifteen-year veteran of the comic industry. He has contributed to comics ranging from *Superman* to the *Silver Surfer*, and his original comic *Joe Boys* depicts the joys of gay life. His illustrations have appeared in *Genre*, *Instinct*, *Unzipped*, *POZ*, *Circuit Noize*, *Odyssey*, *Xodus*, *HX* and *Next* magazines, and his collected work can be seen in the book, *Among Friends*.

INDEX

Underscored page number indicates illustration.